The Mood Cure

Also by Julia Ross

The Diet Cure

The Mood Cure

**Take Charge of Your
Emotions in 24 Hours
Using Food and Supplements**

JULIA ROSS, M.A.

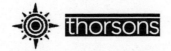
thorsons

Thorsons
An Imprint of HarperCollins*Publishers*
77–85 Fulham Palace Road,
Hammersmith, London W6 8JB

The website address is: www.thorsonselement.com

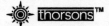

and *Thorsons* are trademarks of
HarperCollins*Publishers* Limited

First published by Viking Penguin,
a member of Penguin Putnam Inc. 2002
First published in the UK by Thorsons 2003

© Julia Ross 2002

Julia Ross asserts the moral right to
be identified as the author of this work

A catalogue record of this book
is available from the British Library

ISBN-13 978-0-00-732369-2

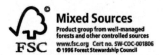

To all those who have sought help
and not found it.
And to Emmanuel.

Author's Note

The nutritional repair tools described in this book are not intended as substitutes for any needed psychotherapy, spiritual guidance, or medical care. They are intended to provide *additional* relief, where appropriate.

If you have a known or suspected medical condition, or are taking medication of any kind, or have specific health concerns, you should consult a qualified health care provider before following any of the suggestions in this book. Supplement and pharmaceutical dosages are intended only as guidelines. Dosage and results will vary according to the specific needs of each individual. Because this book cannot respond to individuals' needs and circumstances, as we do in our clinic, you should ask a qualified health care professional to help you assess and apply *The Mood Cure*. Particularly where mood symptoms are severe or there is a known sensitivity to supplements or medications, it is critical that expert advice be sought before any of the nutrient supplement suggestions are followed, as they could make some conditions, such as bipolar disorder, worse. Although we did our best to provide sound and useful information, we cannot and do not promise results to a reader, nor can we or do we accept liability to anyone who may use the book.

Acknowledgments

I am grateful to all the members of the gifted team that worked together so beautifully on my first book, *The Diet Cure*, and rallied itself once again to produce *The Mood Cure*:

Eugenia Clift Dreyfus, with her acute nutritional intuition, her tender and almost limitless patience, her incredible capacity for detail-tending, her sense of humor, and her dear friendship.

Nutritional research queen Krispin Sullivan, N.C., who unearthed most of the jewel-like references that stud the text of *The Mood Cure*, and offered support on many other fronts.

Jared Dreyfus, master wordsmith, who unraveled the worst of the prose, and keen-eyed and -minded copy editor Sona Vogel, who wrestled the manuscript to the mat.

Sharna Rose, chef extraordinaire, whose culinary contributions have been so helpful, once again.

The visionary Janet Goldstein and her associate Susan Hans O'Connor, who have adroitly shepherded me home again editorially (with the much-appreciated encouragement of Susan Petersen Kennedy).

My delightful and fierce agent, Faith Hamlin, who effortlessly conjured yet another winning book proposal, and still responds immediately to all calls and e-mails, even in extremis.

I also salute Lynn Ferar and Kris Alderton, who joined the fray near the end and got us over the finish line, and our vigilant production editor, Kate Griggs, whose sure hand guided the book into print.

In addition, I've had tremendous support from all the Recovery Systems clinic staff: from Sharon Brusman and Tish Stanney, who run the place so seamlessly and are such a pleasure to work with, and from nutritionist Diane Osborne, who relieved me so ably and with such rare spirit.

Tim Kuss, our senior nutritionist, earned his latest dose of my gratitude by writing the first draft of the "Sex Hormone Tool Kit" and working so hard on our training and certification project, not to mention his role in developing some of the nutrient formulations that have been most helpful to our clients and readers.

Final thanks go to little Charles, who brought joy in dark times, and to Fred and Margo for their steady love and support.

Acknowledgements to the British Edition

Special thanks to Antony Haynes of the Nutrition Clinic in London for his help in compiling the British resource details and to the editorial staff, particularly to Susanna Abbott and Wanda Whitely, at Thorsons for their support and courtesy.

Foreword

We certainly need a *Mood Cure* in the United States, but do you need one in the United Kingdom? Let's compare the emotional facts of life in the U.S. with those in the U.K. They're similar, but there are some interesting differences.

U.S. rates of depression and anxiety have tripled in the past ten years, with more than one in five adults now affected. The use of antidepressants is increasing so rapidly among both adults and children that Prozac (Fluoxetine) has become one of the ten top-selling drugs in the country.

How does the mood climate in the U.K. compare? According to the World Health Organization, depression is the second most common disability, after heart disease, throughout Europe, including the U.K., just as it is in the U.S. Within the U.K. itself, more than one in six adults were found to be either depressed, anxious, or both, in a large government survey published in 2001. As a result, Britons are also using antidepressants routinely, but not at quite the U.S. rate. In 2000, Fluoxetine became the seventeenth largest selling drug in the country and Efexor the eighteenth.

What accounts for the British having a serious, but somewhat less alarming, incidence of mood malaise than we have in the U.S.? There are three major factors at work here: food quality, exercise frequency, and access to bright sunlight. The food quality in the U.K. is slightly superior to that in the U.S., with more fresh food and less packaged food eaten, though that quality is steadily declining as it follows U.S. trends. On the other hand, British weather is much worse and Britons are almost as sedentary as Americans. This means that the dietary advantage that you in Britain still have is partly counterbalanced by lack of sunlight and lack of exercise, so you must vigilantly safe-guard it.

The Mood Cure is intended to help you discover mood-healthy foods and avoid mood-toxic foods by learning from our Yankee mistakes. For example, as you read about the low-fat experiment that failed in the U.S., you can consider enjoying butter on your potatoes once again.

This book will also recommend some wonderfully helpful nutrient supplements. Take Vitamin D, for example. It can be a powerful mood enhancer and is especially critical for you in the U.K. because you don't get enough sunlight to stimulate its natural production. In 2002 the results of a study on the use of supplements made headlines all over the U.K. In it two groups of prisoners in a maximum-security prison were given identical meals three times a day. One group was given vitamins, minerals and essential fats as supplements, including 800 IU's of Vitamin D, the Sunshine Vitamin. The other group was given dummy capsules. Those given the supplements committed 40% fewer violent crimes than those who were not.

Our experience at the U.S. clinic that I run is similar to that of the clinicians who administered the U.K. prison study: we have observed that, even when people adopt a relatively nutritious diet (most Americans subsist on diets inferior to the prison diet in the U.K. study!), it's often not enough to reverse the deeper nutrient deficiencies that can trigger feelings like irritability, depression, anxiety and stress. The use of therapeutic dietary supplements, for a few months, is usually critical for the effective relief of these kinds of mood problems.

If you decide that you'd like professional help in your mood repair project, you're in the right country. Fortunately, as you'll see in The Mood Cure's Resource Section pages 289–348, Britain is rich in practitioners trained to use specific supplements and dietary strategies to eliminate mood problems. Antony Haynes, whose busy London Nutrition Clinic is regularly featured in the national media, Patrick Holford, author and founder of The Institute for Optimum Nutrition, and Amanda Geary, author and head of The Food and Mood Project are three of the leading figures in this field, but there are many other holistic nutritionists throughout the U.K. Many are members of the British Association of Nutritional Therapists, whose contact information you'll find on page 290.

Unfortunately, the British public's access to many mood-saving nutrient supplements is threatened in the European Union by two international directives in particular, operating under the umbrella of CODEX. These are the Food Supplement Directive and the Traditional Medicines Directive. Should these be passed as law, nutrients such as 5-HTP and herbs such as Saint-Johns wort would be under threat. These two supplements feed and stimulate the area of the brain that produces serotonin, our most important natural anti-depressant. As I explain in Chapter 3 the use of these two specific nutrients can be essential for those of you experiencing depression or anxiety and who are looking for an alternative to drugs like Fluoxetine.

I wish you all the best in your personal and collective attempts to retain your access to mood and health-vital supplements. I include, in the Resource Section, specific U.K. sources for the supplements I recommend in *The Mood Cure*. However I also refer to many resources in the U.S., so that you can be guaranteed of your Mood Cure no matter what local restrictions you may encounter.

Contents

STEP 3

Creating Your Nutritherapy Master Plan

STEP 4

Getting Help with Special Mood Repair Projects

The Mood Cure Tool Kits

Step 1

Gaining a
New Perspective
on Your Moods

CHAPTER 1

Are Your Emotions True or False?

I f you're often feeling depressed, anxious, or stressed, you're not alone. We're in a bad-mood epidemic, a hundred times more likely to have significant mood problems than people born a hundred years ago.[1] And these problems are on the rise. Adult rates of depression and anxiety have tripled since 1990,[2,3] and over 80 percent of those who consult medical doctors today complain of excessive stress.[4] Even our children are in trouble, with at least one in ten suffering from significant mood disorders.[5] Our mood problems are increasing so fast that, by 2020, they will outrank AIDS, accidents, and violence as the primary causes of early death and disability.[6]

It's clear that our moods are deteriorating at unprecedented rates. What isn't so clear is why. What is this tidal wave of emotional malaise all about? Are our lives so much more unhappy than they were a hundred years ago, or even ten years ago? It's true that we're facing some unprecedented adversity in the twenty-first century. But even if it *is* the high pressure, or the absence of family support, or the terrorist threat, for example, why are we now so unresponsive to traditionally reliable remedies like long vacations, psychotherapy, and spiritual counsel? Why are we forced to turn more and more to medication for solace?

In this book, I'm proposing that much of our increasing emotional distress stems from easily correctable malfunctions in our brain and body chemistry—malfunctions that are primarily the result of *critical, unmet nutritional needs*. More important, I am proposing a complete yet easy-to-implement nutritional repair plan that can actually start to eliminate what I call our "false moods" in twenty-four hours.

TRUE EMOTIONS VS. FALSE MOODS

Some negative feelings are unavoidable and even beneficial. They're what I call "true emotions." These true, genuine responses to the real difficulties we encounter in life can be hard to take. They can even be unbearable at times, depending on the kinds of ordeals we face. But they can also be vitally important. True grief moves us through our losses, true fear warns us of danger, true anger can defend us from abuse, and true shame can teach us to grow and change. These true emotions typically pass, or diminish naturally, and even when they get repressed or misdirected, they can usually be relieved through counseling. But when we suffer for no justifiable reason; when the pain of a broken heart doesn't mend like a broken bone; when rest, psychotherapy, prayer, and meditation can make little impact—then we must suspect the emotional impostor, the meaningless biochemical error—the "false mood."

Figuring out the difference between false moods and true emotions is the first step in your Mood Cure. Once you've mastered that, you can move on to *eliminate* the fraudulent feelings, of depression, anxiety, sadness, and irritability, that are interfering with your natural capacity to enjoy life.

Learning to Spot a False Mood

➤ When your boss cancels a long-scheduled vacation, you may get justifiably angry, and the next day you won't have any trouble remembering what triggered your anger. At other times, you just seem to "snap" when your child forgets to take out the garbage. Later you say, "I don't know what got into me." The first case is a genuine emotion, the second is a definite counterfeit.

➤ Thinking of a loved one who has died may make you teary, but if every sad or sentimental TV commercial brings you to tears, you're in the grip of false pain.

➤ PMS is notorious for its bad moods. If you're reasonably even-tempered the rest of the month, but become teary and nasty before your period, you're experiencing a clear-cut case of hormonally disrupted emotional balance—a false mood.

➤ We all make mistakes and beat ourselves up from time to time. But if you are finding fault with your behavior or appearance almost every day, it's likely that false feelings of low self-esteem are responsible.

You shouldn't have to live with these kinds of distorted moods on a regular basis. It's like having an engine that sputters, preventing you from having a smooth emotional ride. When your brain's emotional equipment needs a tune-up, you get clues: you don't sleep well, you worry too much, you start feeling overwhelmed, you lose your enthusiasm or your ability to concentrate. You might also start depending on chocolate, wine, or marijuana to get some relief. If you experience these kinds of symptoms frequently, you may have just come to accept them, assuming them simply to be unfortunate features of your basic personality. But chances are you're wrong. Now you have an opportunity to discover your true emotional nature.

The Primary Cause of Your False Moods

Your brain is responsible for most of your feelings, both true *and* false. In concert with some surprisingly brainlike areas of your heart and gut, it transmits your feelings through four highly specialized and potent kinds of mood molecules. If it has plenty of all four, it keeps you as happy as you can possibly be, given your particular life circumstances. But if your brain runs low on these mood transmitters—whether because of a minor genetic miscue, because it's used them up coping with too much stress, or because you aren't eating the specific foods it needs—*it stops producing normal emotions on a consistent basis*. Instead, it starts hitting false emotional notes, like a piano out of tune.

After more than thirty years of intensive, worldwide investigation, most of the false moods and their causes have been identified by one of the fastest-growing fields of science—neuroscience, the field that studies the workings and effects of the brain. Drug companies have been using this information to create products that can give our emotional equipment a quick charge. But that's not the same thing as a real repair job. Fortunately, the emotional tune-up that we need so badly now is readily available. In fact, the repair tools we need for this crucial effort are shockingly simple.

They're specific foods and nutrient supplements that are so exactly what the brain needs that they can begin to correct emotional malfunctions in just twenty-four hours.

HOW I DISCOVERED THE MOOD CURE

I am the director of a clinic that's been doing nutritional mood repair for over fifteen years, but I've actually been a professional dealing with emotional disorders and mood problems since 1975. Early in my career I worked in residential psychiatric settings; later I worked with individuals and families, led intensive therapy groups and workshops, and ran treatment programs for adults and adolescents with addictions and eating disorders. Now I run my own clinic, Recovery Systems, in Mill Valley, California, just across the Golden Gate Bridge from San Francisco.

In 1980, as director of my first counseling program, I began to suspect that poor nutrition was playing a role in the cases that did not respond to our intensive programs of psychotherapy and spiritual support. Our less successful clients were often "emotional eaters." They either consumed lots of cookies, ice cream, chips, and fast food or skipped meals altogether and drank lots of coffee and caffeinated sodas. I started hiring nutritionists to explore the possibility of a food-mood connection, and we soon realized that we were on the brink of a powerful breakthrough. Clients who could be persuaded to eat plenty of protein and fresh vegetables three times a day and avoid caffeine, sweets, and refined starches, like white bread and pasta, felt *much* better emotionally (as well as physically). When they ate well, even those who had major psychological work to do were able to make steady advances in counseling with much less anguish and backsliding. However, the clients who did *not* make the nutritional changes—despite new communication skills, exercise, long vacations, and moderate work hours—did not do nearly as well.

I was encouraged by these results, but I also had to admit that it took the clients who were able to stick with it about ten weeks to fully withdraw from their bad-mood junk foods. For most of them, this was ten weeks of food cravings, fatigue, headaches, and only very slowly diminishing mood swings. More important, too many of our clients just couldn't wait it out and went back to their old junk foods and debilitating moods.

We needed something more.

THE AMAZING AMINOS

Around this time, in the mid-1980s, I read about the work of neuroscientist Kenneth Blum, Ph.D., at the University of North Texas. A prolific researcher, Dr. Blum was studying the brain chemistry of alcoholics and drug addicts. In the course of this work, he'd identified a few genes that could hardwire the brain to *under*produce its most potent "feel good" brain chemicals and instead produce the "feel bad" mood chemistry that made his subjects so vulnerable to addiction. His research explained the perplexing feelings of anxiety, anger, and depression, the chronic insomnia, and the lack of a sense of well-being that plagued so many addicts even in recovery. He called it the "reward deficiency syndrome." This finding was fascinating all by itself, but Dr. Blum made another, even more remarkable discovery. He found that he could override the bad-mood genes by giving his research subjects a few supplemental nutrients. These brain foods, called amino acids, are concentrates of common proteins found in food. They were able to jump-start the addicts' genetically misprogrammed brain chemistry and radically improve their moods. The bottom line: The addicts who took the amino acids were able to stay away from drugs and alcohol. Those who took no aminos had four times higher relapse rates![7]

I was very excited after reviewing Dr. Blum's studies. I had a sense that the amino acids were the missing ingredients in my fledgling nutritional therapy program. Since these supplements were identical to nutrients found in food and, unlike drugs, not foreign to the human body, my nutritionists and I felt comfortable recommending them. It was certainly worth a try.

COMBINING NUTRITHERAPY
WITH PSYCHOTHERAPY

Early on, I decided to give the aminos to three women struggling with bulimia, an eating disorder that is normally very difficult to treat. When they came to our clinic, all of them had been working hard in psychotherapy for some time with no improvement. Like most bulimics, they were depressed, obsessive, and self-critical. All were professionally well established, though, and all were married. One was a happily married 26-year-old, one was 35 and very unhappily married, and the third, at 48, needed marital help, but she and her husband were both determined to work things out.

In addition to taking the aminos, these women committed themselves to following our standard program of protein-and-vegetable-rich, reduced-carbohydrate foods and psychotherapy. I was astonished at how the aminos accelerated each client's progress. Mood improvements that would normally have taken months to achieve began for these women in days. In two weeks on the aminos, all three women had freed themselves of their obsessions with food and most of their associated mood problems. And it kept getting better. After a few months on aminos, the happily married woman, having met all of her goals, graduated from therapy free of both bulimia and mood swings. The unhappily married woman began to do deep and productive therapy after years of being too weakened by her bulimia to use psychotherapy constructively. After her nutritional overhaul, she was able to work through her fears, leave her husband, and establish a happy life for herself. The third woman no longer felt much need for individual therapy (she'd been at it for years) but started couples therapy with good results. All three women were still making excellent progress six months later and starting to go off their aminos. Their psychotherapist was dumbfounded, and so were we.

More than fifteen years and several thousand clients later, the amino acids are still our most effective weapons for fighting false moods. We have consistently found that they not only improve mood almost instantly, but speed up psychotherapy as well. A well-nourished person who has had a brain chemistry tune-up with amino acids gets beyond psychological and emotional obstacles faster, deeper, and more successfully. Not only have our brain-tuned clients had quicker access to critical memories, but they've coped better with those memories, no longer paralyzed by biochemically exaggerated feelings of fear, guilt, or pain.

The effects of nutritionally stabilized moods on our clients' relationships have also been extraordinary. I'll never forget the first family that we treated with both psychotherapy and nutritherapy. A father and mother came to see us, concerned about their 14-year-old son, who was having attention problems and depression plus headache pain so severe that it often kept him at home from school. It soon became clear that Dad had some serious problems, too. He was obsessively controlling and verbally abusive. Though they had received family counseling many times in the past, nothing had ever improved. When it became clear, after a few sessions, that Dad was actually deeply devoted to his family but simply *unable* to control his critical, angry feelings, I suggested that he meet with the same staff nutritionist who was seeing his son. He agreed because he could see that his son's headaches were responding to dietary changes and that his mood and ability to concentrate were improving on the amino acids. When Dad began taking amino acids himself, the change was immediate and powerful: his obsessive, explosive behavior evaporated entirely, much to the amazement and relief of his wife and son. Family therapy proceeded very constructively, since all family members were finally able to listen and respond to one another free of their false moods. Interestingly, Dad also needed some private psychotherapy to adjust to his new emotional style, especially in the business world, where his abrasive personality had become his trademark.

In 1995, our staff began suggesting that our clients try potentially helpful aminos right in the office, during their initial assessments. As a result, we've actually been present as the amino acids have taken effect, typically within fifteen minutes. We've watched and cheered as hundreds of clients shed their false feelings of tension, apathy, irritability, and emotional pain right before our eyes. The word that our clients always use to describe this experience is "amazing." What's more, our clients typically need to take the aminos for only three to twelve months. After that, their mood chemistry repairs are usually complete. They must, however, continue eating plenty of protein, vegetables, and other fresh whole foods and taking their basic vitamin, mineral, and fatty acid supplements.

HOW DO THE AMINOS ELIMINATE FALSE MOODS AND REVIVE TRUE EMOTION?

This is the secret: There are twenty-two different kinds of amino acids in high-protein foods like chicken, fish, beef, eggs, and cheese. You may have heard them referred to as the building blocks of protein. Each amino has its own name and unique duties to perform, but only a few very special aminos can serve as fuels for the brain's four mood engines. Just five or six of these amino acids, taken as supplements, can effectively reverse all four of the brain deficiencies that cause false moods.

Each of the four mood engines in your brain needs a different amino acid fuel. The lower your access to amino fuel, the more false mood symptoms you can develop. The question is how much "gas" do you have in each of your engines? How do you know when you've run too low? How can you fill 'em up? Which amino brain fuels do *you* need? Where can you get them? How long will it take? You'll soon learn what the best brain foods are *for you* and how to find and use the amino acid supplements that will jump-start all of your emotional engines and keep them fired up.

The four emotion generators in your brain are called "neurotransmitters." Some of their specific names will probably be familiar to you: serotonin, catecholamines, GABA, and endorphin. Each of these four neurotransmitters has a distinctly different effect on your mood depending largely on the availability of its particular amino acid fuel.

A well-stocked brain produces true emotions: depending on your life circumstances, you'll generally feel emotionally positive if your key neurotransmitter levels are high.

A poorly stocked brain produces false moods: If you drop too low in any of the key neurotransmitters, you'll tend to develop a specific set of defective moods as a result.

Your Brain's True and False Emotional Chemistry

⊞   If you're high in *serotonin*—you're positive, confident, flexible, and easygoing.

⊟   If you're sinking in *serotonin*—you'll tend to become negative, obsessive, worried, irritable, and sleepless.

⊞   If you're high in *catecholamines*—you're energized, upbeat, and alert.

⊟   If your *catecholamines* have crashed—you can sink into a flat, lethargic funk.

⊞   If you're high in *GABA*—you're relaxed and stress-free.

⊟   If there's a gap in your *GABA*—you'll be wired, stressed, and overwhelmed.

⊞   If you're high in *endorphins*—you're full of cozy feelings of comfort, pleasure, and even euphoria at times.

⊟   If you're near the end of your *endorphins*—you may be crying during commercials and overly sensitive to hurt.

Once any of the false moods evolve, their standard symptoms may come and go, become more or less intense, or remain constant. Whatever the case, the appropriate amino acid fuels, taken as supplements, can reliably, safely, and quickly dispel every vestige of all four false mood types by raising the levels of all four vital neurotransmitters.

Fortunately, every amino acid you'll need can be easily found at your neighborhood health food store or drugstore or by phone or on-line.

WHY ARE YOUR MOOD ENGINES RUNNING ON EMPTY?

Did You Inherit False Moods? Some of us tolerate the same adverse circumstances with much more serenity than others. My mother endured fifty years of marital stress, polio, cancer, heart disease, gallbladder disease, thyroid disease, and more with relish, grit, high comedy, courage, and selflessness. She was rarely depressed, irritable, or fearful. What was her secret? She had two—she'd inherited her own mother's nicely balanced brain chemistry, and she always ate lots of the protein that maintained it.

Did you inherit good-mood genes? Many of us didn't. Over the years, numerous clients have brought in parents, siblings, and children with false mood symptoms very similar to their own. A brief tune-up with amino acids and a dietary "adjustment" was often all that was required to set them right. These experiences taught me how often false moods run in families.

Did you think that your father was hard to be around *on purpose* or that your mother cried at any upset because she was so *weak*? These are the kinds of questions that I have learned to ask when exploring the types of negative moods that run in families. My clients have often found the answers to be unexpectedly liberating: *Although Anna hated to compare her irritability with her father's rages, when she realized that they shared a common brain chemistry deficiency, she ended up having new compassion for him and less of a hurtful sense that his abusiveness had been personal to her.*

We all know families in which everyone is laid-back and others where no one can slow down; outgoing, cheery families and shy, quiet families; worried, perfectionistic, families and sloppy, low-energy families. Ask yourself as you go through this book, "Do my family members share any of my mood traits?" "Are we the same false mood type?" But you won't need to worry about being a stick-in-the-mood. Although we used to think that genetic traits were intractable, when it comes to moods, even genetic programming can be reprogrammed remarkably easily by amino acids and other nutrients.

Is It Your Diet? Regardless of your genes, but especially if your mood-programing genes are inefficient, good nutrition is essential. It's no coincidence that our grandparents' generation had a more cheerful disposition than ours, although they certainly had their share of wars, depressions, diseases, and other hardships to deal with. The fact is that their diets were better. They were lucky enough to grow up before the junk food invasion and before low-calorie dieting had become a way of life. They ate "three square-meals" a day, including plenty of protein-rich foods like beef, chicken, fish, eggs, and cheese. Why are these particular foods so important? Because our four neurotransmitters can be made only out of the amino acids found in high-protein foods.

But protein is not all we need. We also need a good supply of vitamins and minerals to make this magic happen. They're found in fresh fruits and vegetables, which your grandparents ate in abundance but which are lacking in the standard American and British diet.

And there's something else that you may be shocked to learn. If we don't eat enough of the right kinds of *fats*, we will not be able to utilize these natural mood-boosting fuels. Our grandparents ate gobs of the fats we're no longer eating, like butter, and they had much less heart disease, cancer, and depression than we have. (More on this intriguing story in chapter 8.)

Then there's the junk food factor. Commercial food processing strips food of the vital nutrients needed to make and operate your brain's neurotransmitters. These bad-mood foods—including white bread and pasta, sugar-laden cereals and snacks, fried and hydrogenated fats, caffeine, and even the artificial sweeteners in diet soda—can actually *interfere* with your brain's efforts to create good moods. You can't pour sugar or any of these other stressful substances into your mood tanks and expect a smooth emotional ride.

Is It Your Lifestyle? Our modern lifestyle must share some of the blame for our epidemic of mood imbalance. Too much stress—particularly of the unique twenty-first-century variety—can deplete the brain of its "feel good" neurotransmitters, literally wearing it out. A good night's sleep, adequate relaxation, and appropriate "down time" are critical to restoring optimal levels of good-mood chemicals, but these simple restorative remedies are getting lost in our "go till you drop" culture.

Is It Your Hormones? At our clinic, we've continued to learn new ways to improve false moods as we've bumped into new mood problems that have stumped us. Our biggest lessons, beyond how to fuel the brain's four emotion-generating neurotransmitters, have been the lessons we've learned about hormones. Whether it's the two thyroid hormones, the thirty-plus adrenal hormones, or the three sex hormones—estrogen, testosterone, and progesterone—their effects on your mood can be powerful. Without enough of all these hormones operating in concert, the neurotransmitters can be stymied. Liberating your brain's emotional chemistry may require you to launch into a hormone-balancing campaign to eliminate whatever may be holding up the mood show. But don't be intimidated; I'll show you how.

WILL THE MOOD CURE REALLY WORK FOR YOU?

On November 13, 2000, I made a presentation to a scientific conference held in San Francisco on mood and the brain.[8] My staff and I had been asked to review the files of one hundred randomly selected clients who had come to our clinic with significant mood problems. Of the one hundred, ninety-eight had reported major improvements in mood within two weeks, most within twenty-four to forty-eight hours, using the amino acids, the basic nutrient supplements, and the good-mood foods that you'll be reading about in this book. Twelve weeks later, eighty-three had sustained or exceeded those improvements. *The depression, anxiety, oversensitivity, and stress that had brought them to us in the first place had disappeared.*

You can expect to experience the same kind of relief from your own false moods, just as quickly. After all, you'll be using the same techniques. As you've seen, many of the nutritional strategies I've discovered were developed while I was directing treatment programs for people with addictions and eating disorders. As a result, they've been honed on some very serious false moods. If the Mood Cure worked for them, it's very likely to work for you.

But the Mood Cure is not for everyone. I would love to be able to say that at our clinic we've learned how to eliminate *all* false mood problems, but I can't. We do not specialize in, and have very little experience with, severe false mood states such as autism, psychosis, bipolar disorder, violent rage, or paranoia—the biochemical imbalances commonly referred to as mental illnesses. Other clinicians have had experience treating these conditions with natural therapies, sometimes very successfully. Suggestions on finding practitioners, clinics, books, and Web sites that can advise you on how to deal naturally with mood disturbances that *The Mood Cure* does not address can be found in the "Resource Tool Kit," page 289. If you have such problems, please do *not* use the supplements suggested in this book without expert guidance. They could actually make your particular biochemical imbalances worse.

MOVING INTO YOUR OWN MOOD CURE

The first step in your Mood Cure, like the first step in any successful repair job, is to *identify what needs fixing*. In the next chapter, you can start getting down to particulars by filling out the Four-Part Mood-Type Questionnaire. After you've completed this false mood profiling, you can move on to the specific repair chapters and the excitement and relief of experiencing your own personal Mood Cure.

Once you've actually shed your false moods for good, you'll be able to use psychotherapy for any remaining *true* emotional problems stemming from your early life or from more current difficulties. You'll certainly be much better equipped to do effective work if you do decide to go into counseling. You'll also find it much easier to pray and meditate and to exercise, rest, and relax. With this full array of emotional, spiritual, *and* physical resources available to you, you'll be able to face whatever lies ahead with strength, serenity, and a sense of humor.

CHAPTER 2

Identifying Your False Moods

The Four-Part Mood-Type Questionnaire

There's a large chart mounted on the wall of our clinic that lists all the symptoms of the four false mood types. As soon as our clients walk through the door, their eyes are drawn and then glued to this chart. They're fascinated by the four different groups of symptoms, exclaiming, "Yeah, that type is me, but that one isn't," or, "Wow! I have symptoms of more than one type," or, "What does it mean if I have *all* the symptoms on the *whole* chart?" This deceptively simple chart was fifteen years in the making and is based on the thousands of client interviews and hundreds of research papers that enabled us to gradually identify each of the symptoms of the four false mood types. The questionnaire that you are about to fill out was adapted from this chart.

To identify your own false mood symptoms, start by circling the number next to any of the symptoms on the questionnaire that apply to you. Don't minimize! Really think about it. If you're in doubt about whether a certain symptom applies to you, ask someone honest who knows you really well. And don't be frightened if you have most, or even all, of the mood symptoms on the entire questionnaire. Many of our clients do. It won't be a problem. You'll address them all at the same time, using a combination of amino acids and other nutrients.

When you've gone through all four parts of the questionnaire, go back and score each part to see which false mood type (or types) you seem to fit.

THE FOUR-PART MOOD-TYPE QUESTIONNAIRE

Circle the number next to each symptom that you identify with. Total your score in each section and compare it to the cut-off score. If your score is over the cut-off, or if you have only a few of the symptoms described in a section but they bother you (or those close to you) on a regular basis, turn to the chapter indicated.

Part 1. Are You Under a Dark Cloud?

3 Do you have a tendency to be negative, to see the glass as half-empty rather than half-full? Do you have dark, pessimistic thoughts?

3 Are you often worried and anxious?

3 Do you have feelings of low self-esteem and lack confidence? Do you easily get to feeling self-critical and guilty?

3 Do you have obsessive, repetitive, angry, or useless thoughts that you just can't turn off—for instance, when you're trying to get to sleep?

3 Does your behavior often get a bit, or a lot, obsessive? Is it hard for you to make transitions, to be flexible? Are you a perfectionist, or a control freak? A computer, TV, or work addict?

3 Do you really dislike the dark weather or have a clear-cut fall/winter depression (SAD)?

2 Are you apt to be irritable, impatient, edgy, or angry?

3 Do you tend to be shy or fearful? Do you get nervous or panicky about heights, flying, enclosed spaces, public performance, spiders, snakes, bridges, crowds, leaving the house, or anything else?

2 Have you had anxiety attacks or panic attacks (your heart races, it's hard to breathe)?

2 Do you get PMS or menopausal moodiness (tears, anger, depression)?

continued

3 Do you hate hot weather?

2 Are you a night owl, or do you often find it hard to get to sleep even through you want to?

2 Do you wake up in the night, have restless or light sleep, or wake up too early in the morning?

3 Do you routinely like to have sweet or starchy snacks, wine, or marijuana in the afternoons, evenings, or in the middle of the night (but not earlier in the day)?

2 Do you find relief from any of the above symptoms through exercise?

3 Have you had fibromyalgia (unexplained muscle pain) or TMJ (pain, tension, and grinding associated with your jaw)?

2 Have you had suicidal thoughts or plans?

Total _____ *If your score is more than 12 in part 1, turn to chapter 3, page 25.*

Part 2. Are You Suffering from the Blahs?

3 Do you often feel depressed—the flat, bored, apathetic kind?

2 Are you low on physical or mental energy? Do you feel tired a lot, have to push yourself to exercise?

2 Is your drive, enthusiasm, and motivation quota on the low side?

3 Do you have difficulty focusing or concentrating?

3 Do you need a lot of sleep? Are you slow to wake up in the morning?

3 Are you easily chilled? Do you have cold hands or feet?

2 Do you tend to put on weight too easily?

3 Do you feel the need to get more alert and motivated by consuming a lot of coffee or other "uppers" like sugar, diet soda, ephedra, or cocaine?

Total _____ *If your score is more than 6 in part 2, turn to chapter 4, page 53.*

continued

Part 3. Is Stress Your Problem?

3   Do you often feel overworked, pressured, or deadlined?

1   Do you have trouble relaxing or loosening up?

1   Does your body tend to be stiff, uptight, tense?

2   Are you easily upset, frustrated, or snappy under stress?

3   Do you often feel overwhelmed or as though you just can't get it all done?

2   Do you feel weak or shaky at times?

3   Are you sensitive to bright light, noise, or chemical fumes? Do you need to wear dark glasses a lot?

3   Do you feel significantly worse if you skip meals or go too long without eating?

2   Do you use tobacco, alcohol, food, or drugs to relax and calm down?

Total _____ *If your score is more than 8 in part 3, turn to chapter 5, page 77.*

Part 4. Are you Too Sensitive to Life's Pain?

3   Do you consider yourself or do others consider you to be very sensitive? Does emotional pain or perhaps physical pain really get to you?

2   Do you tear up or cry easily—for instance, even during TV commercials?

2   Do you tend to avoid dealing with painful issues?

3   Do you find it hard to get over losses or get through grieving?

2   Have you been through a great deal of physical or emotional pain?

3   Do you crave pleasure, comfort, reward, enjoyment, or numbing from treats like chocolate, bread, wine, romance novels, marijuana, tobacco, or lattes?

Total _____ *If your score is more than 6 in part 4, turn to chapter 6, page 100.*

True-Life Stories of the Four False Mood Types

Cara had a typical case of the "dark clouds." She'd been low in confidence all her life. She was a doer, though—her underwear drawer was a work of art, and her boss adored her perfect projects and reports (not that she was ever satisfied herself). She worried a lot and woke up in the night feeling panicky at times. She had recently started to feel really depressed and had tried an antidepressant but hadn't liked its side-effects, though it had lifted her mood a bit. She'd tried therapy, but hadn't had much to talk about—she'd come from a close, warm family, and her adult life had gone fairly well. She was out of luck till she came to our clinic and completed her mood profile, which showed that she had almost every symptom in part 1! She left with some targeted brain repair supplements and the next day called to report the best night's sleep and the best morning mood she'd had in years.

Emma was too lethargic to clean up her underwear drawer. She had "the blahs," the kind of low-energy depression that too often made her unmotivated, unexcited, and unfocused. She was sick of being an emotional flatliner, but she had no idea what was wrong or what to do about it. We did, though. We could see that she needed our most brain-stimulating nutrient supplements. Fifteen minutes after she took them, we could see that she was feeling more like the person she was meant to be: humorous, sharp, and more alert. This became a permanent state of being for her after a few months of nutritional brain repair work and a revitalization of her thyroid function.

Rob had plenty of drive and energy, but he was a real "stress" type. Years of sixty-to-eighty-hour workweeks, too much coffee and fast food, and too many skipped meals, plus a drawn-out child custody battle, had turned him into a tense, wired, and tired mess. He was clearly sinking into adrenal burnout. On his new antistress supplements and regular meals, he was able to cut out his coffee without a backward glance, cut back his work hours, and begin to feel like a new man.

Sam was "too sensitive." He teared up whenever he talked about anything painful. He avoided hashing out problems with his wife because it was just too uncomfortable for him. Instead, he tuned out with a beer or a bowl of ice cream in front of the TV. Things started to change when we recommended some supplements that allowed him to tolerate pain more easily and enjoy life a lot more (without either the beer or the ice cream). Then, when he was no longer overly sensitive, we recommended couples therapy, which he was then able to tolerate and even enjoy.

HOW TO USE THE MOOD CURE

Now that you've completed and tallied the questionnaire, you've taken the first step in your Mood Cure: you know which false mood type (or types) you are. Having this crucial information will allow you to move on to step two, "Eliminating the Four Most Common Mood Imbalances." There you will discover what is causing you to have a particular set of false moods and what you can do about it. At the bottom of each part of the questionnaire, next to your score, you'll find the page number of the chapter that will tell you more about your symptoms and all about the solutions to that particular mood type's problem. For example, if you find yourself checking off symptoms in part 1, "Are You Under a Dark Cloud?" you'll turn to chapter 3, "Lifting the Dark Cloud." Each chapter ends with "Action Steps" that summarize all its suggestions, to make them easy to follow.

If you recognize significant symptoms in two, three, or all four parts of the questionnaire, you'll read each of the corresponding chapters. If your score is under the cut-off number in any part of the questionnaire and the symptoms you do identify with are significant, look over the relevant chapter to explore further.

Next you'll move on to step three, "Creating Your Nutritherapy Master Plan." There you'll learn about the good-mood foods that will become the heart of your diet and about how to avoid the bad-mood foods. I'll make it easy for you by providing simple and tasty menus and recipes.

Step three also features a master supplement plan that will provide you with several key pieces of your Mood Cure. First, it describes the basic vitamins, minerals, and other nutrients that I want you to make a permanent part of your life. Second, it warns you of anything that might make it unwise for you to take a particular supplement. Finally, it provides a master list of all the special repair supplements recommended in each chapter of the book. You'll copy this list and check off just the items you'll be using for your own supplement plan. Then you'll take your list to the store, get your supplies, start taking your supplements, eat your good-mood foods, and watch your false moods slip away.

As you work through steps two and three of *The Mood Cure*, you may find that you have other mood-related troubles beyond the big four and a mood-poor diet. Step four, "Getting Help with Special Mood Repair Projects," provides the answers if you have questions about sleep difficulties, addiction problems, or alternatives to antidepressant medications.

The Mood Cure concludes with five tool kits. The "Resource Tool Kit" will help you locate all the products and services described in the book. The next three tool kits give you the detailed, technical advice you'll need in order to deal with any hormonal imbalances that may be holding up the mood repair process. Finally, the "Food Craving Tool Kit" will outline effective options if "emotional eating" is a particular problem for you.

When Are You Cured?

You should start *feeling* cured in the *first week* as your nutritherapy program begins to take hold. At some point, in a few weeks or months, depending on your unique biochemical needs, your repair process will be complete. You will have corrected the underlying imbalances that had produced your false moods in the first place. After that, you'll be able to travel on your own true emotional power, so you'll stop taking the special repair supplements and continue to feel just as good without them. All you'll need to do to maintain your new sense of well-being and prevent a relapse into false moods after that will be to keep eating lots of *good-mood food* and taking a few basic nutrient supplements.

I wish you a very smooth and rapid shedding of your false moods and the enjoyment of discovering your true emotional self!

Step 2

Eliminating the Four Most Common Mood Imbalances

CHAPTER 3

Lifting the Dark Cloud

Eliminating the Depression and Anxiety
Caused by Inadequate Serotonin

Serotonin deficiency is far and away the most common mood problem we see at our clinic. Serotonin starvation is a virtual epidemic in the United States, inflicting its unique brand of dark cloud misery on people of all ages, sexes, and walks of life. One researcher estimates that more than 80 percent of adults in the United States suffer from this deficiency.[1]

The reason that serotonin is so emotionally vital is that it is our primary defense against both depression *and* anxiety. Serotonin deficiency is a factor in many seemingly unrelated psychological and physical symptoms, ranging from panic and irritability to insomnia, PMS, and muscle pain. Some "dark cloud" types have only a few of the possible deficiency symptoms, but many have almost all of them. Yet they tend to function well, typically getting more done, because of their tendency toward perfectionism, than other, less mood-impaired people. As a result, they often assume that they're just stuck with some unfortunate but indelible personality quirks and try to work around them. Some try serotonin-boosting drugs, like Prozac, with mixed results, and resign themselves to a somewhat better, but still limited emotional life.

Let's take a close look at the mechanics of this mood type. You already know from the questionnaire in chapter 1 that your brain contains four different emotional zones. Its serotonin quadrant needs to be brimming with molecules at all times. When it is, your brain can cheerfully fire away with this ready fuel supply, transmitting positive feelings and thoughts. If not, these happy reactions are blocked. But that does not simply leave you feeling emotionally blank. A decrease in serotonin can produce the reverse of every warm, happy feeling that adequate serotonin would normally allow you to experience: instead of seeing your glass as half-full, you see it as half-empty. Instead of feeling proud of your accomplishments, all you can think of is what you *haven't* accomplished. Instead of a sound sleep, you get insomnia. Instead of enjoying your family members, you're irritated by them. Instead of peace, you have anxiety. Instead of looking forward to life, you may regard it with dread and even have thoughts of suicide.

Precious serotonin is synthesized in your body from tryptophan, an amino acid (protein building block) found in foods like turkey, beef, and cheese. Tryptophan first converts into a substance called 5-HTP (5-hydroxytryptophan), which then converts directly into serotonin. This crucial three-step process can be short-circuited by a number of things. For example, if there isn't enough tryptophan in your diet—a problem for many of us—your body can't manufacture enough 5-HTP or serotonin to keep you happy. Or your natural production of serotonin may be inhibited by chemicals in your food such as caffeine, alcohol, or the artificial sweetener aspartame. Your serotonin production can even be disrupted if you are pregnant or not getting enough sunlight or exercise. Bouts of extreme stress can also dry up your pool of this emotionally vital brain chemical. Finally, you may have inherited a genetic tendency to underproduce serotonin, one that can be aggravated by all of the above.

No matter what the cause of your drop in serotonin, it does not mean that you are doomed to languish in this particular mood pit for the rest of your life. Even the saggiest serotonin levels can be quickly elevated, allowing you to experience the full range of emotion that nature intended for you. Later in the chapter I'll be telling you all about the nutrient repair strategies that can lift your dark cloud and bring out your emotional sun in less than a day. First, though, I'd like to tell you more about why your cloud is dark and about how it feels to live under the influence of serotonin deficiency.

WHY ARE YOU SEROTONIN STARVED?

Are You Eating a Pro-Serotonin Diet?

Serotonin, like everything else in your body, is made out of the foods you eat. You really can't feel "right" if you don't provide your emotion-producing sites with plenty of the specific fuels they need. Low-calorie

---

Where You Might Have Lost Your Serotonin

➤ *In your diet*—if you're not eating pro-serotonin foods like protein and healthy fat or if you are eating antiserotonin foods such as caffeinated sodas, coffee, or "diet sweetened" drinks or foods.

➤ *Under stress*—as your brain struggles with overwhelming or chronic demands.

➤ *In your genes*—if you inherited "false mood" brain programming.

➤ *In the evening or in winter*—when there's not enough bright light to signal your brain to make serotonin.

➤ *By lack of exercise*—when you've underestimated the brain-enhancing effect of physical activity.

---

diets and skipped meals, for example, can quickly reduce vital serotonin-making supplies.

Few foods contain 5-HTP or serotonin themselves, so everything depends on your getting enough tryptophan from your diet. Where do we get tryptophan? *From high-protein food.* Unfortunately, tryptophan has been diminishing from our food supply for the past one hundred years, about as long as our rate of depression has been climbing!

Tryptophan is still found in foods like turkey, beef, pork, dairy products, chicken, and eggs; but, in proportion to the other twenty-one aminos that compose protein foods, it is the runt. These foods have three times more of many of the other amino acids than they do of tryptophan. But this wasn't always so.

Wild game, like the venison our forebears ate, was higher in tryptophan than the meat we eat today. The difference is largely the result of how the animals we eat now are fed themselves. Rather than the grasses and other plants that wild animals grazed on, our modern stockyard animals are fed low-tryptophan grains like corn. This fattens up the animals in record time, but as a result, the meat from these animals is much lower in tryptophan. To compound the problem, we humans have also increased our consumption of low-tryptophan, grain-based carbohydrates like bread, pasta, bagels, cookies, and so on, which has further diminished our access to tryptophan.

If you are a vegetarian, you're at a greater risk of developing tryptophan malnutrition. Even if you never touch a piece of meat, you do get some tryptophan from foods like nutritional yeast, milk products, nuts, seeds, bananas, and pumpkin. But other than the milk products and yeast (which many vegetarians don't eat), most vegetarian foods contain *much* less tryptophan than animal-derived foods do. And that's important to remember, because decreases in the amount of tryptophan you consume can so easily prevent your brain's serotonin stores from increasing.

Numerous studies have shown how easy it is to create a serotonin deficiency in depressed people within a few hours simply by feeding them protein shakes that contain the other amino acids but no tryptophan. That's why skipping meals or eating meals without protein is almost guaranteed to reduce your serotonin-derived happiness. Our clinic recommends a minimum of 4 ounces of a protein food per meal (that is, at least a chicken-breast-size portion three times a day).

Unfortunately, though eating more protein will help, it is no guarantee that you'll get enough tryptophan into your brain. That's because of the blood-brain barrier, which protects your brain against the mayhem of nutrients in the bloodstream. It's a selective filter that allows only so many amino acids to get into the brain at any given time. Because there's so much less of it to begin with, tryptophan can easily get lost in the shuffle—no matter how badly it's needed—leaving you serotonin deficient.

You may also have been put at risk of serotonin deficiency from the start by being fed infant formula that did not contain the high human breast milk ratio of tryptophan to other aminos. Breast milk has a higher proportion of tryptophan than either cow's milk or soy milk. The net result is reduced serotonin in formula-fed babies. Were you one? One study, reported in a book that I recommend to you, *The Crazy Makers: How the Food Industry Is Destroying Our Brains and Harming Our Children*, focused on sleep and found that supplementing infant formula with tryptophan safely resulted in more and better sleep.

Believe it or not, getting too little healthy fat may be another way in which your diet has contributed to your low serotonin state. Increasing fat intake increases the availability of tryptophan in the brain.[2] Did you notice on the Mood-Type Questionnaire that anger and negativity are reliable symptoms of serotonin depletion? Both emotions increase on low-fat diets. A study comparing a 41 percent fat diet with a 25 percent fat diet found that subjects' moods deteriorated with reduced-fat intake.[3]

Last, and certainly not least, our fast foods and skipped meals have depleted us of many of the vitamins and minerals that assist in the magical

---

Serotonin's Enemies

Don't inadvertently sabotage your serotonin defense efforts. Here are some tips on how to avoid common anti-serotonin substances:

1. *Stimulants like caffeine* (also ephedra, diet pills, ma huang, cocaine, and the like)—They stimulate rather than relax, narrow rather than broaden focus, and inhibit rather than promote sleep. They are serotonin's number one enemies. If the idea of doing without them appalls you, turn to chapter 4 for better natural ways to get more alert and energized.

2. *Aspartame,* alias NutraSweet, is enemy number two. One of its primary ingredients, the amino acid phenylalanine, converts to the stimulating substances tyrosine, dopamine, norepinephrine, and adrenaline. Aspartame also contains aspartic acid, one of the most "excitatory" of nutrients. Both aspartic acid and L-phenylalanine compete with and trounce tryptophan and serotonin. If you are low in serotonin, you will need help relaxing and, in the evening, drifting toward sleep, so you should avoid aspartame as well as caffeine, particularly any time after lunch, when serotonin levels always begin dropping for the day.

---

conversion of tryptophan to 5-HTP and then to serotonin. Without enough calcium, magnesium, vitamin D, and B vitamins, for example, the neurotransmitters can't be made consistently. With so many of us eating far from enough fresh, whole vegetables, fruit, beans, and grains, we've become deficient in many mood-crucial nutrients, which is why it is important to eat good-mood foods and take the basic supplements laid out in the master plan in step three.

Is Stress Sapping Your Serotonin?

Chronic exposure to high-stress situations can sap your brain of serotonin as it quickly uses up your serotonin supplies trying to keep you calm and centered. Although all of the chemicals responsible for your sense of well-being are exhausted by too much stress, serotonin is often the first and most significant causality.[4] And stress, these days, can be never-ending.

Is It Your Genes, Gender, or Sex Hormones?

Like all the other mood chemistry deficiencies that I discuss in this book, a deficiency in serotonin function can be inherited. Through genes that under-program serotonin-producing activity, you can inherit a tendency to be shy, angry, depressed, obsessive, or sleepless. Look around at your family members and chances are you'll see the same symptoms that you circled in part 1 of the Mood-Type Questionnaire. The good news is that these symptoms can all be eliminated using the nutritional suggestions in this chapter. We used to think of genes as immutable, but now we know that they are capable of changing their messages in response to changing circumstances, such as their nutritional environment.[5] Regarding gender and sex hormones: *Females simply produce less serotonin than males do, as much as a third less.* This is a primary reason why women are almost twice as likely to have mood problems as men, though many men are now becoming serotonin deficient as well. In women, PMS and menopausal mood problems result when levels of sex hormones, notably estrogen, which help program serotonin production in the brain, fall too low. One of our clients suddenly became suicidal and her periods stopped, though her life circumstances were at an all-time high. Neither our nutrients nor her MD's antidepressants helped till she got a hormone level test and an estrogen patch. In males, depression and anger are common symptoms of andropause (male menopause). But they are tied to lowered testosterone levels and raised estrogen levels and the role of serotonin is unclear. (See the Sex Hormone Tool Kit for more.)

Are You Getting Enough Light, Especially in Winter?

Serotonin is one of the few body chemicals that is stimulated by light. And not just any light will do. How you feel may vary, depending on the type and amount of light available to you at each season of the year *and even* at each hour of the day. For lower-serotonin people, the late afternoon tends to be the beginning of the "unhappy hours." Many of them hate the fall, the winter, the twilight, and the night, for good reason. More than 25 percent of Americans suffer from a special sensitivity to the natural decrease in sunlight that occurs during the fall and winter.[6] Technically known as "seasonal affective disorder" (or, appropriately, SAD), this condition's "dark cloud" symptoms significantly increase when the angle of the sun drops and serotonin levels drop along with it.

But don't fret if you know or suspect that you suffer from winter depression. You can raise your serotonin levels *any* time of the year with the amino acids and other supplements I'll be describing later. These nutrients are especially effective if you combine them with some bright light. At least half of SAD sufferers respond well to bright lamp therapy.[7] And then there are supplements of vitamin D, the sunshine vitamin, which can be even more effective than bright light in helping relieve SAD.

Part of the problem is that even on a summer day, we may not get enough light. Natural sunlight ranges from 2,000 lux (a standard unit of illumination roughly equivalent to 125 watts) on a cloudy winter day to 100,000 lux on a clear summer day, but most of us spend our days indoors and get less than 100 lux a day! Being exposed to bright natural or artificial light during the day may raise your mood by raising your serotonin levels, but only if the light gets bright enough. That translates to at least thirty minutes a day within three feet of a light bulb burning 150–200 watts, which is equal to 2,500 lux (or lumens). There are stronger light boxes, but we've generally found 2,500-lux lamps very effective without the potential side effects of stronger lamps, including anxiety, nervousness, or even eye damage.[8]

If your spirits are not lifted by nutritional supplements alone, plan to spend a total of thirty to sixty minutes a day under your lamp without glasses or contacts on. Try to have your sessions before three P.M., as bright light later might suppress your sleep. Start with ten to fifteen minutes under your lamp and increase as needed.[9] Make sure that the light can reach your pupils while you read, talk, or work on your computer. You should be able to feel the benefits right away.

We worked with a whole family, born in Mexico but living SADly in Northern California, who fell in love with the 2,500-lux Ott lamp in our office during their family education session. They each bought one to take home and extras to ship to other relatives also stranded too far north in the United States. The lamps, designed by John Ott, a pioneer in the study of the effect of light on behavior and health, contain full-spectrum fluorescent bulbs, providing natural as well as intense light.

Interestingly, exposure to bright light during the day not only improves your emotional outlook, it also helps your sleep. Bright light in the morning decreases your daytime levels of the hibernation-and-sleep-promoting brain chemical melatonin, but it will *raise* your nighttime levels, helping you to sleep well. In fact, poor sleepers with SAD respond best of all to light therapy.

In the "Resource Tool Kit," you'll find details on how and where to find anti-SAD lighting equipment.

Are You Getting Enough Exercise and Oxygen?

Ever notice that you feel better after you've been hiking, cycling, or working out? Exercise can definitely raise your serotonin levels. Even brief and moderate workouts will do it for most of us. You may already have developed exercise routines that you can count on to keep you going moodwise. You can probably feel the difference when you don't get to the gym or out for a brisk walk or a swim, as your serotonin levels quickly sag again. Or are you one of those who don't exercise much at all and miss out on this healthy, natural antidepressant activity? If so, see chapter 4 on how to increase your energy so you *can* get out there and enjoy it.

Here's how exercise can increase your serotonin stores: When your muscles get to working, even during moderate exercise, they put in a routine call for amino acids for muscle repair. Your bloodstream always carries an assortment of amino acids for just such contingencies and delivers them quickly to the muscles in need. That's true for all aminos except one—tryptophan—the only one that can be used by your brain to make serotonin. While the other aminos are being diverted, tryptophan gets a free ride right through the blood-brain barrier! Once through, it quickly converts into enough 5-HTP and then serotonin so that in half an hour or so you can go humming out of the gym, smiling out of the pool, or floating off the dance floor.

Exercise also helps raise serotonin by increasing your intake of *oxygen,* which is critical to the formation of serotonin from amino acids. All that huffing and puffing really pays off! (That's probably one of the reasons why taking deep breaths when you're angry or upset is so helpful, too.)

Exercise diminishes depression just as well as light therapy, so why not do both? Get outside and walk or jog in the sunlight whenever you can. On a clear day, even the winter outdoor light is often brighter than a therapeutic lamp and, combined with exercise, can really improve your mood. By the way, both exercise *and* light raise oxygen levels in the brain.[10]

Unfortunately, exercise-stimulated serotonin works only in the short term. (The same is true for light therapy.) You may have come to depend on exercise to keep your mood up, but you can lose this thin edge if you can't exercise enough to keep your serotonin levels high—if you're too tired, or too busy, or break your leg, or get sick. Fortunately, as you'll soon see, there are other, even better ways to build and guard your serotonin stores. But if you can, get exercise outdoors during the day at least three times a week.

GETTING CLEAR ABOUT
YOUR OWN DARK MOODS

Before we go into detail about how to use which nutrients to quickly optimize your serotonin levels, let's look at how a lack of serotonin may be specifically affecting *your* mood, *your* behavior, and *your* life. A good baseline understanding of where you are mood-wise when you begin will give you an effective way to measure your progress. This is a good time to review the symptoms that you checked off in part 1 of the Mood-Type Questionnaire. Which symptoms did you *really* identify with? Which ones are you unclear about? Which ones are you unaffected by? Go through the following section and read more about the symptoms and how they do or might apply to you. You'll come away with a clear picture of your own low-serotonin symptom state. You'll also get a good idea of how your symptoms can change, based on the examples I'll give you of how our clients felt and acted before, and after, they started their serotonin building programs.

Relieving Depression—How and When
Do You Get Depressed?

All of the drugs, like Prozac, that stimulate serotonin activity are called "antidepressants," so you may have wondered why I haven't mentioned the word *depression* much so far. I haven't because I've found the word *depression* to be much too vague to be very useful. If you think of yourself as depressed, what do you mean, *exactly*? Do you have the low energy slumps, or are you overly anxious and negative? Or do both descriptions fit you? Do you sleep too much or not enough? Only these kinds of specifics can tell you exactly what kind of depressive state you're dealing with, and they're the only clues that will lead you to real solutions.

I'm alerted to dark cloud depression by a distinctively gloomy yet agitated mental outlook. It's not just bored and flat (that's the province of what I call the blahs and discuss in the next chapter). Rather, it's worried and obsessive. The negative feelings and thoughts can just keep on coming, unfazed by real-life circumstances no matter how pleasant they might actually be. When real-life circumstances are *not* pleasant, this kind of depression can be a heavy emotional load to carry. Typically, though, you're experiencing more inner negativity than your real life warrants, one that says, "No, my life will never be happy or fulfilled," or, "What if my daughter gets really sick and can't finish college?" or, "I *know* my evaluation is going to be bad." Both the present and the future can look quite hopeless when serotonin is low and the "what ifs" take over.

Dark-cloud types may see life as looking so hopeless that they may think seriously of suicide or even take suicidal action. This is obviously the blackest kind of depression possible. We have had a few clients who have been suicidal when they came to us and many others who had been suicidal during one or more previous periods in their lives. Most were relieved of their deep depressions by serotonin-building nutrients along with psychotherapy and an improved diet, but not all. If you have suicidal thoughts, it's very important that you seek professional help immediately. There may well be more than a brain chemistry imbalance involved, or you may have an imbalance that the nutritional methods suggested here will not correct. Do not attempt to treat this problem by yourself!

The majority of the low-serotonin clients we see usually start to look on the bright side very quickly. It happened in ten minutes for one of our depressed clients who tried one of the pro-serotonin amino acids in our office and suddenly started noticing the flower arrangements on the desk and her nutritionist's pretty red hair. More significant, clients typically report within forty-eight hours that they've stopped dreading their days and started looking forward to them instead.

Struggling with Low Self-Esteem?

Like most psychotherapists, I have spent many long hours struggling to help people with shyness and low self-esteem. I have usually started with assertiveness training and backed it up with a deep exploration of the past and present circumstances that might be contributing to a lack of confidence. My female clients have hated their bodies. My male clients were more likely to doubt their ability to be competent on the job. All of them were much too hard on themselves, with frequent inner self-scoldings and unnecessary guilt or shame. Sound familiar? The trouble was that psychotherapy didn't always help. Self-critical thoughts and feelings often continued to dog my clients, no matter how hard we worked. I couldn't understand it.

But when those same clients changed their diets and began using pro-serotonin supplements, something amazing happened—as their serotonin levels rose, so did their self-confidence. One of the most dramatic trans-formations in self-esteem I've ever seen involved Fleur, a jazz musician who had been a bulimic for fifteen years. Research confirms that bulimics are low in serotonin and that they stay marginally low even in recovery, which is why their thoughts and moods tend to continue to be so negative and why they so often relapse.

Fleur was in psychotherapy and went to Overeaters Anonymous meet-ings regularly, but she'd been unable to stop bingeing, purging, and overexercising. Her self-esteem was completely tied to the size of her thighs. She was measuring her thighs with a tape measure several times a day and taking desperate steps, like abusing laxatives, if she found the numbers going up. We immediately designed a supplement protocol to re-build her nutrient-stripped system.

When she came back the next week, she reported feeling much better and being free of her urges to binge and purge. Then I asked her, "What about the tape measure?" She looked blank for a minute, then a shocked expression came over her face and she answered, "I completely forgot about that. I haven't done it all week!"

This example makes a point that is especially poignant to me—Fleur had been convinced that she was just an ugly, inadequate mess *at the core.* But the *real* Fleur was able to blossom into her true self with the correc-tion in serotonin chemistry that a few nutrient supplements could pro-vide. Once Fleur's brain chemistry was corrected, she became much more active and productive in therapy, too. Until then, she'd just been going over and over the same senseless feelings of self-hate and the same empty body image issues that her low serotonin had forced on her. She was actu-ally a very strong, positive woman, who easily learned to assert herself ap-propriately when her biochemical confidence was restored by certain amino acids, the basic supplements, and her good-mood foods.

Are You Overwhelmed by False Guilt? Do you feel guilty too often? Even when you've done nothing wrong, do you feel that you have? If your own behavior *does* get out of line, do you get upset out of all proportion? Because many low-serotonin sufferers condemn themselves without a trial, it's no wonder that violent suicides are just as likely as violent crimes to be associated with low serotonin levels. Raising your serotonin levels will leave you with a *healthy* conscience, not a toxic one.

Are You Obsessive or Controlling?

Are you a perfectionist? Many of our clients have always felt driven, unable to relax about grades, looks, or work. Do you wonder about, or have other people commented on, your tendency to focus on a single worry: your weight, your work, or a problem that you perceive in someone else? This tendency to be obsessive is a quality that typically disappears with adequate serotonin. Often these symptoms are so familiar that you think of them as normal. Like the repetitive worries that keep you awake at night or being too "anal" about your school or work projects or your housekeeping. But that's not really you: it's low serotonin. Even with more compulsive behaviors and rituals, like hand washing and hair pulling, it's usually the same story.

"Controlling" is another name that you might be called if your serotonin is low. You may be hypervigilant and critical about how other people do things. You may take over and do things for them, creating a codependent cycle in which they come to depend on you but resent you for not letting them work it out for themselves.

Whatever your personal serotonin-depleted style may be, increasing your serotonin levels will allow you to start to move more gracefully and graciously from one stance to another, to try new things, to be more creative and less rigid. And don't forget that the symptoms of low serotonin tend to run in families. Does anyone else in your family come to mind regarding these traits? For example, we've had dozens of clients whose mothers obsessed about their own weight, constantly dieting and making critical remarks about themselves. Often they obsessed about their children's weight as well, overmonitoring their food intakes and taking them to diet doctors at very young ages.

Obsessiveness may appear or get worse after pregnancy, if already marginal levels of serotonin fall too low. The baby may be affected, too. We worked with a young mother who had been part of a study testing the effects of the medication Paxil on obsessive-compulsive disorder (OCD). She twisted her hair obsessively and had to go back to check that her door was locked three times before she could leave the house. Paxil had made her tired, caused her to gain unneeded weight, and had only taken the edge off her OCD. She was looking for a better way, now that the study was over, for herself and her 5-year-old son. Her little boy was obsessive in several ways, but his outstanding obsession had to do with the movie *101 Dalmatians*. It was the *only* thing he talked about and the only thing he'd been able to think about for quite a while. A few weeks later, while on the supplements, she reported considerable relief from her own obsessions and told us the following story about her son: He had come up to her about a week after starting his supplement and said, "Gee, Mom, it's kind of fun thinking about something besides *101 Dalmatians!*"

You, too, can become more flexible, relaxed, and obsession-free once your serotonin levels have been nutritionally shored up.

Are Angry Feelings Getting in Your Way?

If you have low serotonin levels, you are likely to be experiencing feelings of impatience, edginess, and unreasonable irritability. For example, violent criminals have much lower serotonin than do nonviolent criminals. And while you may not be given to violent rages, were you prone to tantrums as a child? Is anger affecting your relationships now?

Most (but not all) people with subnormal brain serotonin do feel irritable too often. Whether they're able to control the expression of their angry feelings is another matter that may relate to how low their serotonin levels have fallen. For example, some of our female clients become much more irritable, even violent, during PMS than at any other time of the month.

One of the worst aspects of sapped serotonin is how it can harm your relationships. I've had many clients whose marriages improved dramatically as they became less irritable and critical. Other relationships can heal as well. My client Clara was appalled by her outbursts at her young son, because she had been badly abused by her own father. She had never forgiven her father, though he had mellowed as he'd gotten older. She had always seen him as sadistic but felt that she was in an entirely different category, because she knew that she loved her son. I asked her to consider that her father's behavior, like hers, might have been involuntary—the impersonal expression of a malfunctioning brain. This relieved her of some of the hurt and anger that she still harbored toward her father. Although he will probably never apologize to her and fully mend their relationship, her new perspective on his past behavior has helped.

If you have been harmed by a parent's or sibling's irrational anger, dealing with the same kinds of feelings in yourself can be a very bitter frustration. Understanding the brain chemistry of anger can be a powerful force for healing old family wounds and putting an end to the wounding pattern.

I've been intimidated by my own angry clients at times. A real standout was a 16-year-old giant brought in by his mother, who adored him but cowered in the corner of my office in our first session while I tried to figure him out. Since he sulked and snarled much of the first hour, it wasn't easy. But I finally got enough information out of the two of them to confirm that his disposition included depression, insomnia, and low self-esteem, along with chronic irritability. He'd been in an outpatient counseling program for a year, because he'd been caught with marijuana at school. As a result, he'd tried to stop using marijuana, but he hadn't been able to resist the mood boost that it gave him. His mom thought we might be able to help get him back on track. After gleaning this information, I consulted with one of our nutritionists and gave him 2 capsules of 5-HTP. About ten minutes later, he began to smile and actually volunteer information about himself. He wasn't aware of the extent of the change (he usually felt that his anger was everyone else's fault), but his mother was thrilled by it. She recognized that her true son was emerging from the hell that serotonin deficiency had created for them both. *Note:* There are certain kinds of extremely angry behavior that seem to have more to do with imbalances in the minerals copper, zinc, manganese, or other nutrients in the body than with serotonin levels. I recommend the book *Depression-Free Naturally,* by Joan Mathews-Larson, if your anger does not dissolve upon using the supplements recommended in this book.

Is Fear or Anxiety Ruining Your Life?

You may be experiencing a cluster of traits that all have to do with a single annoying or even tormenting symptom of low serotonin: false fear. Whether you experience it as *shyness, anxiety,* or *panic,* your fear quotient is a good gauge of how deficient in serotonin you are. You may have tried to accept your disorder as "just the way I am" if it's mild or fought it with therapy, medication, and behavior modification if it's crippling.

I always ask my clients what their moods were like when they were children. Many of them tell me that they've always been shy or a worry-wart. But what is shyness? It's just a way of describing chronic, low-level fear combined with another classic low-serotonin symptom: low self-esteem. And *worry?* It's usually an unproductive mental reflex that is actually a combination trait in which three low-serotonin symptoms gang up together: fear, obsessiveness, and negativity.

Panic and *phobia* are obviously the most fearful symptoms of low serotonin. They can start early in life or develop later. Are you excessively afraid of heights, airplanes, spiders, or enclosed spaces? Has fear about exams, interviews, or public performance swelled into full-blown terror, complete with heart palpitations and difficulty breathing? Do you wake up with panic attacks in the middle of the night or have nightmares on a regular basis? (Remember that the night is the lowest serotonin production point of your twenty-four-hour cycle.) Even these extreme symptoms can usually be dissolved nutritionally by raising serotonin with a few key nutrient supplements.

A handsome 24-year-old actor came to see me because he'd been having unrelenting anxiety (including stage fright) and frequent panic attacks since he was 5 years old. He'd tried everything, including too much alcohol, to no avail. Yet a few weeks on his nutritherapy program and he was volunteering for cold script readings in his acting classes!

Serotonin deficiency is the most common cause of both anxiety and panic attacks in our experience, but thyroid or adrenal malfunctions can also be significant factors. If the nutritional supplements recommended in this chapter don't eliminate your panic, see chapter 5's suggestions for using calming amino acids like GABA. If no supplement helps, it's time to consider testing your thyroid and adrenal functions: first look at the symptom list on pages 66 and 79 to see if either problem sounds like yours. If so, follow the testing and treatment suggestions in the "Thyroid Tool Kit" and the "Adrenal Tool Kit."

Important *Physical* Clues That Your Serotonin Is Deficient

In addition to affecting your emotions, low serotonin can also affect your *body*. I want to alert you to these *physical* symptoms, because you may not realize that they have a connection with your mood states. The most common are (1) gut and heart problems, (2) sleep problems, (3) fibromyalgia and other pain conditions, and (4) cravings for carbohydrates, alcohol, and certain drugs.

Gut and Heart Problems

If you've lived with your stomach in knots because of low-serotonin worry or anxiety, it might help you to know that 90 percent of the serotonin in your body is not in your brain; it's in your gut. When you raise your sero-tonin levels, your digestive tension (including constipation) can often dis-solve along with your mental constriction. Your heart is also partly serotonin dependent; it's well known that low-serotonin-style negative moods, including fear and anger, are closely associated with heart disease. Nourishing all three emotional centers—your brain, your gut, and your heart—with the right pro-serotonin supplements and diet can result in big improvements in your health as well as in your mood.

Sleep Problems

More than half of the low-serotonin clients we see at our clinic have some kind of trouble sleeping. Many of them obsess and worry instead of get-ting to sleep, while others wake up in the night or too early in the morn-ing. If you, too, have sleep problems along with low-serotonin false mood symptoms, then those sleep problems can be easily solved, using the sug-gestions for supplements, food, light, and exercise made in this chapter. If not, turn to chapter 12 for several sleep solutions beyond those I described here.

Pain and Low Serotonin: Do You Have Fibromyalgia, TMJ, or Migraines?

Fibromyalgia is the name of a painful affliction that can cause mild to se-vere discomfort throughout the muscles of the body, with the worst areas of diffuse pain and stiffness usually concentrated in the upper and/or lower back. At least ten million Americans, mostly women, suffer from it.[11] More and more people are also suffering from closely related TMJ (teeth grinding, painful tension in the jaw). If you are one of them, you can ex-pect good or complete relief within a few weeks. These conditions are un-questionably associated with low serotonin. Fibromyalgia can have other causes, too, including low thyroid, but we've found that it usually re-sponds very well to nutrient therapy, as does TMJ.

Raising serotonin levels not only has a powerful muscle-relaxing effect, it can also powerfully stimulate our natural painkillers, the endorphins. That's part of why the serotonin-specific nutrients I'm about to reveal can be so effective with painful conditions like migraines and arthritic pain, particularly in combination with a good-mood diet, the basic supplements, and the elimination of allergy foods.

Do You Have Afternoon and Evening Cravings for Ice Cream, Sweets, Cereal, and Other Artificial Serotonin Boosters—Especially in the Winter?

Do you find yourself eating high-carbohydrate snacks in the late afternoons and evenings when both the light and your serotonin production start to sink? Does this really get out of hand during the darker months between Halloween and Valentine's Day? Most of these SAD calories are nutritionally empty, or worse than empty, and they are as potent as drugs in the way they can manipulate your brain and body. They can set off bodywide stress, causing your pancreas to release insulin in order to remove the excess carbohydrates from your bloodstream and store them as fat. The insulin sweeps most of the amino acids out of your bloodstream, along with the carbs. Only one amino gets left behind—tryptophan—and it goes right into your brain, unimpeded by the other aminos that usually crowd it out.

Ice cream, cereal and milk, and hot chocolate are favorite nighttime fixes because they contain tryptophan (all milk products do) as well as sugar. Unfortunately, these sweet foods are also highly addictive and can quickly turn into unneeded pounds. More important, they also raise blood sugar levels too high and can put you at real risk of developing diabetes. Hundreds of our clients have inadvertently developed Type II diabetes, or come close to it, as a result of using sweets to raise their serotonin levels.

Whether you start to yearn for a Snickers bar at three P.M. or ice cream at nine P.M., the real question here is: are you craving carbs because your serotonin levels have dropped with the sun? If you're a regular afternoon or evening craver, I'd bet on it. If you wake up in the night and eat carbs, it's a dead certainty. Swallowing one or two pro-serotonin nutrients right before you'd ordinarily crave carbs will typically knock out these cravings on the spot and spare you the negative mood that may have directed you to the fridge in the first place.

Alcohol is another carbohydrate commonly used as compensation for low serotonin levels. Do you find yourself needing a beer, a glass of wine, or a cocktail before dinner, when serotonin levels start to drop rapidly? You won't need to when you've raised your serotonin levels naturally. (Ironically, alcohol and other drugs actually *reduce* serotonin levels in the long run.)

Marijuana can alter many brain functions, including serotonin levels, which is why so many people smoke pot in the evenings to relax and get to sleep. But marijuana, like alcohol, ends up *inhibiting* serotonin production and can become addictive. It also has negative effects on brain, lung, heart, and reproductive functions.

One of the extraordinary virtues of *natural* serotonin boosting is that it breeds neither dependence nor diabetes. You'll be pleased, as so many of our clients have been, to enjoy its safe, effective, and legal relaxation without any negative consequences. If you suspect that low serotonin has made you, like so many others, dependent on alcohol or pot, please also look into chapter 13.

THE SPECTACULAR SUPPLEMENTS THAT POWER SEROTONIN

The Twenty-four-Hour 5-HTP Transformation

The almost instant solution to most low-serotonin problems is an inexpensive nutrient supplement made from an African bean. It can be found in most health food stores. It's 5-HTP (5-hydroxy trytophan). Your body can make its own 5-HTP to convert into serotonin, but there's one catch: It must have enough tryptophan on hand from food to make it out of, and chances are it doesn't. If you take a 5-HTP supplement, though, your serotonin production will no longer be dependent on the tryptophan you may or may not get in food. That means that you can quickly yet naturally replenish your serotonin stores and begin to feel the return of your true emotional self in minutes.

Although 5-HTP has been studied and used extensively in Japan and Europe since before 1980, our clinic began using it only when it became available in the United States in 1997. Since then, we have seen hundreds of almost instant transformations in mood as a direct result of its use.

As an antidepressant, 5-HTP is so effective that it has repeatedly matched or *outperformed* many of the most established antidepressant drugs, including Prozac, without the negative side effects so often associated with these drugs. In a 1980 study of ninety-nine patients who had been deeply depressed for an average of nine years, *almost half achieved complete recovery,* while others experienced significant improvement after being given 5-HTP supplements. The study's author, Dr. J. J. Van Hiele, had this to say about the benefits of 5-HTP: "I have never in 20 years used an agent which: (1) was effective so quickly; (2) restored the patients so completely to the persons they had been and their partners had known; [and] (3) was so entirely without side effects."[12]

Numerous other studies also attest to 5-HTP's remarkable safety and effectiveness, even when compared to prescription antidepressants:

➤ The manufacturer of Prozac, Eli Lilly, recently conducted a study combining 5-HTP with Prozac. Serotonin activity was increased 150 percent on Prozac alone. It was increased 615 percent after 5-HTP was added.

➤ In studies comparing 5-HTP with Luvox, a potent antidepressant drug similar to Prozac but more popular in Europe, (1) 5-HTP improved 68 percent of depressed patients as compared to 62 percent of those on Luvox;[13] (2) both 5-HTP and Luvox improved depression levels about 50 percent, but 5-HTP had an 11 percent lower failure rate than Luvox.[14]

➤ In another study, 5-HTP eliminated anxiety symptoms in 58 percent of patients as opposed to 48 percent on Luvox.[15]

➤ In terms of side effects, serotonin reuptake inhibitors (SSRIs) like Prozac and Zoloft cause sexual dysfunction in 50–75 percent of users, while 5-HTP studies show *no* sexual dysfunction and few other side effects.[16,17] In one study, 5-HTP had fewer side effects than the placebo!

My staff and I have been amazed at how quickly 5-HTP can lift the spirits of clients who had been depressed for so long that they had forgotten what it was like to be cheerful and optimistic. Within a day or two after starting their 5-HTP, they typically report that their feelings of anxiety and negativity have evaporated, that their sleep has improved, and that their self-esteem has been restored. Amazingly, we have seen these 5-HTP transformations take place before our very eyes, in as little as ten minutes. We have watched as surly teens turned into friendly humans, cranky adults turned into comedians, and shy, self-conscious people turned into real charmers.

One of my favorite 5-HTP success stories was told to me by Lynne, a driven, accomplished, and edgy advertising executive who came to see me after she'd been terminated from her job owing to a company merger. Although she initially came because of depression over her job loss, after we'd talked for a while, she realized that she had actually been living under a dark cloud for almost as long as she could remember. Lynne realized that even during the height of her professional success she had not felt good about her accomplishments and was too concerned with the negative possibilities in her life to focus on the positive realities. Like other dark-cloud types, Lynne also stayed up late at night, either worrying or working on projects. As a result, she'd wake up tired and drink several cups of coffee to get going, which further depleted her precious serotonin stores. The only time Lynne smiled easily was when she mentioned tennis, which she played almost daily after work and on weekends. (And a good thing, too, since exercise raises serotonin levels.)

Within minutes of talking to Lynne, it was obvious that she was a perfect candidate for 5-HTP. In addition to suggesting 5-HTP in the afternoon and at bedtime, our staff advised her to eat more protein and take the basic supplements. A week later, when Lynne came back into the office, she was a different person. The previously worried, irritable woman was now smiling and joking. I wasn't surprised to hear that she was also getting to sleep earlier and waking up so alert that she didn't need her coffee. Three weeks later, she reported that her mood and sleep were still great, but that another totally unexpected benefit had kicked in. Her tennis game had improved so much that she found herself winning against higher-ranked opponents because she was so much more relaxed and rested. No mean feat at 56! After a few months, Lynne found that she no longer needed her 5-HTP. All of the benefits she'd received by using it were holding, despite the fact that she still had no regular job.

About 85 percent of our dark-cloud clients who have tried 5-HTP, like Lynne, have experienced a remarkable improvement in mood and outlook. The odds of it helping you are overwhelmingly in your favor. However, 5-HTP doesn't work for everyone. If you don't feel better after a week on up to 300 milligrams a day of 5-HTP, you can use one of the other super-serotonin-elevating remedies that I discuss next.

Another Serotonin Savior—Tryptophan

Some people need additional nutritional help, beyond what 5-HTP can provide in the serotonin-building department. About 15 percent of our clients have found that 5-HTP either did nothing or made them sleepless, queasy, or mildly uncomfortable in some other way. (*Note:* If you get any adverse symptom from 5-HTP or any other supplement, stop taking it!) If you turn out to be one of the few who does not respond well to 5-HTP, there are two excellent backup remedies. One or both should work beautifully for you.

The first is the amino acid I've already mentioned as being the unique food source of both 5-HTP and serotonin. It's the amino acid tryptophan.

You know that high-protein foods contain this very special amino, but you probably don't know that tryptophan is *also* available as a supplement. Taken between meals in this concentrated form, it is converted much more quickly than it is from food, where it's less concentrated and has to compete with all the other aminos in the bloodstream to get into your brain. Our clients find that tryptophan supplements work as quickly as 5-HTP does and research shows it to be equally impressive:

➤ Over and over, studies have shown that removing tryptophan from our diet lowers serotonin and increases depression (including winter depression), insomnia, panic, and anger and also triggers bulimia and chemical dependency. In contrast, adding it as a supplement can raise serotonin 200 percent[18] and prevent or reverse all of these dark cloud problems.[19]

➤ The beneficial effects of tryptophan on sleep are legendary, and studies have demonstrated its powers in PMS[20] and fibromyalgia,[21] as well.

➤ In my favorite study, tryptophan stopped obsessive birds from plucking themselves bare of their own feathers.[22] (There's a tryptophan product based on this study called Avian Tranquility that is popular among veterinarians who treat obsessive-compulsive parrots!)

➤ Some psychiatrists, desperate to help patients not benefiting from anti-depressant medication alone, have added tryptophan with positive results: in a British study of depressed patients who had been untouched on medication alone, tryptophan was added and the depressive symptoms suddenly dropped more than 50 percent.[23] In another study, when combined with Prozac, tryptophan increased the speed of antidepressant effects and eliminated the sleep disturbances that Prozac caused.[24]

Actually, tryptophan has had an even longer and more illustrious history as a serotonin savior than 5-HTP, but it was taken out of circulation for several years and has only recently been returned. (For a full recounting of the tryptophan saga, see page 222.)

Tryptophan is harder to find and more expensive than 5-HTP, but it's a godsend for those who don't do well on 5-HTP. Tryptophan not only converts to 5-HTP and then to serotonin in minutes, it can also be used to make the important B vitamin niacin and many other valuable enzymes in the body. It is available by prescription (from compounding pharmacists only), mail order, and through some health practitioners. We've carried it in our clinic since 1999. You'll find ordering suggestions in the Action Steps at the end of this chapter.

The Happy Herb: Saint-John's Wort

Aside from 5-HTP and tryptophan, the only other really effective natural serotonin booster I know of is the ancient herbal remedy Saint-John's wort. Much of the research on Saint-John's wort has been done in Germany, where this herb outsells Prozac as an antidepressant. The reason is that it's been found to work as well as or better than Prozac and similar drugs, with few side effects:

> ➤ In a study comparing Saint-John's wort with Prozac, the two were exactly equal in effectiveness. Both provided 48 percent improvement in symptoms of depression.[25]
> ➤ In another study comparing the herb to Prozac, both provided slightly over 50 percent improvement.[26]

We've found that Saint-John's wort often helps to raise serotonin levels when the amino acids somehow do not. One of our clients, Nan, was always irritable and sleepless. Unfortunately, she was very sensitive to foods and supplements, and she got headachy and spacey on 5-HTP and tryptophan, so we tried a tincture (liquid extract) of Saint-John's wort. That did the trick, reducing most of her angry feelings and helping her get to sleep. It wasn't quite as complete a solution as we're used to getting from 5-HTP and tryptophan, but she was definitely feeling and sleeping better because of it.

While we understand how nutrients like 5-HTP and tryptophan work in the brain, Saint-John's wort, like most herbs (and the drugs often derived from them), is mysterious in action. We sometimes successfully combine Saint-John's wort with 5-HTP or tryptophan. Mostly, though, we rely on it as a safe alternative when the other two supplements just don't work. This typically happens only when thyroid function is sluggish. For example, we discovered that Nan had thyroiditis, a not uncommon autoimmune disease of the thyroid gland. (More later on the thyroid factor.)

SAM-e Sometimes

There's one other nutrient that sometimes helps when serotonin levels are low and the other supplements don't work. SAM-e, a natural antidepressant used and researched extensively in Europe, became a sensation in the United States when it appeared on the cover of *Newsweek* magazine in 1999. It has been researched and used successfully for many years in Europe for depression, and it helps with a variety of other ailments, including arthritis and liver damage as well.

SAM-e (S-adenosyl-L-methionine) is a chemical found naturally in every cell of our bodies and is key to many crucial cellular functions, including the production of serotonin and the three other mood-regulating neurotransmitters in our brains.

We all have some SAM-e, but SAM-e levels in depressed people are typically low. Our supplies can become badly depleted by poor diet, specifically when the vitamins B_{12} and folic acid required for its production are lost, as well as through alcohol and stimulant drug addiction or simply by aging. We find that very few of our clients need SAM-e because the aminos, combined with B vitamins, usually work so well, but those people who have benefited from it have done so in a big way!

We recommend SAM-e if the aminos or Saint-John's wort don't completely relieve depressive symptoms, particularly in people over forty; or where alcohol, cocaine, or other stimulants have been a problem; or where arthritis or liver function is a problem. It is not as quick to show results as the aminos, but if you try it, stick with it for at least one bottle's worth to see if it will help.

Melatonin for Sleep Aid

If sleep is a problem for you, melatonin supplements may be very useful temporary adjuncts to your pro-serotonin supplement program. As you'll see in detail in chapter 12, melatonin is made out of serotonin. Taking melatonin supplements can relieve the drain on your serotonin store, leaving it more available to shore up your mood. Often, though, 5-HTP, tryptophan, or Saint-John's wort supplements provide enough serotonin to improve both mood and sleep.

Tips on Taking
Serotonin-Boosting Supplements

At first, when you take your 5-HTP, tryptophan, or Saint-John's wort, you'll feel the difference, typically within fifteen minutes, but your mood will be noticeably elevated for only a few hours. That's why most people need to take these supplements at least twice a day. Middle or late afternoon and nine to ten P.M. are usually the best times to take them, but take them earlier if your symptoms trouble you in the mornings. *For children, use one-fourth to one-half the adult dose to start, depending on age.*

As you nourish your brain's serotonin zone with these amino fuels, your serotonin levels will rise, eventually to capacity. After that you'll be able to count on improved moods all the time, yet you won't need any more supplements to keep them that way. At some point in the next few weeks or months, your brain will give you a signal to let you know that you've done it—you've filled up on serotonin. How will you know? Maybe you'll get too relaxed, even sleepy during the day; maybe you'll get a mild headache after a dose. Most people, though, just forget to take their 5-HTP or other supplements after a while and realize that they feel fine without them. Yet those same people, in the first few weeks, would immediately have felt their moods plummet if they'd skipped a dose. Carefully check your low-serotonin symptoms on the Mood-Type Questionnaire over the next few weeks and months to see if your brain has normalized. It could happen surprisingly soon. For example, we've had a few clients whose irritability disappeared on 5-HTP, only to come back a few weeks later. When they cut back on their 5-HTP, their mood improved again. Their serotonin depletion was minor, and the 5-HTP had corrected it very quickly. This reverse effect is called "serotonin syndrome," but it's actually a phenomenon that can happen with any nutrient: when you take the nutrient, at first, if you're deficient, you feel better. Later, if you get too much of the nutrient, the symptoms that result are the same as those you had when you were deficient.

Once something like this happens to you, you'll take your pro-serotonin nutrients only on an as-needed basis. That's assuming that you've been, and continue to be, eating plenty of tryptophan-containing protein foods. If not, you'll end up taking supplements for a longer period of time, and your overall health will suffer from lack of protein. I suggest that you briefly stop taking your 5-HTP after you complete each bottle to see if you still need it or not. If your dark cloud rolls back in, you're not yet ready to stop. Check again after the next bottle.

If you get *no reaction,* good or bad, from these supplements, your *thyroid* may be too sluggish to perform its job of converting nutrients into serotonin in your brain. Low thyroid is a well-established factor in depression. To explore the possibility in your own case, read the thyroid section in chapter 4, on page 65. In this case you may do best on Saint-John's wort, which, like antidepressant drugs, does not require the assistance of thyroid hormone to raise serotonin levels. If even Saint-John's wort does not help, the only alternative I know of is antidepressant medication, which you might need to use at least until you get your thyroid repaired.

You might also need to explore another condition called "pyroluria," which can make it hard for the brain to utilize pro-serotonin nutrients. You can read more about pyroluria on page 303 in the "Resource Tool Kit."

Note: The solution to any adverse symptom that crops up after you've started a supplement is to *stop taking the supplement right away* and review the suggestions in chapter 10 on page 207.

ACTION STEPS

The Action Steps that follow will guide you in designing your serotonin building plan. *Your dark clouds are doomed!* The following steps recap all the specific suggestions made in this chapter. Check off the supplements that you feel you'll want to try, and note the amounts and timing that seem indicated for your specific needs. Then insert them into a copy of the blank master supplement schedule on pages 202–205.

Before you purchase or swallow any supplements, though, remember that your serotonin-enhancing supplements are only part of your Mood Cure; you'll need to combine them with the basic supplements on that master schedule and good-mood foods to get the results I've promised.

To check for any contraindications, study the "Caution Box" on pages 199–200 before you decide to add 5-HTP, tryptophan, Saint-John's wort, or SAM-e to your master supplement schedule.

Hormones, Sleep, and Panic

If the following symptoms do not abate on the special repair supplements plus the basic supplements and good-mood foods, follow the directions indicated:

Hormones: If PMS and menopausal moods linger, see the "Sex Hormone Tool Kit."

Poor Sleep: If you aren't sleeping better immediately, and perfectly in two weeks, see chapter 12.

Panic: Read chapter 5 if it continues.

If you are generally disappointed in your response to your program, please read the section on low thyroid on page 65 in chapter 5.

Light, Exercise, and Oxygen

Exercise moderately for at least thirty minutes, outdoors, during the day, three to four times a week as you are able. If you have SAD, you may need to use a therapeutic lamp as well, especially in winter. (See the "Resource Tool Kit" for sources.)

SUPPLEMENTS

5-HTP

	AM	B	MM	L	MA	D	BT*
50 mg (*not* 100 mg)	—	—	—	—	1–3	—	1–3

Start with one 50 mg capsule in midafternoon. Go up to two (100 mg) if you don't get much benefit from one in an hour. Add a third, if needed for maximum effect, in about an hour. Now you've established your dose. Take the same dose at nine-thirty at night if you have sleep problems. If moodiness (or craving for carbs or alcohol) occurs only in the evening before bedtime, move your midafternoon dose up closer to dinnertime or take your bedtime dose earlier (an hour or two after dinner). You can also take 1 or 2 more capsules if you wake up in the night and don't drop right back to sleep or if you wake up anxious and worried in the morning. (More on sleep remedies in chapter 12.) Between 4 and 6 (50 mg) capsules a day is all that our clients typically require. Larger or more depleted people sometimes need more.

---

*AM=on arising; B=with breakfast; MM=midmorning; L=with lunch; MA=midafternoon; D=with dinner; BT=at bedtime.

continued

Tryptophan

	AM	B	MM	L	MA	D	BT*
500 mg	—	—	—	—	1–3	—	1–3

The above directions apply to taking tryptophan, if you take it instead of 5-HTP, except that a tryptophan capsule contains 500 mg. It's available only by mail order or on-line. Call my clinic at 800-733-9293 (www.dietcure.com), look at the Resource Tool Kit section on page 289 or Bios Biochemicals at 800-404-8185 (www.biochemicals.com) in the US.

Saint-John's Wort

	AM	B	MM	L	MA	D	BT*
300 mg	—	—	—	1–3	—	1–3	1

Take 1 capsule (300 mg) three times a day. This is the dose used in over twenty-five successful studies on Saint-John's wort and mood. Use a glycerin tincture if you prefer drops. Drops seem to be more effective, as are all supplements that get absorbed through the mouth. For sleep problems, take your last dose by nine-thirty P.M.

SAM-e

	AM	B	MM	L	MA	D	BT⁴
400 mg	—	2	—	2	—	—	—

If you get no improvement after one bottle, discontinue. If you do get improvement, you may be able to cut your dose in half after one or two bottles.

---

*AM=on arising; B=with breakfast; MM=midmorning; L=with lunch; MA=midafternoon; D=with dinner; BT=at bedtime.

continued

Melatonin

Take 1 to 6 mg at bedtime. See chapter 12 for more on melatonin dosage.

When to Stop

Stop if you have any adverse effects from your supplements. Otherwise use your original part 1 score from the Four-Part Mood-Type Questionnaire as a baseline. Review your symptoms regularly to make sure they're disappearing. If some, but not all, symptoms disappear, increase your dose of 5-HTP or try tryptophan or Saint-John's wort. Check for a thyroid problem (page 65) or pyroluria (page 303) if no supplement is totally effective. Stop after you've finished each bottle of 5-HTP, tryptophan, or Saint-John's wort to see if your low-serotonin symptoms come back. If not, you do not need to take any more of the supplements. Your serotonin buildup may be complete for now, but keep your supplements around for the occasional low day, especially in winter.

RECOMMENDED READING

Murray, Michael, N.D. *5-HTP* (New York: Bantam Books, 1998).

Mathews-Larson, Joan, Ph.D. *Depression-Free, Naturally* (New York: Ballantine, 2000).

Norden, Michael, M.D. *Beyond Prozac* (New York: Regan Books, 1996).

Seiden, Othniel, M.D. *5-HTP: The Serotonin Connection* (Rocklin, Calif.: Prima Publishing, 1998).

Sahelian, Ray, M.D. *5-HTP: Nature's Serotonin Solution* (New York: Avery, 1999).

CHAPTER 4

Blasting the Blahs

Rebuilding Your Energy, Motivation, and Capacity to Focus

Our clinic has had a major impact on the local coffee merchants. Because of us, they've lost hundreds of their former hard-core customers. Our secret? Being able to restore animation, energy, and focus *naturally*. If you can't get going in the morning without caffeine, if you can't remember the last time you were genuinely excited about things or able to concentrate easily, this chapter is for you.

In "Lifting the Dark Cloud," I described a type of depression known for its symptoms of negativity, irritability, anxiety, sleeplessness, and obsessive behavior. That syndrome arises from a lack of the neurotransmitter serotonin. In this chapter, I talk about a different brand of depression (although you could have both)—a state in which, rather than too little sleep, you may get too much sleep and have trouble dragging yourself out of bed. One in which you may often wish you *were* obsessive, because you don't seem to have enough focus and concentration to get things done. Rather than feeling emotionally agitated, you may not feel much of anything. Rather than getting angry or upset at people, you may just nod and give in because you can't summon up the energy to react. Rather than being full of dark clouds, your mental sky may be colorless. I call this type of depression "the blahs."

There are two obstacles that could be at the root of your problem, and their mental and emotional effects can be almost identical: one is a lack of a group of vitalizing brain chemicals called "catecholamines." The second is a lack of vitalizing thyroid hormones. Since, like many people, you could be lacking in both, be sure to read this entire chapter to sort through each of the possible causes of your blahs, as well as each set of solutions I propose. But don't be discouraged. Even if you have the double blahs, you'll find that getting revved back up on a permanent basis is quite doable.

THE THREE CATS: HOW BRAIN SLUMP HAPPENS

Let's start with brain stall. If your brain is producing lots of the catecholamines, you should feel energized, upbeat, and alert. If your system is underproducing any one of them, you will suffer from some form of the blahs. There are three kinds of catecholamines: dopamine, norepinephrine, and the best known of the trio, adrenaline. Since there are more similarities than differences among the three, and to spare you repetition of these awkward names, I'm going to call them collectively the "cats."

Your sparkle—the feeling of zest and excitement that may be missing from your life—is derived from this trio of supercharged brain chemicals. All three cats can arouse and excite you emotionally, mentally, and physically if they're working up to speed. Dopamine, the parent cat, produces the other two and is the most prolific in your brain. Its two offspring, norepinephrine and adrenaline, are very active in your brain as well, but they're also famous for their activity in your adrenal glands, where they provide the jolts of energy that help you respond to stress.

"Attention!" is the cats' marching call. Cats are intended to make you alert to all of the important events taking place around and within you, so that you can act on them quickly and decisively. They enthuse you in the face of positive news and alarm you in the face of threats. They prime you to take action and even program your physical movements. They are your internal cheering squad and drill sergeant combined.

The extent to which you are extroverted or introverted likely depends on how much cat activity your brain is producing. If you tend to be the quieter one—more the listener than the outgoing conversationalist—it could be a cat issue. Watch and see if you don't start taking up more verbal space, sharing more of yourself, when your biochemistry becomes more extroverted.

The cats are particularly active under high-stress conditions, but any exciting prospect can elevate their levels: the anticipation of a meal, a run, or a vacation, for example. If you're low in the cat department, though, you may not react strongly to anything. Having too few cats is also why you may have trouble with focus and concentration. Are you deficient in the number one cat function: attentiveness? Even when paying attention involves being physically still, extraordinary mental activity may be required. For example, the cats should be *very* busy while you read a book. If you find yourself rereading paragraphs, your distractibility probably has to do with having too few cats on duty.

Easily distracted people have sleeping cats. The areas in their brains that contain the most cats may work pretty normally until they turn to a project that requires concentration. Then the cats can get strangely quiet, and quiet cats can't get your attention.

If you're low in any of your cats, you're almost guaranteed to be drawn to stimulating substances of some kind. How much do you like cat boosters like coffee, chocolate, or NutraSweet? Are you one of the people for whom tobacco, alcohol, or marijuana acts like an "upper" instead of a "downer"? Do you dance on the table or do your laundry while you're on one of these cat substitutes? Or does it take cocaine or some other major stimulant to get you going?

Any of these drugs can temporarily increase your cat levels by as much as 1,400 percent. Cocaine and amphetamines, for example, both force a huge cat release,[1] but the effects are short-lived. These drugs almost inevitably quit giving real satisfaction over time because your brain simply can't produce enough cats to meet the relentless demand. The ultimate result, cat depletion,[2] is what accounts for the long-term withdrawal depression that stimulant addicts experience after they quit taking drugs, and it's what drives 90 percent of them back to their drug use.

Whole classes of antidepressant medications have been designed to try to mimic or amplify the cats' activities in the brain—notably, the popular Wellbutrin (or Zyban), the older tricyclics and MAO inhibitors, and simple uppers like Dexedrine, Adderall, and Ritalin. Even some of the serotonin reuptake inhibitors like Prozac and Zoloft, whose primary job is to enhance serotonin's calming influence, also have cat-stimulating effects. That's why some people, high in cats but low in serotonin, find that SSRIs make them jittery or sleepless.

At our clinic, we've had much better results using nutrients to boost cat levels. One amino acid in particular has worked wonders in helping our clients recover their natural vivacity and focus. It's called "tyrosine."

Tyrosine—Nature's Energizer

Levels of the amino acid tyrosine are known to be low in people with low-cat depressions.[3] Tyrosine, found plentifully in high-protein foods like beef, fish, and eggs, provides the unique raw ingredient that your brain uses to produce all three big cats, dopamine, norepinephrine, and adrenaline. Studies at the Massachusetts Institute of Technology initially demonstrated that tyrosine supplementation could increase the cats dramatically.[4] Many subsequent studies have found that tyrosine could produce impressive antistress,[5] antidepressant,[6] and pro-concentration[7,8] results, just as we've seen firsthand with so many of our clinic's clients.

For over fifteen years we've been successfully using tyrosine to overcome apathetic depression and attention deficits. We've watched as hundreds of flat, tired, easily distracted clients were revitalized soon after taking a few capsules of tyrosine. Typically, it takes only ten or fifteen minutes for this superabsorbable amino supplement to reach the brain and start turning on the lights.

A particularly dramatic example of tyrosine's effects occurred during the initial meeting with a young Native American man, Stan, who was so depressed and unfocused that he could hardly talk, although he had traveled three hours to get to our clinic and clearly wanted our help.

Stan came from a family where low moods and alcoholism abounded. He'd been in counseling for several years but never got much benefit from it. When I asked him to point on the mood type chart to the negative mood symptoms he was feeling right then, he immediately picked out the symptoms of the blahs—apathy, exhaustion, introversion, and poor concentration—and said, "I'm really 'down,' and I'm so tired all the time." I could see that he was not going to be able to proceed with the interview without help, so after quickly conferring with our nutritionist, I handed him a capsule of tyrosine.

As I'd hoped, Stan began to come to life soon after taking his first capsule. Within ten minutes it had him smiling and moving around comfortably in his chair. Most important, he started to *talk*, so we were easily able to complete his work-up. Stan took his tyrosine home and continued to take it and feel much less depressed, and much more alert and focused, from that day on. He did better work on the job and started socializing easily with people for the first time in his life.

One thing puzzled us about Stan's recovery: He got dramatic results from an unusually small amount of tyrosine. The most likely explanation, we later learned, involved his Native American ancestry, which made him by nature a more efficient nutrient absorber than European Americans tend to be. This fact is attributed to a "thrifty" gene that historically allowed Native Americans to extract maximum nutrients from a sparse diet.

While Stan was fortunate in this regard, I can assure you that even with less efficient digestive systems, European Americans also get immediate benefit from tyrosine, they just need to take a little more of it. You'll get a lot more information later in the chapter on exactly how tyrosine supplements work, but now let's take a look at how you and Stan landed in the dumps in the first place.

GETTING CLEAR ON WHY YOU'RE SINGING THE BLAHS

If your cat levels are low, there are several possible reasons. Let's explore these reasons before we go on to how you can remedy the situation.

Is It Your Genes?

About 35 percent of Americans carry an altered gene that misprograms their production of the catecholamine dopamine.[9] Because dopamine parents the other two cats, this inherited foible can easily impact energy, mood, and ability to focus. Do the blahs run in your family? If so, don't be intimidated by the possibility of having this genetic miscue. Although it may sound like an irreparable problem, it isn't. The influence of genes in this case can be counterbalanced by remarkably gentle and natural yet scientifically validated nutrient therapy.

Kenneth Blum, Ph.D., the researcher in the field of brain chemistry and genetics whom I mentioned in chapter 1, discovered that the genetic anomaly in dopamine programming could cause mood and behavior problems—notably "blah"-type depression and distractibility. He also found that this inherited deficiency could lead to stimulant drug addiction. Most important, Blum discovered that these problems could be remedied through the use of certain targeted amino acids, most notably tyrosine.

In my favorite of his studies,[10] Blum succeeded in reducing depressed moods in newly recovering cocaine addicts. Cocaine addicts in early recovery are about the most apathetic people on earth. Why? Because they were low-cat in the first place or they wouldn't have been drawn to the big upper, and although cocaine initially enhances cat production, it ends up stripping it to the bone. Close to 40 percent of the cocaine addicts in the thirty-day treatment program whom Dr. Blum studied became so depressed that they dropped out of treatment during the first few weeks, unable to tolerate their drugless, hopeless, catless emotional state. Using tyrosine and other amino acids I discuss in this chapter, Dr. Blum was able to eliminate their intolerably low moods, and as a result, their AWOL rate dropped from 40 percent to 4 percent! Nutritherapy can be more powerful than debilitating genes *or* addictive drugs.

Are You Too Stressed?

Have you been under so much stress that you've drained your stores of the cats that are so essential for keeping you in good fighting trim? There really is a limit to how many of the cats your brain and adrenal glands can produce at one time. Exceed that limit often enough, and your cat supply is soon in the red. For example, cat deficiency occurs routinely under military battle conditions.

This is how it happens: At the first sign of an impending stressor, your brain sends word to the response center in your adrenal glands. There, cat messengers are made and sent throughout your body to prepare for fight or flight or both. Your heart speeds up, your muscles tense, your breathing slows down. You're ready for action. Over time, with prolonged stress, especially if cat production is not your strong point anyway, you'll run low on supplies. You won't be able to meet the demand for cats.

While your brain and adrenals can still mobilize the cats, you may find that you actually use stress to help you concentrate and get things done. Have you noticed that you "work better under stress"? That's because stress can wake up even sleeping cats, who can then help you get into productive action. But eventually the stress will burn you out.

Are You Feeding Your Cats Well?

Most people who suffer from mood problems are not eating well, and cat-deficient people are no exception. *Low-cal* or *high-carb* diets cause cat depletion because they're low in protein, and protein malnutrition is a leading cause of the blahs. If you don't eat high-protein foods like eggs, salmon, and cottage cheese, you may be stripping your brain of the key amino acids that it needs to make your cats. The more sweet or starchy carbs you eat, the less of these antidepressant aminos arrive in your brain, even if you *are* eating protein, because carbs cause the insulin release that tends to sweep these aminos out of your bloodstream, into your muscles, and out of reach of your brain.

Protein-rich animal-derived foods are very high in the crucial amino acid tyrosine, but vegetable protein is not. For example, there are about 840 milligrams of tyrosine in three scrambled eggs, 400 milligrams in a quarter-pound hamburger patty, and 900 milligrams in a chicken breast, but you'd have to eat twenty-four almonds to get a scant 150 milligrams of tyrosine. If you are *vegetarian,* by the typically low-protein nature of your diet, you run the risk of cat deficiency. If you eat a lot of soy-based foods, you also run the risk of low cat levels because soy tends to inhibit the conversion of tyrosine into the cats.[11]

Within two weeks of the start of a *low-calorie diet,* the cat-feeding amino acid supply can drop so low that cat levels can be cut in half.[12] The amino acids used to make cats are also needed for many other crucial body functions. They're constantly in demand for muscle repair, for example. Only 2 percent of these precious aminos get to the brain under the best of circumstances, and when you're dieting, even less is made available. The depletion of other nutrients by too much dieting, skipped meals, or fast food, notably the depletion of B vitamins, vitamin C, calcium, magnesium, and vitamin D, can also contribute to the problem. Like protein, all are key players in both depression relief and stress reduction and are critical to adequate cat function.

Are You Sedentary?

Physical activity can raise the cat levels, but if you don't have enough cats to begin with, you won't have the energy to start exercising. Don't push yourself, though. Forced jogs or showing up at aerobics classes when your heart really isn't in it can just further exhaust you. It's not that I don't want you to exercise; I certainly do. But I want you to do it when you feel energized and eager, not when you feel tired and overwhelmed. After a few weeks on cat-producing aminos, you should be ready to undertake more physical activity, which can then raise your mood and energy even more. (If not, be sure to check the thyroid section later in this chapter.)

Is It Your Sex Hormones?

Estrogen, progesterone, and testosterone are surprisingly busy in your brain, interacting intimately with all your neurotransmitters, including the cats. When estrogen in particular falls too low, it can trigger the blahs by failing to stimulate the cats. The same is true of low testosterone. In both the male *and* the female "pause," and in the hormonally unstable peri-menopausal years leading up to female menopause, both these hormone levels can drop quite low. If you're going through any of these hormonally unpredictable phases and experiencing mood problems, you should con-sider thorough sex hormone testing. I believe that everyone over 40 should have the best information possible on their sex hormone levels, especially if they have troubling symptoms like severe PMS or prostate worries, in ad-dition to mood changes. Any serious premenopausal symptom (such as en-dometriosis or irregular periods) warrants the same investigation. The best sex hormone testing we've found, by far, is saliva testing. You can find all the

---

ADD: Solving the Case of the Sleeping Cats

If you have ADD (attention deficit disorder), your cats are asleep. Brain images of people with ADD show very little activity in cat-rich areas of the brain. You should be able to wake those cats up with tyrosine supplements, accompanied by a radical diet cleanup (no sugar, flour, or allergy foods) and the other special supplements I recommend in this chapter, along with the basics from chapter 10. Many of our ADD clients have come to us with low adrenal and thyroid functions that needed extra help too. Remember that the cats can be aroused or put to sleep by your adrenal glands as well as by your thyroid gland and your brain. See chapter 5, "All Stressed Out," if you are easily or exces-sively stressed, a sure sign of weakened adrenals.

Both ADD specialist Dr. Daniel Amen, author of *Healing ADD*, and Dr. Eric Braverman, author of *The Healing Nutrients Within*, advo-cate combining cat-stimulating prescription drugs with tyrosine as a second step in ADD treatment, if the aminos alone aren't enough. If you seem to really need stimulants like coffee, phentermine, or Ritalin, try them *with tyrosine* to enhance their effectiveness and protect your-self from drug-induced cat depletion.

details on how to do an accurate exploration of your sex hormone levels in the "Sex Hormone Tool Kit," page 329.

TYROSINE TO THE RESCUE

Tyrosine is a truly phenomenal natural antidepressant. In addition to being the fuel that your brain uses to make its three antidepressant catecholamines, it is one of the basic ingredients that your adrenal glands need to produce their heroic "fight or flight" chemicals. If you are no longer able to handle stress, like a soldier with shell shock, your adrenal glands may have run too low on their own special cats. Tyrosine has been studied and found to be effective in reversing the physical and mental consequences of stress in military and other subjects.[13]

On top of having antidepressant and stress-protective powers, tyrosine is a primary component of your most powerful pleasure-promoting chemicals, the "enkephalins" (cousins of the better-known endorphins). In this role, tyrosine also contributes to an overall sense of well-being.

Last, but far from least, tyrosine is the raw material from which your thyroid gland makes its vital metabolic regulators, the hormones T_3 and T_4, which stimulate every cell in your body, including your cat-producing brain cells. People with low thyroid function typically have low levels of tyrosine,[14] and we've often seen tyrosine supplementation eliminate symptoms associated with this glandular condition, right along with the symptoms of a catless brain.

Note: There is more of the thyroid hormone T_3 in high-cat brain areas than in any other part of the brain. But if your thyroid is sluggish, it may not be able to supply your brain with enough T_3 to produce the cats, even if you take in plenty of tyrosine. When our clients with the flat, tired blahs do not respond dramatically and consistently to tyrosine supplementation, blood testing almost always reveals a low-thyroid condition that requires medicating. You'll need to do some of the thyroid investigation described in the second part of this chapter if tyrosine supplements and a few other supportive nutrients plus increased protein intake don't relieve your symptoms.

Some Tips on Using Tyrosine

Before you take tyrosine, please check for any possible contraindications in the "Caution Box" on pages 199–200 in chapter 10. Then start by taking only *1* capsule of tyrosine first thing in the morning, before drinking any coffee. In fact, try to skip your coffee altogether that day (and, hopefully every day, with the help of tyrosine).

Stan started his antidepressant experiment with one 500 milligram capsule of tyrosine and experienced positive results right away. If you feel no benefit in thirty minutes (it usually takes only ten), take a second 500-milligram capsule. If you still feel little or nothing after another thirty minutes, take a third.

Few people need more than 2 capsules at a time, unless they've been using lots of coffee or other, harder, stimulants like cocaine. But they do need to take them two to three times a day at first: early morning, midmorning, and midafternoon, if they tend to have a three P.M. slump. (If you're a poor sleeper, however, keep your midafternoon dose no higher than 1 or 2 capsules, and take it no later than three P.M. Like coffee, tyrosine might interfere with your brain's efforts to build up your natural sleeping potion, melatonin, as I explain in chapter 12.)

Caffeine and the Cats

If you rely on coffee as your pick-me-up, it is particularly important to take tyrosine supplements and to eat tyrosine-rich protein foods in the morning so that you can make and keep yourself alert without it. Caffeine raises your mood for a short time, only to bring it crashing down later. To make matters worse, it robs you of the crucial morning appetite that would otherwise lead you to eat a good cat-stimulating breakfast (not to mention impairing your sleep, your blood pressure, and the other things I mention in chapter 7). You'll be surprised at how well substituting tyrosine for caffeine will work for you. (Plan on going through the usual caffeine withdrawal headache at first, though.)

Don't overdo tyrosine or it can make you jittery or even raise your blood pressure too high. Let me give you an example of what can happen when you take more tyrosine than you personally need. David and his daughter Sharon were experiencing the blahs after years of demanding careers and unrelenting family-related stress. They read about tyrosine in *The Diet Cure*. It sounded so good that they decided to take 4 capsules three times a day—much more than the recommended starting dosage—because they assumed that more would be better and they were so run-down. Both did have overnight increases in energy and a complete elimination of their depressive symptoms.

After two weeks, however, David started to feel unusually tense and to wake up a little *too* early. When he went for a physical, his doctor told him his blood pressure was too high. David came to see us soon afterward and we told him to stop his tyrosine and read the warnings he'd apparently overlooked in *The Diet Cure*; too much tyrosine can cause headaches, elevated blood pressure, and a wired, jittery feeling.

David reported that his mood and energy slumped as soon as he stopped taking tyrosine, but his blood pressure went back to normal. A few weeks later, we suggested that he take 1 tyrosine capsule in the early morning and again at midmorning for a while, monitoring his blood pressure as he went along. His apathy disappeared again right away, but this time his blood pressure stayed down.

David's daughter Sharon, on the other hand, could initially handle 4 capsules of tyrosine at a time just fine. She loved them. After six weeks she cut back to 3 capsules (three times a day). In her third month, she settled at 2 capsules three times a day; and after six months, she no longer needed tyrosine *at all*.

Your body's reactions must be your guide in determining how much tyrosine you'll need and when you can start cutting back. If, for any reason, you feel discomfort or no benefit after starting tyrosine, but you clearly have the symptoms associated with cat deficiency, do the following:

1. Stop taking your tyrosine and review the amino acid warning signs in the "Caution Box" on pages 199–200.
2. Read part 2 of this chapter starting on page 65 to see if you have a low-thyroid condition.

The Amino Acid Phenylalanine

Most low-cat people will experience wonderful results with tyrosine; however, a small minority may not respond to tyrosine alone. Tyrosine can be converted from another amino acid, called phenylalanine, which is also plentiful in high-protein foods. Phenylalanine converts into tyrosine and several other important brain- and body-regulating biochemicals. Like tyrosine, it is available as a supplement and can be used instead of tyrosine, if tyrosine turns out, after a day or so, not to be as helpful as you'd like. You might do better on one amino than the other, or do best combining the two. If you want to try phenylalanine, start with a 500-milligram capsule and increase as needed. Stop taking it if it also causes any discomfort or does not provide benefits.

Other Cat Boosters

There are several other natural cat boosters that you'll want to add to your supplement regimen if you feel that you need a bit more support than either tyrosine or phenylalanine, or both, can provide you.

Actually, all of the basic vitamins, minerals, and fats described in chapter 10 help your brain to convert tyrosine into the catecholamines. The following basics are particularly pro-cat:

Omega-3 fish oil—You'll certainly need this one. By correcting fatty-acid imbalances in your brain (the brain is 60 percent fat), this supplement can usher out low-cat depression and increase concentration in a hurry. By eating more fish and taking omega-3 fish oil supplements, you can raise your cats by 40 percent! And you may feel the effects very quickly. Fish oil contains DHA and EPA, the brain-activating form of omega-3 fats. (Flax oil is also a good source of omega-3 fats, but less helpful, especially *in the brain,* for most people than fish oil, because it doesn't readily convert to DHA or EPA.)

In addition to taking omega-3 fish oil supplements, I recommend that you reduce your intake of vegetable oil (except for olive oil, which is fine), because doing so will help protect your brain's supply of the vivacious omega-3s. Soy, corn, canola, and other omega-6 vegetable oils compete with the omega-3s for space in the fatty walls of your brain cells and are typically rancid and brain harmful anyway (as you will learn in chapter 7).

Vitamin D—This fat-soluble vitamin is actually a hormone that directs the conversion of tyrosine to cats in both your brain and your adrenal glands. Vitamin D orchestrates much of this action through its relationship with calcium, which is literally at the controls in your brain cells (as well as in your bone cells). Your basic supplement plan, laid out in chapter 10, will explain how to use the omega-3 fats, vitamin D, and minerals like calcium.

Pycnogenol and OPCs—These pine bark or grape seed extracts encourage cat activity in the brain and can be helpful with focus and concentration problems. Try them if you have attention deficits and if tyrosine, phenylalanine, the basic supplements, and eliminating bad-mood foods aren't enough.[15] Take 100 milligrams twice daily.

SAM-e—SAM-e is world-famous for its pro-cat antidepressant effects. We've found that about 5 percent of our clients have needed it. This crucial natural chemical is used throughout the body and brain and tends to be too low in some people—for example, in those who have used stimulant drugs. Add 800 to 1,600 milligrams of SAM-e per day, if tyrosine, the omega-3s, and dietary protein don't perk you up in a week or two.[16,17] (SAM-e can also be marvelous for the liver and joints.) If it doesn't take effect after one bottle's worth, though, it probably won't.

You'll find a recap of all the above supplement suggestions in the Action Steps at the end of the chapter. But before you drop the book and rush to your local supplement supplier, please read the next section and give some thought to whether or not your thyroid is part of what's giving you the blahs.

IS YOUR THYROID BRINGING YOU DOWN? MEET THE NUMBER TWO CAUSE OF THE BLAHS

There's one prescription antidepressant that you may never have heard of, though it outsells most other medications in America, far outstripping even Prozac in sales. That drug is the synthetic thyroid hormone Synthroid.

Psychiatrists have been using Synthroid and similar thyroid-promoting medications to treat depression for many years, either alone or to improve the effectiveness of antidepressant drugs.

According to Professor Ridha Arem, M.D., chief of endocrinology at Baylor University's Ben Taub Hospital and author of *The Thyroid Solution*, one in ten of us, over twenty million of us, suffer from thyroid dysfunction. He calls the depression and mental fog typically associated with this dysfunction "the common cold of emotional illness."[18] Based on his estimate and our clinic's experience, at least one-third of the people suffering from symptoms of the blahs are having trouble with their thyroid gland.

Your thyroid gland sits at the base of your throat, just above your breastbone. From this perch it directs the metabolic action of every cell in your body. Notably, thyroid hormones are critical to the digestive breakdown and absorption of all amino acids, including tyrosine. In your brain cells, thyroid hormones direct tyrosine's magical conversion into the antidepressant cats. If either or both functions falter, tyrosine does not arrive abundantly in the brain, and what does come in can't be converted effectively into cats. The result: mental, emotional, and physical apathy and, often, unneeded weight gain, among other things.

We learned from one of our clients how intimately thyroid function could be associated with depression. Sheyna, a gifted artist who had been depressed for many years, had noticed an improvement in her mood from tyrosine and a high-protein diet, but a stubborn layer of depression combined with fatigue, chilliness, and unaccountable weight gain had continued to plague her. She hadn't been able to get in to see our medical consultant until a month after she'd started the program, but when she did, her symptoms and blood test results led him to a diagnosis of *hypothyroidism*. He prescribed careful doses of thyroid hormone to mimic the natural output of a healthy thyroid gland. Voilà! The lights turned on. She had a new and unmistakable "emotional glow," along with more sustained energy and nice warm hands.

After taking her thyroid medication, Sheyna experienced other new benefits as well. Her amino acids started to work twice as effectively for her in eliminating her junk food cravings, so she was able to lose more unneeded weight and begin exercising regularly. In addition, her overall health continued to improve dramatically from the time she started to get help for her thyroid. Since then, we've never ignored the thyroid when it comes to mood, and we continue to learn more about the thyroid-mood connection every year.

Do You Have These Symptoms
of Low Thyroid Function?

Take a moment to scan the following list to see if you identify with these symptoms. Depression is only one of the many negative effects that you may be facing if your thyroid is malfunctioning.

Common symptoms of low thyroid function:

- Low energy, fatigue, lethargy, need lots of sleep (more than eight hours), trouble getting up and going in the morning
- Depression (including postpartum or after the start of menstruation or menopause)
- Tendency to feel cold, particularly in hands and feet
- Poor concentration and memory, mental sluggishness
- Family history of thyroid problems
- As a child, played quietly rather than physically and/or now have trouble getting exercise without a guilt trip
- Weight gain began when you got your period, had a miscarriage or an abortion, gave birth, began menopause, or worsened after low-calorie dieting
- Chubby or overweight since childhood
- Tendency to excessive weight gain or inability to lose weight despite normal eating
- Hoarseness, gravelly voice
- Low blood pressure/heart rate
- Menstrual problems, including excessive bleeding, severe cramping, irregular periods, severe PMS, scanty flow; early or late onset of first period (before 12 or after 14 years old); premenopausal cessation of menstruation (amenorrhea)
- Reduced sexual drive
- Swollen eyelids and face, general water retention
- Thinning or loss of outside eyebrow hair
- Tendency to have a low temperature
- Headaches (including migraines)
- High cholesterol, atherosclerosis, or excessive homocysteine
- Lump in throat, trouble swallowing pills
- Slow body movement or speech

Additional possible symptoms:

➤ Goiter; enlarged, swollen, or lumpy thyroid (look at the base of your throat, under your Adam's apple and above your sternum)

➤ Coarse, dry hair

➤ Bulging eyes

➤ Infertility, impotence

➤ Weak, brittle nails

➤ Anemia, low red cell count

➤ Adult acne, eczema

➤ Dry, coarse, or thick skin

➤ Pale skin

➤ Hypoglycemia

➤ Constipation

➤ Hair loss

➤ Labored, difficult breathing

➤ Swollen feet

➤ Nervousness, anxiety, panic

➤ Enlarged heart

➤ Premature graying

➤ Gallbladder pain

➤ Pain in joints

➤ Autoimmune conditions often associated with thyroiditis: diabetes, rheumatoid arthritis, multiple sclerosis, lupus, Addison's disease, allergy, candida overgrowth, and pernicious anemia

➤ Angina, heart palpitations, irregular heartbeat

➤ Muscle weakness

➤ Atherosclerosis

➤ Extreme flexibility (double-jointed)

➤ Strong-smelling urine

➤ Tongue feels thick

➤ Vision, eye problems

➤ Excess earwax

Checking off your symptoms on this list is a solid start. But go beyond it to make an even stronger case. Ask yourself, "When did my symptoms begin? What illnesses or upsets was I experiencing at that time? Have my symptoms always been there?"

Quite a few of our clients report the start of symptoms after a tonsillectomy (the tonsils are close to the thyroid). The start of menstrua-tion, menopause, or a pregnancy is perhaps the most common trigger in women, but the incidence of thyroid problems among women doubles after menopause, and up to 30 percent of women with PMS have some kind of thyroid problem. Among men, the rates of thyroid dysfunction climb steeply after age 60, but we've seen many younger men with thyroid malaise, often starting with unusual weight gain in childhood. Most of our low-thyroid female clients began to gain unneeded weight and lose needed vitality in puberty.

If you've found that you have many of the symptoms on the list above, check them off and take the list to show to your physician. Thyroid mal-function is easily overlooked by many doctors, who simply run a single test, read the results with outdated reference ranges, ignore the symptoms thoroughly, and tell you to see a therapist or a diet doctor. For this reason, I recommend a very specific strategy for demanding attention for your thyroid. Otherwise you may never get any. I detail this technical strategy, from finding an effective doctor to testing your thyroid, to successful treatment, in the "Thyroid Tool Kit," page 306.

What Can Interfere with the Thyroid-Brain Connection?

Your thyroid makes two primary hormones: one is called T_4 and the other is called T_3. "T" stands for the amino acid tyrosine, and the numbers 4 and 3 stand for the number of molecules of the mineral iodine in each hor-mone. Through these two hormones, your thyroid literally ignites every cell of your body and brain by activating its genetic coding.

Within the cells of the brain, your thyroid converts T_4 (its more pas-sive, storage hormone) into T_3 (its activator hormone). This, for example, transforms the sleeping cats into a vigorous, healthy depression-fighting force. Without proper thyroid function, specifically in regard to T_3 activa-tion, the brain's neurotransmitters cannot alter your moods effectively. You may have the blahs because without enough T_3 your brain's nerve cells cannot transform the tyrosine you ingest into enlivening cats. In fact, the areas of the brain that should contain the most T_3 also contain the highest concentration of cats.

Without adequate T_3 your brain cells not only can't produce adequate amounts of the cats, they can't effectively produce enough of other key neurotransmitters, like serotonin, either. If you identify with symptoms anywhere on the Four-Part Mood-Type Questionnaire, but the aminos don't work for you, it's very likely your thyroid that's the problem.

Several things can interfere with your having a perfect thyroid-brain connection. Let's look at each possible cause separately.

Could it be genetic programming? If you've inherited a slow thyroid, your brain will become sluggish right along with the rest of you. Do you have a mother or any other relative who has the low-thyroid symptoms listed above or who has been treated for them?

Most of our low-thyroid clients do have family members who share their symptoms of depression, low energy, weight gain, and cold feet. Typically these clues have been ignored, dismissed as inevitable family traits (like blue eyes), and never explored or treated. In other cases, our clients have been amazed to discover that some of their family members had actually been diagnosed and put on thyroid medication for years or had even had their thyroid glands removed surgically. No one had ever mentioned it until they asked.

Give this possibility some thought and talk with your family members about it. Any information you get can help you figure out whether you have inherited an impaired thyroid that may be negatively impacting your mood.

Could it be the food you're not *eating?* If you are dieting or just not eating often enough (that is, less than three meals a day), you may not be getting enough "thyroid food." Low-thyroid depression is a common consequence of *dieting,* when so many nutrients typically get depleted. During the first day on a low-calorie diet, as supplies of all nutrients (including tyrosine and iodine) run low, your body wisely responds by slowing down your thyroid function. With each succeeding day (or diet), your thyroid can turn down another notch. Over time, especially if you tend frequently to diet, skip meals, or eat as little as possible, your thyroid function can forget to turn back up. This is what accounts for the "yo-yo syndrome": your thyroid may no longer keep calories burning efficiently, so you'll tend to gain back all the weight you lose, and more, time and time again. And, of course, your thyroid won't be able to keep your brain working efficiently, either.

We've found that protein and the amino acid tyrosine are particularly helpful to ex-dieters who complain of depression and the other symptoms associated with the blahs. Getting adequate calories and avoiding low-cal dieting is *essential* for keeping the thyroid gland turned on or for turning it up once it's been turned down. According to the World Health Organization, that means approximately 2,100 calories or more per day for females and 2,300 or more for males. We've found that although individual caloric needs vary, this rule of thumb allows our clients to maintain healthy weight and lose unneeded weight.

Iodine deficiency can be a contributor to thyroid problems and has caused big problems in parts of the world where the natural iodine supply is low. The American Midwest, for example, is called the "goiter belt," given the high incidence of disfiguring neck swelling caused by an iodine deficiency in the local soil. Since iodine was added to table salt years ago, and since midwesterners now tend to eat food from many different regions, goiter has become an unusual sight. In fact, these days exposure to *too much* iodine from iodized salt may be a more common thyroid hazard.

Tyrosine is by far the most important thyroid food, but for the thyroid to make and properly use its hormones, it requires other nutrients as well. One of them, vitamin B_{12}, which is made in the gut, is ironically often underproduced when digestion-enhancing thyroid levels are low. Other vitamins and minerals that are crucial to thyroid function are iron, selenium, zinc, folic acid, and the other B vitamins. Are you eating plenty of the colored vegetables and fresh fruits that provide these thyroid-crucial nutrients? When was the last time you ate some sautéed spinach or chard? If not, work more of them into your daily diet.

Could it be the antithyroid food you are *eating?* The foods listed below are well-known goitrogens (can cause goiters or swellings on the thyroid) because they interfere with thyroid function:

Wheat and its cousins rye, barley, and oats These are the most exhausting foods on the planet. They're the only foods that can typically make you sleepy (and bloated) after meals and lower your vitality level all day. They are known to cause thyroiditis, a common and debilitating low-thyroid condition. I talk about these grains and how to know if they're a problem for you, in chapter 10.

Soy foods—As little as 3 to 4 tablespoons of soy per day can powerfully suppress your thyroid function and lower your metabolic rate.[19] This applies to soy-based infant formula and protein powders, soy milk, and tofu. For further discussion of my concerns about soy, see chapter 10.

Cruciferous vegetables—So named for their cross-shaped blossoms, these vegetables include cauliflower, cabbage, collards, broccoli, brussels sprouts, kale, turnips, and swede. These thyroid-suppressing veggies also contain indoles, dithiolthiones, and other chemicals that activate enzymes that destroy carcinogens, so don't eliminate them, just don't eat them daily.

Millet—This is another grain that can be a thyroid suppressor.

Could it be chronic stress or emotional or physical trauma? Any of these things—particularly injury to the head or neck—can reduce thyroid function. Thyroid malaise can be part of the permanent aftereffects of post-traumatic stress disorder. Your thyroid pumps out its T_3 and T_4 as soon as a stressful event begins, and it can get overwhelmed if the stress is intense or prolonged. Some stressors, such as starvation or major injury, actually cause the brain to order a turning down of the thyroid to preserve calories and slow down the metabolic pace.

Chronic or severe stress can also wear out your stress-fighting *adrenal glands,* which are partners with your thyroid in providing energy and a positive attitude, especially during times of adversity. If supplies of cortisol, the adrenals' galvanizing antistress hormone, get depleted, your thyroid can be affected in several ways.[20] The adrenal hormone cortisol is required for converting T_4 to T_3, so if it's not available because your adrenal glands have become too depleted to produce it, your thyroid function also suffers. If your cortisol levels stay high for too long, as they always do in the initial stages of extreme stress, your thyroid may slow down its hormone production to compensate. (Otherwise cortisol could literally tear your body apart, scavenging for nutrients that it takes from your flesh and bones to use for its battle with stress.) Be sure to read up on stress and the adrenals in chapter 6, if high stress has been a problem for you.

Could it be your tap water? If you drink unfiltered tap water, the added fluoride and chlorine can interfere with the proper functioning of your thyroid. Both chemicals can be mistaken for thyroid-vital iodine (all three are similar chemically) and, therefore, displace iodine in your thyroid.

Fluoride has actually been used to suppress thyroid function in people with overactive thyroids. Chlorine is also associated, in both animals and humans, with reduced T_4. [21,22,23] (By the way, no major study has ever found that fluoridation is effective in reducing cavities![24])

Avoiding fluoride and chlorine is a good reason to drink purified water, preferably filtered in your own home. Make sure the filtration system eliminates both fluoride *and* chlorine, as well as the harmful hydrocarbons in unfiltered water that have also been shown to suppress the thyroid.

Could it be your medication? Certain prescription drugs can inhibit the thyroid. Estrogen (including the estrogen in birth control pills) and lithium are the most well-known thyroid-inhibiting drugs. Sulfa drugs and antidiabetic drugs also slow thyroid function.[25] Other drugs can as well, so review any drugs you are taking with a pharmacist and your physician to find out. You can also study the information on the enclosure that should accompany all medication.

How Did You Develop *Your Own* Thyroid Problem?

For some people, only one of the above factors is the key to a thyroid problem, while for others many or all of these factors can contribute. For example, fluoridated drinking water alone may not suppress your thyroid, but in combination with daily soy intake and a genetic vulnerability, it can be part of a gang-up that can finally overwhelm your master gland. We're exposed to so many biochemical bullies these days, it's not always possible to be sure which one lands the final blow.

Reviving Your Thyroid

There are actually three kinds of thyroid malfunction. The most well-known and common is low thyroid, or *hypo*thyroidism, which we've just discussed. The other two kinds of thyroid malfunction are autoimmune (Hashimoto's) thyroiditis and *hyper*thyroidism.

   If your thyroid is a problem for you, finding the right solutions for your particular kind of thyroid problem will benefit you, literally from head to toe. Your mood and mental clarity will improve along with your physical energy. Your heart will be immeasurably strengthened, your digestion and assimilation of nutrients will speed up, and you'll burn calories better.

Pregnancy Alert

If getting pregnant will make you happy, repairing your thyroid may be a godsend. Otherwise, be very careful. Fertility and a healthy thyroid go hand in hand.

Every cell in your body will benefit by getting your master gland back in action.

Most of our clearly low-thyroid clients haven't had much luck with over-the-counter glandular thyroid preparations, perhaps because their potency is so unpredictable. By law, they are supposed to have the truly active ingredients, T_3 and T_4, removed. Fully potent extracts from animal glands can be had by prescription. That's the primary reason we've had to rely on pharmaceutical help for thyroid revival; but if your thyroid problem is mild to moderate, over-the-counter glandulars can be helpful.

The other natural remedy that we have seen be effective with some people is the homeopathic thyroid products which contain potent though submicroscopic amounts of animal thyroid tissue. You may need to find a homeopathic practitioner who is familiar with these types of remedies (called "sarcodes") or one who will research them for you. Or just buy them yourself and see how you respond.

Most of our low-thyroid clients have had to seek holistic medical assistance to get properly tested and to get full potency medication, whether glandular or synthetic. Please see the "Thyroid Tool Kit" for specific guidance in every step of this campaign to revive your thyroid—from finding an effective physician to determining if a course of medication is really working. The reason I'm going to give you such detail in the "Thyroid Tool Kit" is that this information is very hard to come by. It's technical and you'll need to study it, but without it you may never know what your options are and never fully recover from the mental and physical blahs.

ACTION STEPS

Revving Up Your Brain and/or Your Thyroid

Before you focus attention on your special anti-blahs supplement strategy, remember that if you don't use these special supplements in conjunction with the basic supplements and lots of good-mood foods, you'll be disappointed by the results.

Your basic supplements are described in chapter 10 and are listed on page 202, in a daily schedule. This is followed by a list of all the special supplements recommended in every chapter of the book, including this one. Check off the special supplements that you think you'll need from the

Action Steps below, and then transfer them to the master supplement schedule, where you will assemble your entire individualized supplement program.

Be sure to check for any contraindications by studying the "Caution Box" on pages 199–200 before you add nutrients such as tyrosine, phenylalanine, or SAM-e to your master supplement schedule.

	AM	B	MM	L	MA	D	BT
❏ L-tyrosine 500 mg	1–4	—	1–4	—	1–2	—	—
Try one before you increase your dose of tyrosine and cut back on it if you get agitated or experience any unusual symptoms.							
And/or							
L-phenylalanine 500 mg	1–4	—	1–4	—	1–3	—	—
❏ Extra omega-3 fish oil*							
(300 mg combined DHA/EPA)	—	1–2	—	1–2	—	—	—
❏ SAM-e 400 mg	—	—	2	—	2	—	—
❏ Grape seed extract 100 mg	—	1	—	1	—	—	—

*In addition to your basic doses.

Advanced Support for Your Thyroid

➤ Over-the-counter thyroid glandulars, as directed. Look for GF Thyroid by Systemic Formulas, Thyroid by Nutri-Pak, or TG 100 by Allergy Research
➤ Homeopathic thyroid, as directed.
➤ Glandular or synthetic prescription medications (see the "Thyroid Tool Kit" for details)

RECOMMENDED READING

Arem, Ridha, M.D. *The Thyroid Solution* (New York: Ballantine Books, 2000).

Shomon, Mary J. *Living Well with Hypothyroidism* (New York: Avon Wholecare, 2000).

Shames, Richard, M.D., and Karilee Halo Shames, R.N., Ph.D. *Thyroid Power: Ten Steps to Total Health* (New York: HarperResource, 2001).

Langer, Stephen, M.D. *Solved: The Riddle of Illness* (New Canaan, Conn.: Keats, 1984).

Braverman, Eric R., M.D., Kenneth Blum, Ph.D., Richard Smayda, and Carl C. Pfeiffer. *The Healing Nutrients Within* (North Bergen, N.J.: Basic Health Publications, 2002).

Amen, Daniel, M.D. *Healing ADD* (New York: Putnam, 2001).

Taylor, John F., Ph.D. *Helping Your ADD Child* (Roseville, Calif.: Prima Publishing, 2001).

CHAPTER 5

All Stressed Out

How to Recover from Adrenal Overload

What does the word *stress* mean to you? Do you immediately think of the threat of war, the pressure of too many deadlines, too much debt, a bitter divorce, or the death of a loved one? If you do, of course you're right, but these kinds of stressors are only *part* of the problem. Surprisingly, they're sometimes the least of it. There are many less obvious but equally potent factors that can keep us feeling overwhelmed: the biological trauma that can be inflicted upon us by things like a punishing diet, brutal workouts, silent infections, or inherited deficiencies in our stress-coping capacity.

Stress isn't necessarily a bad thing; in fact, we need a certain amount of stress to keep us alert, help us get things done, and add spice to our lives. But when stress is chronic and relentless, it can have just the opposite effect. It can eventually leave us too depleted to enjoy life or even to function normally.

The problem is that the human body was designed to deal with entirely different kinds of stresses from those we're confronted with today. The stress response system we've inherited helped our ancestors flee from the occasional wild animal or warring tribe, but is ineffective for the modern kinds of multiple, nagging, continual pressures many of us must endure.

All stressors trigger the same cascade of powerful biochemical events, and it all begins in the adrenal glands. Small but mighty, your adrenals sit like supercharged golf balls on top of your kidneys in your lower back.

Think of them as your "A Team," and be very grateful that you have them, because without them, life would be literally unbearable.

The adrenals are very hard workers, producing from thirty to sixty different hormones. When confronted with a stressful situation, they immediately increase the production of two—first adrenaline and then cortisol. The adrenaline surge alerts you to imminent danger and prepares you to fight or flee. But this is meant to be a short-lived response. After the initial shot of adrenaline, the adrenals pump out cortisol, which helps subdue the adrenaline rush and infuses you with strength and stamina. Longer-acting cortisol is extremely important for your sense of well-being, particularly in the face of ongoing stress. It's a prolonged cortisol surge, for example, that keeps concentration camp prisoners and anorexics alive through one of its more extraordinary capabilities—that of raiding the body's own muscles, bones, and fat tissues to salvage the nutrients essential for survival. Cortisol is the "can do" hormone, the "bring it on" hormone. It's the hormone that allows you to conquer, rather than succumb, to ongoing adversity.[1] Up to a point.

If continual overtime or an endless lawsuit keep the pressure coming, the levels of adrenaline and cortisol can pump too high, too often, and keep you feeling chronically wired and strained. Surprisingly, though, many of the modern-day stressors that trigger these excessive reactions have nothing to do with upsets, injuries, anger, or fear. For example, a high-sugar, low-protein diet can trigger stress reactions without our even realizing it, and so can any severe or chronic infection.[2] So can caffeine and environmental chemicals we're exposed to on a daily basis. Whatever the cause, constant exposure to elevated stress hormones not only keeps us in an overamped emotional state, it can also lead to significant physical problems such as heart disease, osteoporosis, obesity, dampened immune function, and Alzheimer's disease. It can destroy cells in the center of the brain responsible for the storage and transfer of memory as well. See why I take stress so seriously? And so should you.

WHAT HAPPENS WHEN YOU RUN OUT OF YOUR STRESS-COPING HORMONES?

There's a limit to what your adrenal stress response system can take. Eventually, chronic stress can start to wear out your adrenals and diminish their ability to produce *all* of their precious hormones, notably courageous cortisol. When you begin to feel that you just can't take it anymore, it's a sure sign that your adrenals are no longer producing enough of their stress-fighting gladiators.

When your "A Team" gets too run-down, you no longer have the wherewithal (that is, the cortisol) to deal with even the most pedestrian of stressors. You can be overwhelmed by the sound of the phone ringing or your child's crying, thrown by a challenge, rattled by a crisis. Just when you should be mustering your resources, you get irritable and ineffectual. When your cortisol levels sink so low that you can no longer rise to stressful occasions, you've literally "lost it." The A Team has thrown in the towel—you are a victim of adrenal burnout.

After years of testing day-long cortisol levels in hundreds of people, our clinic has found fewer than ten reports showing excessively high levels and even fewer showing normal levels. The vast majority of the test results we've seen have shown abnormally *low* cortisol levels. Far from showing an ability to meet unusual stress with strength, these test results reflect what may be an epidemic inability to meet even a normal day with anything but anxiety, irritability, and exhaustion. They reveal stress-coping resources that have been broken by overload.

Many studies now confirm that low cortisol is an increasingly common and potentially serious problem. Over 50 percent of those admitted to an intensive care unit in one recent study had below normal, rather than the expected abnormally high, levels of cortisol.[3] A study of 289 men found that low cortisol was the overriding factor in the development of diabetes, stroke, and cardiovascular disease.[4] A study of women with breast cancer found that those with low cortisol had fewer natural immune system killer cells and died earlier.[5] No reserves left to fight the *really* important stressors.

Adrenaline reserves, too, can eventually deflate, as stress-induced exhaustion sets in. More than 70 percent of Americans may be affected.[6]

WHERE ARE YOU ON THE ADRENAL BURNOUT CONTINUUM?

How do you know if you've experienced too much stress? Your score on part 3 of the Mood-Type Questionnaire gave you one indication. For a much more complete picture, look at the following list of the common symptoms of adrenal exhaustion. Think about which of these symptoms in particular apply to you, how often you experience them, and how much they bother you.

- ➤ Sensitivity to exhaust fumes, smoke, smog, petrochemicals
- ➤ Inability to tolerate much exercise, or you feel worse after exercising
- ➤ Depression or rapid mood swings
- ➤ Dark circles under the eyes
- ➤ Dizziness upon standing
- ➤ Lack of mental alertness
- ➤ Tendency to catch colds easily when weather changes
- ➤ Headaches, particularly migraines, along with insomnia
- ➤ Breathing difficulties
- ➤ Edema (water retention)
- ➤ Salt cravings
- ➤ Trouble falling asleep or staying asleep
- ➤ Feeling of not being rested upon awakening
- ➤ Feeling of tiredness all the time
- ➤ Feeling of being mentally and emotionally overstressed
- ➤ Low blood sugar symptoms
- ➤ Need for caffeine (coffee, tea, and others) to get you going in the morning
- ➤ Low tolerance of loud noises and/or strong odors
- ➤ Tendency to startle easily
- ➤ Food or respiratory allergies
- ➤ Recurrent, chronic infections, such as yeast infections
- ➤ Lightheadedness
- ➤ Low tolerance for alcohol, caffeine, and other drugs
- ➤ Fainting
- ➤ Tendency to get upset or frustrated easily, quick to cry
- ➤ Tendency to get a second wind at night
- ➤ Low blood pressure
- ➤ Haven't felt your best in a long time
- ➤ Eyes sensitive to bright light
- ➤ Feeling of being weak and shaky
- ➤ Fatigue and muscular weakness
- ➤ Sweating or wetness of hands and feet caused by nervousness or mood swings
- ➤ Ability, sometimes, to relieve depression and moodiness by eating

- Frequent heart palpitations
- Chronic heartburn
- Vague indigestion or abdominal pain
- Infrequent urination
- Sweet cravings
- Lack of thirst
- Clenching and/or grinding of teeth, especially at night
- Chronic pain in the lower neck and upper back
- Inability to concentrate and/or confusion, usually along with clumsiness
- An unusually small jawbone or chin; lower teeth crowded, unequal in length, or misaligned
- A chronic breathing disorder, particularly asthma
- An excessively low cholesterol level (below 150 mg/dl)
- Bouts of severe infection

DO YOU REMEMBER WHAT LIFE WAS LIKE PRE-BURNOUT?

Before we get into stress-liberation strategies, I'd like you to pause for a moment and try to recall the time before you started having these symptoms, when you could really handle, or even enjoy, stress. Do you remember when you could still face deadlines, confrontations, and long commutes with gusto and a sense of humor? Do you remember when you used to see difficulty as an exciting challenge: all-nighters in college, running marathons, your first job, your first diet? Do you remember making jokes about setbacks instead of becoming short-tempered and edgy? When was the last time your neck and shoulders didn't feel tight and achy? When was the last time you regularly enjoyed an hour of peaceful daydreaming, a warm fire with no TV on, a whole weekend of lounging around with your family or friends, or a quiet stroll through the neighborhood at twilight?

This is an important exercise because it can help you gauge how long you've been burning out and give you a concrete sense of your goal: How you'll experience life when the feeling of being overwhelmed is a rare, instead of a constant, sensation. How I hope you'll soon feel after you've followed the recommendation that I'm going to make later in the chapter about how to use effective nutritional peacemakers. But first, let's look into the root causes of your adrenal burnout.

GETTING CLEAR ABOUT YOUR STRESS-COPING CAPACITY OR LACK OF IT

It's easy for stress overload to creep up on us. Our society rewards the busy, high-flying multitasker. We can get so caught up in the challenges of juggling all the complex demands in our lives that we don't recognize the very real risk of burnout. Looking at all the factors that are affecting your personal stress-coping capacity will help you identify exactly what you'll need to change in order to meet life's challenges with eagerness and strength once again.

How Much Genetic Fortitude Got Passed On to You?

We're all built to handle stress, but each of us has a unique, partly inborn stress-coping capacity. Some of us are born with a fragile sensitivity to stress and wear out early in life. Others can muscle through quite a bit of adversity before they wear thin. Then there are those remarkable people who really seem to thrive on constant challenge and action, powerhouses of energy and stamina into old age.

To get a better idea of what kind of person you were born to become, consider your parents and other close relatives. How have they handled stress? Have they needed tobacco, alcohol, or chocolate to cope with it? Have they gotten weepy, testy, or even explosive under fire? Our clients often describe parents or grandparents who couldn't tolerate stress without a drink or a scapegoat.

How Many External Stressors Do You Currently Face, and How Do You Cope with Them?

Among all the various factors contributing to adrenal burnout, the most obvious ones are the external stressors: the overwork, illness, injury, pain, cruelty, privation, fear, and loss that life so often presents us with. Relationships at home and at work are our primary sources of this kind of stress, and this has probably always been the case, but some new factors, unique to the twenty-first century, explain why up to 90 percent of all visits to primary care physicians are now prompted by stress-related problems:[7]

> ➤ We are eating the most stressful diet ever known. Ironically over 70 percent of us eat the very worst junk foods in order to *relieve* our emotional stress![8]

> ➤ Today, over 75 percent of our households are single-parent families, many living far from extended family members.[9] This means that both adults and children are now impacted as never before by too little time and too little support.

> ➤ Pressures in the workplace have skyrocketed. There's been a *700 percent* increase in workmen's comp claims for mental stress since the 1980s in California alone, and 25–40 percent of American workers now report stress burnout, particularly women with children. Stress ranks second only to family crisis among problems in the workplace.[10]

> ➤ The chemical pollution that is overwhelming our food, soil, air, water, and even our buildings adds a whole new dimension to the stresses we face.

> ➤ Rising rates of adolescent suicide, the third leading cause of death among teens, are closely tied to stress, and even children complain of stress now, with up to one in ten suffering from a serious anxiety or panic disorder.[11]

It all adds up to an extraordinary new, specifically Western, style of stress.

The nutritional suggestions I'll make in this chapter can help you cope with these external stressors. However, they cannot take the place of an honest assessment of your life, of the draining realities that you may need to eliminate or learn how to handle more constructively, or of the counsel and prayer that you may require in the process. Sometimes changing your job or getting counseling with your spouse can miraculously return you to your old self. Other times something as simple as learning to cry can help tremendously. In an early study on stress, the parents of children dying of leukemia had their stress levels tested. The parents who did not cry had much higher levels than those who were able to cry. We now know that crying serves a very specific biological purpose. Human tears, unlike the tears of any other animal, contain a substance called ACTH, the hormone that actually sets off the stress response and is literally washed away by a good cry.[12]

In counseling you can learn to cry and to breathe deeply, to assert yourself, to express anger appropriately, and to simplify your life. But if your stress has gone on for too long, you may recover only part of your natural vitality by changing your circumstances. If that's the case, you can find the rest of it by following the suggestions in this chapter. And if you haven't yet been able to make those stress-reducing changes in your life, you may need to get in shape first. Big changes (even good ones) do cause more stress, so you'll be much more effective if you get into nutritional training now.

Are You Nourishing the A Team? Nutritional catch-up really should be your first priority. Why? Because something else has been increasing, right along with on-the-job pressure, pollution, and our private ordeals. It's the junk food epidemic. We're undernourished as never before, burdened with an unprecedented fear of food and calories combined with an inability to limit our consumption of stressful sweets, caffeine, and other fast foods. Too often we have no time to prepare fresh food. Too often we don't eat at all. It turns out, though, that the more stress we're under, the *better* we have to eat, to literally "keep up our strength." Instead, partly because we've run out of time and energy, under stress, we've taken to eating more poorly than ever before in history. Most fast food is low in nutrients and high in system-shocking sugar, rancid fats, and chemical additives, so it actually *adds* to our stress level instead of subtracting from it.

The one thing that may be harder on us than eating stressful foods is not eating *anything*. Skipping meals and going on low-cal diets create an inner emergency state (called starvation) that is highly stressful. If you frequently feel exhausted at the end of the workday, it may be because you're not eating enough. In a recent study, two groups of department store workers were assessed for signs of stress by comparing them after a forty-seven-hour workweek and after a thirty-two-hour workweek. All felt much more stressed after the longer workweek, but those who experienced the worst stress were those who skipped meals or underate.[13] I know that many of you are pressed for time during the day, but I'm willing to bet that you'd not only feel a lot better, but would actually be more productive if you fortified yourself with three meals made from good-mood foods that I describe in chapters 8 and 9.

Let's take a look at how *you're* doing personally in the food department. How are you fueling yourself for the daily onslaught?

In the morning: Do you start your day with a jolt of sweetened coffee, plus a bowl of sweetened cold cereal, and perhaps some sweet frozen or packaged juice? Or maybe you grab a sugary latte with a sweet scone or a doughnut? Or do you have nothing at all except coffee?

At lunch: Is your midday meal something like this: soda, crisps, sandwich, burrito, a container of instant soup mix, or a burger? You're probably too hungry to skip lunch entirely, unless you really get too busy—in which case, do you have a diet soda, more coffee, and maybe a candy bar?

Dinner: Do you end the day with a heaping plate of pasta with a little cheese? Are you so tired that you bring home a pizza and top it off with ice cream? Or are you too tired for anything—do you go to bed (if you can sleep) after crackers and cheese or a bowl of sweetened cereal?

Why *not* eat this way? Because, as I mentioned earlier, if you're eating this way, you're eating the most stressful food ever known.

Hypoglycemia: Are You Poisoning the A Team?

The A Team is specially trained to keep your blood sugar (or glucose) levels steady and constant. Too much or too little sugar in your bloodstream can give you diabetes or put you into a coma, so regulating your reaction to sweet and starchy carbohydrates is one of your adrenals' most critical responsibilities. Typically, the A Team is running down the field to rescue a *low* blood sugar situation (otherwise known as "hypoglycemia"). This is our most common blood sugar problem, though it often leads to high blood sugar ("diabetes"), which is now an epidemic in the West. Up until one hundred years or so ago, these blood sugar problems were rare because we ate regularly, heartily, and relatively sweetlessly. On the farms and in towns and even in the cities, big meals were standard, but big servings of sugar were not. Americans ate 25 pounds of sugar a year in 1900. We now eat over 125 pounds a year, five times *more* sugar a year than we did then. We also eat lots more starchy white flour products (white bread, bagels, pasta), which act almost exactly like sugar in the body.

Sweets of all kinds and their white flour twins can raise blood sugar too high within minutes. Then adrenaline alarm bells go off, and insulin is sent out to scoop up all that alarming excess blood sugar and store it as fat.

That leaves the blood with very little of the glucose that it needs to distribute as fuel to keep the body going. If your blood's sugar supply drops critically low, the A Team rushes out again, this time with cortisol, to salvage some precious stored sugar from emergency fuel depots in your liver and muscles. This effort takes a lot out of the A Team, leaving it much less able to protect you from serious stressors, like a redundancy letter, a sick child, or an infection.

With our current diet so full of sweets and starches, the adrenals are tremendously overworked. On a normal day the adrenals produce an average of about 20 milligrams of cortisol, but any illness, even the flu, requires a surge of cortisol many times above normal levels.[14] With the constant distraction of high-carb foods to deal with, from breakfast cereals to daytime sodas to nighttime desserts, cortisol supplies can begin to shrink along with your health. Remember: Sugar is a highly adulterated druglike food that not only causes debilitating stress, but is also the number one fuel for cancer cells!

Common Symptoms of Low Blood Sugar

> Nervousness
> Exhaustion, weakness
> Faintness, dizziness, tremors, cold sweats
> Drowsiness
> Forgetfulness, confusion
> Constant worrying, unprovoked anxiety
> Craving for sweets *or* alcohol
> Heart palpitations, rapid pulse
> Indecisiveness
> Lack of coordination
> Lack of concentration
> Muscle twitching and jerking

> Sighing and yawning
> Irritability
> Depression
> Headaches
> Insomnia
> Internal trembling
> Numbness
> Crying spells
> Leg cramps
> Blurred vision
> Itching and crawling skin sensations
> Unconsciousness

More Obvious *and* Surprising Causes of Stress

Unbalanced sex hormones. In PMS, especially as women get closer to menopause (any time after age 35), a stress-generating theft may be under way. An interesting and vital role of the sex hormone progesterone is that of controlling the release of the most relaxing chemical in the brain: the neurotransmitter called GABA. In fact, progesterone literally turns GABA on. In *women,* levels of progesterone and GABA are supposed to be at their highest in the week before menstruation. But progesterone levels tend to drop too low in PMS and every day as menopause draws nearer. One big reason is that stress can redirect the hormone-producing adrenal glands. Instead of progesterone, they're busy overproducing stress response hormones like adrenaline and cortisol. If you feel unusually stressed as part of PMS, chances are your progesterone and GABA levels are low. *Men* can suffer from depleted progesterone, too. It's a factor behind certain kinds of insomnia, for example. See the "Sex Hormone Tool Kit" for information on how to test and, if necessary, safely rebalance your sex hormones.

Infection. Any prolonged or frequent illness, infection, injury, or pain is an adrenal stressor that causes a rise in cortisol. But if the elevation goes on for too long, it can weaken your immune system, eventually making you vulnerable to more illness and a vicious cycle of stress and re-stress. Eventually you can run so low in cortisol that its protective surges no longer rise to your needs. Cortisol levels need to be flexible and moderate. If they are too low or too high for too long, you'll get into trouble.

Intestinal intruders. No malignant presence is too small to attract the attention of the A Team, which can be out, day and night, waging a hidden but exhausting war against microscopic invaders, foods that you may not even know you're allergic to, or toxic exposures of various kinds. At our clinic, we've found overgrowths of yeast or parasites to be surprisingly common contributors to adrenal burnout. *Yeast or fungal overgrowth* can spread throughout the body as a consequence of taking too many antibiotics, steroids, or birth control pills, and eating a high-sugar, refined-carb diet. *Intestinal parasites* can be picked up in exotic travel or from pets, unwashed produce, or infected food handlers. Both kinds of pests can cause bloating, itching, bowel problems, low energy, and many other problems, and they're extremely depleting of the adrenals. See the "Adrenal Tool Kit" for more on these tiny ravagers.

Allergens. Anything that you're allergic to is an adrenal stressor: grass, cat dander, wheat, milk products, shellfish, soy. If you're regularly exposed to and reacting to these or any other allergens, your A Team is overworking. Dealing with the kinds of inflammation associated with allergic reactions is an adrenal specialty. That's why asthmatics (asthma is usually a response to a food or inhalant allergen) end up having to use a powerful synthetic cortisol steroid like prednisone: their supplies of the natural anti-inflammatory steroid cortisol are not up to the job. See chapter 7 for how to decide what foods you may be allergic to. This can be an important first step toward recovery, as my client Roger recently learned.

At age 57, after twenty long, stressful years of supervising sales in a twelve-state territory, Roger had exhausted his adrenals and his cortisol output was in the dumps. From his health history, we learned that Roger had been dealing with sinus infections on and off for years. Suspecting that an allergy was the cause of these sinus woes, we recommended that Roger eliminate wheat from his diet along with any sweets. Going off wheat and sugar gave Roger new energy and vitality. Once he felt better, we suggested that he try wheat again to verify that he had a true allergy to it. Sure enough, he felt exhausted soon after eating two slices of bread, and from that point on, he stopped eating wheat altogether. His ability to handle stress *and* avoid sinus infections improved substantially as well.

Note on stressful soy foods: Not only is soy a common allergen, it is also known to interfere with the production of stress-coping hormones in the adrenals. See the soy section in chapter 7 for more on this surprising villain.

Exercise. Moderate exercise is a stress fighter, but the adrenals can be overworked if you overdo it. If exercise leaves you feeling tired rather than invigorated, your adrenals are probably worn out. In fact, post-exercise fatigue is a classic diagnostic sign of low adrenal function. Marathons, too much working out, or any exercise addiction can push you beyond the "healthy" levels of exercise your body actually needs. Be very careful to stop pushing past your balance point, no matter how little exercise it means you'll need to do for a while.

Toxic stress. Some degree of chemical contamination in our air, food, soil, and water is now a constant reality both at work and at home. Environmental illness—when toxins suddenly overload even people who may never have previously been reactive—is a growing problem. All of us are vulnerable, and a good part of whether we succumb to or survive the toxins that surround us has to do with our adrenal health. Cleaning solvents, hairsprays, insecticides, mercury fillings, and other toxins can provide the straws that break the A Team's back. Testing for and eliminating toxic chemical exposure may be necessary. (See details in the "Adrenal Tool Kit.") Meanwhile, keep it to a minimum.

ADRENAL REVIVAL: STRESS-FIGHTING SUPPLEMENTS AND FOODS

Nutritional repair can make all the difference to the A Team's ability to protect you from the ravages of stress. Remember, the A Team has up to sixty hormones to produce and distribute. It needs the right raw materials in the right amounts to manufacture all these hormones, including lots of good cholesterol. Your job is to keep your adrenals supplied with enough cholesterol and the other nutrients they need by eating at least three meals a day full of healthy proteins, fats, carbohydrates, vitamins, and minerals. You're also going to need some nutrient first aid.

GABA—Nature's Stress Buster

GABA (gamma-aminobutyric acid) is your brain's natural Valium. Actually, Valium is one of many tranquilizers designed to mimic or amplify GABA's naturally calming effects.

GABA is unique in that it is both an amino acid (that is, a building block of protein) *and* a potent mood enhancer. I don't know of any other common nutrient that can act directly as a mood regulator the way GABA can. Biochemists call it an "inhibitory neurotransmitter," one that turns *off* certain kinds of brain reactions, specifically the production of "excitatory" chemicals like adrenaline that can become so overwhelming when you are under too much stress. But the demands of dealing with too much stress can deplete our GABA supplies. Taken as a supplement, GABA can help us not only turn off stress reactions after an upset, it can even help *prevent* a stressful response when taken prior to an expected ordeal.

I've seen GABA supplements restore blessed biochemical calm in a matter of minutes, as they did for my client Abby. Abby had been full of vitality growing up and had brought that vibrant spirit into her adult life. She'd enjoyed raising her two children and helping her husband run an international business at the same time. But when her husband contracted a crippling ill-ness, Abby was alone, afraid, grieving, caring for both him and their children, and simultaneously running the business single-handedly.

By the time Abby got to my office, her tension level was so palpable that her hair was almost standing on end. She was in constant fight or flight mode, with adrenaline pumping out of control. She had been spiral-ing like this for over a year when I met her, despite having an excellent therapist and many supportive friends. I gave her a 100-milligram peppermint-flavored GABA tablet and told her to let it dissolve under her tongue. The sublingual forms of nutrients work very quickly because they bypass the stomach and go directly through the bloodstream into the brain. Amazingly, within five minutes, Abby felt calm and grounded.

Like so many of us, Abby was not able to escape her stressful circum-stances. What she *was* able to do was escape her *reactions* to them by calm-ing the agitated brain chemistry that was compounding her real-life problems. In her follow-up appointments, Abby reported that her calm-ness continued. The instantly relaxing GABA supplements, backed up by a much improved way of eating, kept her excessive stress reactions perma-nently under control.

We usually recommend starting with the lowest potency GABA avail-able, 100 milligrams, one to three times a day. But you might need to take as much as 500 milligrams. When you no longer need extra GABA to calm things down, it will just make you tired rather than relaxed. *Note:* Take your first, experimental dose of GABA at home in case you get too relaxed or tired (to drive, for example).

Relaxation Aids Beyond GABA

Two other aminos can neutralize overamped states in ways similar to GABAs. One of them, "taurine," is the soothing nutrient that can actually turn off brain seizures![15] The other, "glycine," helps to relax muscles, and for some people it can be even more generally relaxing than GABA. Many supplements combine these three soothing aminos in formulations that are easy to find. (See the Action Steps at the end of the chapter.)

Calmes Forte, a popular homeopathic remedy, can be another effec-tive antidote to too much stress. Homeopathic remedies, popular world-wide, contain submicroscopic amounts of herbs or other substances and work on the vaccination principle. My mother used Calmes Forte to forestall or reduce her stress reactions from the time she was in her 70s until she died at 84. She lost her stress-coping adrenal reserve at 30 when she got polio (a well-established adrenal destroyer) and never recovered her ability to handle stress well. Calmes Forte was a blessing for her as it has been for many people who've been buying it for years in health food stores. Another tranquilizing balm is the B vitamin inositol, taken as a powder (1–4g per day with meals).

Supplements to Lighten Up Your Stressful Private Thoughts and Feelings and Help You Sleep

The supplements 5-HTP, tryptophan, and Saint-John's wort, praised at length in chapter 3, can eliminate certain private stresses that are generated by depleted brain serotonin. If you checked off symptoms in part 1 of the Mood-Type Questionnaire like anxiety, low self-esteem, sleep problems, and obsessiveness, your negative inner thoughts and feelings may very well be unnecessarily compounding the more tangible stresses in your life. Have you felt driven and pressured all your life—perhaps since childhood? Have you been a high achiever, a perfectionist, rarely satisfied with any accomplishment? Have you, too often, been uptight, frightened, or at least worried beyond reason, your stomach tight, unable to relax even when you've had the opportunity? Have you had trouble getting to sleep or staying asleep? This kind of inner tension can become a constant, stressful goad, pushing you toward adrenal exhaustion.

After GABA, serotonin is your brain's most important anxiety buffer, and too much stress can use up both your serotonin and GABA stores. If you were born deficient in serotonin, stress can be a real emotional disaster, depleting you even further. When the brain's serotonin fuels, tryptophan and 5-HTP, are in short supply, the stress response gets triggered and your cortisol and other stress chemicals rise. But all this can be quickly reversed when you take these serotonin-boosting nutrients as supplements.

One of my clients, now a successful banker, was so anxious as a child that he had panic attacks every time he arrived at his elementary school. Later in life, he continued to suffer from insomnia and extreme anxiety every time he had to speak at a meeting. In his case, and in the cases of *many* others, stress from life circumstances is often not the only, or even the worst, problem. Like them, your past may have been relatively trauma-free, but your mood or sleep chemistry may have been killing you.

Fortunately, this kind of stressful brain chemistry can be improved in a day. Take the banker. He'd come to rely on the cocktail hour for relief from the anxious thoughts that otherwise kept him awake at night. But he was permanently freed of his anxiety, his sleeplessness, and his cocktails soon after he began using 5-HTP along with GABA, good-mood foods, and the basic nutrients.

Pyroluria: Some people with very special chemistry may need another set of supplements in addition to GABA and 5-HTP. These people have an inborn error in metabolism that causes them to convert vitamin B_6 and the mineral zinc into unusable compounds. Because B_6 and zinc are part of the nutrient team that creates serotonin and other neurotransmitters in the brain, pyrolurics are prone to chronic inner tension as well as intolerance to outer stress and other unique symptoms, like knees that crack and a tendency to sunburn and stretch marks. See page 304 for a pyroluria questionnaire and suggestions for help.

Be Alert and Recharged with Amino Energizers

Has stress burned out your vitality and stamina and your ability to concentrate? Are you using too much caffeine instead, trying to cope? Your levels of the highly energizing chemicals adrenaline and norepinephrine (or noradrenaline) are always released and sometimes used up by chronic responses to stress.

Experiments using the amino acids tyrosine and phenylalanine in stressful conditions, including battle conditions, when stress is at its maximum, have found that they can both quickly restore adrenaline and norepinephrine levels, reverse battle fatigue and shock, and promote clear thinking and action, even "under the gun."[16,17] Try these natural energizers in the morning instead of coffee, and later in the day, if this sounds like you. (See chapter 4 for more on this topic.)

Repairing Post-Traumatic Stress Disorder (PTSD) and Other Severe Adrenal Deficiency Conditions

Severe stress can sometimes leave a biochemical brand, dooming us to a semipermanent state of code red. One of the elements common to people with this condition, called "post-traumatic stress disorder" (PTSD), is low cortisol—that is, exhausted adrenals. People with PTSD literally can't "get on with it."

As we've begun to understand the imprint of PTSD on the brain, we've begun to learn how to correct the biochemical imbalances that create it. Our clients with PTSD have all had low cortisol levels and been low in GABA and serotonin. PTSD is also sometimes associated with a deficiency of the stimulating fight or flight chemicals. Some people with PTSD have all of the above.[18] We have seen a combination of GABA, 5-HTP, and tyrosine raise those depleted brain levels, reduce excess stimulation, and restore energy and verve in many people with PTSD. This combination can provide some emotional flexibility and allow psychotherapy to be more effective in helping people with PTSD move beyond the past. But if you have PTSD, you'll probably also need to measure and aggressively support your adrenal function with the methods described in the "Adrenal Tool Kit."

Holocaust survivors diagnosed with PTSD have been found to have very low cortisol levels. No one knows what their pre-Holocaust cortisol levels were like, but we do know that they passed on their weakened stress-coping capacity to their children. Their children had similarly low levels of cortisol and a similar inability to tolerate stress.[19] The more life stress these children were exposed to, the weaker their defenses against it became as their cortisol levels fell even lower. We can imagine the stress-coping legacy that they'll pass on to their own children without a lot of the kind of help you're getting in this chapter.

Your Basic Stress-Reducing Supplements plus the Special Two That Stop Carb Cravings and Hypoglycemia

The basic supplements that I recommend for *everyone* who needs a Mood Cure are listed in chapter 10. They are vital for any antistress campaign. After even a single high-stress week, your supplies of vitamins and minerals can drop by 30–40 percent. That's what the U.S. Army learned in a study of the effects of "hell week" on recruits who were actually eating pretty well. You'll need all of the basic nutrients and then some, to make up for what you've lost to past stress and poor diet. For example, your adrenals use up about 90 percent of the vitamin C you take in and require a constant rich supply of the B vitamins as well. Our clients can really feel that mid-afternoon B-complex lift. Your basic calcium, magnesium, and vitamin D are also used up at a tremendous rate by your adrenals during stress. Your adrenals need plenty of both vitamin D and omega-3 fat in order to make their stress-fighting adrenaline and norepinephrine. Many people report significantly increased energy as well as peace of mind when they take these two nutrients as part of their basic supplements.

At the same time that you start taking these basic antistress supplements, if you find that you cannot easily give up sweets and starchy, white-flour based foods, you're going to need (and love) using the special supplements chromium and glutamine.

The mineral *chromium* helps keep blood sugar levels stable, but it gets used up by a high-carb diet. Putting more back into your body as a supplement restores blood sugar stability (even for diabetics). It also eases the cravings for carbs that erupt during blood sugar drops, saving your A Team from further exhausting heroics.

Glutamine is an amino acid that your brain can use as an emergency substitute fuel when you haven't eaten recently or have been eating too many carbs and your blood sugar level is too low. This glucose stand-in stops the impulse to run to the candy machine when it's low blood sugar time. This, of course, saves your adrenals from overworking. L-glutamine can stop carb cravings and get you feeling steady and even within ten minutes (less if you open a capsule and place the contents under your tongue).

If the basic supplements and these two anti-carb-craving supplements don't eliminate your taste for sweets and starches, please turn to the "Food Craving Tool Kit." This is crucial. Unless you're able to cut your excess carb intake, you'll continue to exhaust the A Team's priceless resources by the gruntwork of having to clean up after a junk food fest.

ANTISTRESS FOODS

Even with all your antistress supplements, you're still going to need to eat the best-quality food possible to keep yourself adequately fueled in the face of twenty-first-century strife. But don't worry about how you're going to make the shift to three great meals and a few hearty snacks a day. I'm going to make it easy. And please don't worry about gaining weight. The high-carb processed food you're probably eating now is the most weight-promoting food on the planet. In fact, our fast foods are reaching more and more of the planet's population and causing unheard-of weight gain as they become popular and replace healthier local foods.

Protein and Fat—Top Stress-Busting Foods

Eating protein is crucial for keeping your blood sugar balanced and the A Team in shape: 20 to 30 grams or more of it three times a day makes people feel stronger and more energized partly because it stimulates a nice rise in cortisol. If you're burnt out, your depleted cortisol levels are probably pretty saggy, so this dietary boost can be very welcome. You should feel the difference within two days.

Most high-protein foods provide the wonderful combination of protein and saturated fat that the A Team really loves. Certain fats, the saturated, shorter-chain ones, will keep your blood sugar more stable than any other foods. That's why we all enjoy butter on our food so much: it satisfies our bodies and lets us know we can stop eating because our blood sugar won't drop precipitously the way it does with high-carb, low-fat foods. Think turkey *and* swiss, chicken with the skin on, full-fat cottage cheese. No stressful energy dips can befall you if you've eaten healthy fat with your protein at least three times a day.

You'll probably need to increase your protein and, if you've been restricting your fat, add more extra-virgin olive oil, butter, whole eggs (not just the whites: the yolks contain half the protein and all of the good fat and other bountiful nutrients in an egg), and dairy products (ideally organic, raw, and whole).

If your fear of fat has become entrenched, understandable after years of antifat brainwashing, turn to chapter 8 for more clarification. Plan to spend a lot of time in that chapter getting used to what stress-free eating really means.

Sample Low-Stress Menu

Breakfast: Three-egg spinach omelet with potatoes cooked in butter or 1 cup or more of full-fat cottage cheese and fresh fruit. *Lunch:* A Cobb salad; or a turkey or tuna and cheese sandwich with salad. *Dinner:* Chinese chicken stir-fry with rice; or a steak with a baked potato, and a nice big salad. *Snack:* Fresh fruit with a few nuts or a yogurt smoothie. You'll feel the difference right away, and you can find or take food like this even on the road.

ADVANCED ADRENAL BURNOUT

Testing

If you make all of the improvements in diet and take the supplements I've just suggested, yet still have many of the symptoms on the adrenal burnout list, you're likely to be in an advanced stage of adrenal burnout. Please be sure to get your adrenal function *tested* as soon as possible. Saliva testing is by far the most accurate way to measure how much fight is left in your adrenals. In fact, it's the most accurate testing I've ever seen. If your test results show that your levels of stress-coping cortisol and DHEA are below normal, you'll need to follow the ultimate adrenal repair strategies laid out for you in detail in the "Adrenal Tool Kit," along with detailed information on testing. Please take this tool kit's very complete but technical information to holistic health practitioners for help in ordering the tests, interpreting the results, and renovating your adrenal function. Suggestions for finding such practitioners can also be found in the tool kit. For example, you'll find out why acupuncturists can be so helpful and when medical help is essential.

Please use the Action Steps that follow and the "Adrenal Tool Kit," if needed, as your guides in your stress recovery campaign. I wish you all the best in finding your way out from under the pressure, but really, with these tools you can't miss!

ACTION STEPS

Supplements

Before trying any of the supplements recommended in this chapter, check the "Caution Box" on pages 199–200 for any contraindications.

The basic supplements you'll be taking are described in chapter 10 and listed on page 202 on the master supplement schedule. This is followed by a list of all the special repair supplements recommended in every chapter of the book, including this one. Note the following special supplements and doses that you think you'll need and add them to the master supplement list to create your individualized master supplement plan.

And don't forget that your antistress campaign will flounder if you don't dump the stressful foods, eat lots of good-mood foods, and take your basic supplements.

Frontline Stress Beaters

To relax your mind and body:

➤ GABA 100–500 mg, one to three times a day at or before your high-stress times, typically midafternoon and/or bedtime.
➤ Or try a combination of GABA with the aminos taurine and glycine, for example.
➤ GABA Calm by Source Naturals, True Calm by NOW Foods, or Amino Relaxers by Country Life.
➤ Homeopathic Calmes Forte 1–2 capsules, as needed.
➤ Inositol powder, 1–4g a day, with meals.

To stop excessive sweet and starch cravings:

➤ Glutamine 500–1500 mg early morning, midmorning, and midafternoon and at bedtime if you tend to wake up in the night hungry.
➤ Chromium 200 mcg three times per day with meals and at bedtime (not needed if you take the True Balance Multiple as per chapter 10).

For inner mental stress (if you have symptoms in part 1 of the Mood-Type Questionnaire) and carb cravings that occur in late afternoon or evening that the above supplements don't stop, and for trouble sleeping:

➤ Read chapter 3 and try 5-HTP, 50–150 mg midafternoon and at bedtime or try 500–1,500 mg tryptophan at the same times.
➤ Or if that doesn't do it, try Saint-John's wort, 300 mg (standardized) three times a day with meals.

For pyroluria:

➤ Take the questionnaire in the "Resource Tool Kit"; if your score is over 15, follow the directions there for taking a home urine test to confirm the problem. Also test your zinc levels as recommended there and follow the suggestions for dealing with the problem.

For energy and alertness:

➤ Tyrosine (if you feel depleted or exhausted, but not jittery) 500–1,000 mg in early morning and midmorning. You can take it midafternoon, too, but try to take it before three P.M. to avoid disrupting your sleep (and stop if it does get disrupted). You might also try a combination of tyrosine and phenylalanine in formulas like TrueFocus by NOW.

Food

Eat three meals, no more than five hours apart. You may also need between-meal and bedtime snacks. Emphasize protein, fats, and vegetables at meals and as snacks before you add whatever healthy carbs you need (such as fresh fruit, potatoes, beans, whole grains). See chapter 8 for details. *Avoid sweetened foods, refined (white) starches, and caffeine.* Also be sure you eliminate any foods you might be *allergic* to (such as wheat or milk products), as per chapter 7.

Testing

A one-day, four-sample saliva test for cortisol and DHEA levels is a must. *See the "Adrenal Tool Kit" for testing details.*

Ultimate Adrenal Repair Strategies

If the saliva testing shows you to be below normal in cortisol and DHEA at any time of the day, work with a health practitioner in using the ultimate antistress supplements and medications discussed in the "Adrenal Tool Kit."

Exercise

Do *not* push yourself. Workouts should make you feel better, not more tired. Start with gentle walking. Increase to moderate levels as your tolerance builds.

RECOMMENDED READING

Wilson, James L. *Adrenal Fatigue: The 21st-Century Stress Syndrome* (Petaluma, Calif.: Smart Publications, 2002).

Peeke, Pamela, M.D. *Fight Fat After Forty* (New York: Penguin, 2001).

CHAPTER 6

Too Sensitive to Life's Pain?

How to Amplify Your Own Comforting Endorphins

Some people take great pleasure in life. Everyone they meet is a potential treat. A song, a sunrise, a hot bath, an apple—many things delight them. Even when painful things happen, they seem to rebound well, without too many emotional scars or prolonged suffering.

These lucky people are loaded with the brain chemicals that transmit enjoyment, contentment, and euphoria. They're blessed with high levels of naturally comforting substances that are many times more powerful than morphine or heroin. These inborn wonder drugs are called "endorphins," and they are actually a complex of at least fifteen potent brain and body chemicals that all amplify pleasure and make pain tolerable.

There's a special smile that I think of as the "endorphin smile." Maybe you'll light up with it when I mention the word *chocolate*. Most of my clients do. My assistant breaks out in it when I mention her boyfriend's name. Most people grin this way when I ask them if they've ever been to Hawaii or Paris. It's the "love smile."

Think of something that you love and tune in to how you feel. "I *love* that man," or that woman, that beach, that CD, that movie, that book, that dress, that team. These are the feelings this chapter is all about.

The nerves in the skin can trigger a release of endorphins, making a massage or a sunbath heavenly. A brain capable of transporting lots of endorphins can provide the "happy" to a happy memory, the glow to a new love. A hug, a kind word, even deep breathing can raise endorphin levels.

Many different foods can raise endorphin levels, too, although as you will see, some can give you a longer-lasting lift than others.

The question is: Do *you* have enough endorphins to boost in the first place? How high and how often can they soar? Do you find it hard to locate enough natural enjoyment or comfort in *your* life? Do you find that even major treats give you only brief or dim pleasure? If so, you may be endorphin deficient.

If your endorphin levels are low, you're one of many of us who were born low in the joy department or have run low after expending too many of our endorphins coping with too much of life's pain. If you identify with this particular false mood type, you have probably discovered some ways to hide it or get around it. Do you have a protective veneer of toughness or joviality? Do you avoid emotional intimacy or confrontation? Do you look for comfort in chocolate or other foods? In alcohol? In painkilling drugs? In an activity? In sex? If you are deficient in endorphin and too vulnerable to pain as a result, you can easily be driven to painkilling substances, activities, and even people.

A lot of what we know about the endorphin connection comes from naloxone, a drug that actually shuts down endorphin activity. When naloxone plugs into endorphin sites in the brain, it prevents endorphin levels from increasing. It also keeps counterfeit endorphins, like the painkillers heroin and Vicodin, from plugging in. But that's not all. Naloxone also blocks the pleasurable effects of alcohol, marijuana,[1] and chocolate, as well as tobacco,[2] sweet and fatty foods,[3] activities like sex[4] and gambling,[5] and even of beloved people like Mommy.[6] It turns out that all of the above can get a significant rise out of endorphin. Meditation and running are also effective endorphin-level raisers,[7] and bungee jumpers can count on a more than 200 percent endorphin increase![8] For obvious reasons, the lower in endorphins we are, the more drawn we are to these substances and activities.

My client Paula is a good example of how depleted endorphin levels can distort appetite as well as mood. Paula, who was an actress, came to see me about her mood problem because, as she said in exasperation, "I'm sick and tired of overeating and gaining weight every time I get hurt and upset. And I've been doing it all my life." Although Paula initially presented herself in a dynamic, upbeat way, a few minutes after we started to talk, she began to wipe away a trickle of tears that continued to flow on and off throughout our two-hour assessment. As I listened to Paula describe her life, it became apparent that she could not shake off the disappointments and slights that many of us can let roll off our backs.

Paula's life had actually gone fairly smoothly until a few years before, when her husband had begun to drink too much. Then she'd found herself deeply affected but unable to even talk to him about it. When we looked at her Mood-Type Questionnaire together, it became clear that she was an "overly sensitive type." She'd checked off most of the symptoms in part 4, the low-endorphin section. From what she said about her gentle alcoholic father, I suspected that Paula was genetically wired to underproduce endorphins, and when I met her adolescent daughter, Amy, the next day, my guess was confirmed.

When Amy came in for her own assessment, she brought in a Mood-Type Questionnaire identical to her mother's and had the quivering chin and welling eyes to go with it. Paradoxically, Amy's life was going very well. She was excelling in school and at work and going out with boys she liked. After talking with Amy, I could see that, like her mother, she also took things too much to heart and had the same trouble rebounding from everyday setbacks. It was obvious that Amy had inherited her mother's biochemical mood type. Fortunately for both Paula and Amy, their genes did not have the final word. With the aid of endorphin-boosting supplements and a dietary tune-up, Paula and her daughter were soon able to laugh about their former teariness. Their lives hadn't changed, but they'd become relatively pain-free and completely tear-free since their first day on their nutritherapy programs.

I watch carefully for people like Paula and Amy who get a bit (or a lot) teary during their first appointment with me. Almost everyone who comes in to see me has painful experiences to relate, but those who feel the most pain often reveal it through their tears. They turn out to be, not necessarily the most injured, but the least able to tolerate injury.

Tears are not the only low-endorphin clues I watch for. Frequent feelings of what I think of as unnatural sadness are common symptoms as well. Sad feelings naturally come with grief and loss, but if they are unbearably painful, go on for too long, or appear without any obvious life circumstances to justify them, low endorphins are usually the reason. I'm often told by incoming clients, "I just feel sad a lot, for no reason," or, "I've always felt sad, I think." They also talk a lot about being overly sensitive: "Even as a child, I was always told I was too sensitive."

This kind of emotional rawness should be shielded by a soothing layer of endorphins, but each of us has a unique supply of this natural sensitivity buffer. Some people have emotional skins so thick with endorphins that it takes a sledgehammer to get through to them. Others have emotional skins so thin that they bruise with the slightest pressure. Fortunately, even the most endorphin depleted people can fortify themselves by using certain nutrients to boost their endorphin levels and quickly begin to better tolerate life's pain and enjoy its pleasures.

HOW DID YOU BECOME ENDORPHIN DEFICIENT?

There are several paths that could have led to your becoming deficient in your natural anesthetics. Read this section to identify which factors have had the most impact on you.

Is it your genes? You could have been born with an endorphin deficiency and discovered it when you faced your first major emotional injury. Some people discover it early, but other people have such nice families and early childhoods that they don't really discover their deficiency till their teens. What about you? Were you one of those whose genetic vulnerability was so severe that early on even the most mundane upsets were too much for you? Did your family call you a "crybaby" or "just too darned sensitive" growing up? Was your first romantic or other rejection terribly hurtful? What are the other members of your family like? Is emotional sensitivity a common trait? Does a need for anesthetics like chocolate or alcohol run in the family? A yes to any of these questions could indicate a genetically low endorphin supply.

Has too much stress drained you of your endorphins? Maybe your genes were not the problem, and your early childhood was pain-free. You might once even have been endorphin-rich, emotionally happy and resilient, but later used up too much of your endorphin reserve in dealing with prolonged or repeated abuse or other emotional or physical pain or distress.[9] Do you feel that you "just can't take any more"? It may be quite true that, though you once had enough, you may now have run too low in this natural means of making a hard life worth living. Chronic pain can have concrete, biochemical repercussions (especially if there is a genetic trapdoor ready to drop open under you).

Any kind of prolonged stress can wear down your endorphin levels. You use up quite a bit of endorphin every time you are upset, injured, sick, scared, or even excited. Whether you're in labor or pushing past the strain of a long-distance run (both of which require an equal amount of endorphin!), you're subtracting from your painkilling treasury.

Adrenaline and endorphin are released together by your pituitary and adrenal glands to help you deal with significant stressors.[10] A rise in endorphin is meant to prepare you for any injury that may be about to befall you during a stressful event and to soothe you afterward. Endorphin levels can get so high during a major calamity that you might not experience significant pain, even from a serious physical injury, for as long as an hour afterward. Raised endorphin levels are what can actually calm you down *after* an upset, too, forcing a 50 percent drop in cortisol, your most powerful stress hormone.[11]

Have you had too much emotional or physical pain? Studies have found endorphin levels to be abnormally high in people who have suffered past emotional trauma.[12] If you have enough endorphin, you may be able to repress emotional pain sometimes even for years, expending a constant supply of endorphin to keep up the denial. Several University of California at Irvine studies have found that high self-deception is accompanied by high endorphin levels.[13] When endorphin levels run low, denial may run out until only synthetic painkillers like sugar, alcohol, or drugs can keep the numbness going and the painful truths on ice.

The way we get through the stages of grief after a major loss has a lot to do with how well supplied we are with endorphins beforehand. Within minutes of a traumatic event like the death of someone close, the levels of endorphin in our brains increase and stay high for differing amounts of time. Most of us experience the early pain as coming "in waves" as our endorphin levels rise and fall. At some point, endorphin levels descend for good and a new phase of grief ensues as we face our feelings without as much anesthesia. Hopefully we are left with enough endorphin to bear it. Those who aren't look for help from alcohol, drugs, food, sex, and anything else that will stimulate their endorphins a little.[14] Fortunately, the nutritional tools you'll be trained to use in this chapter can usually do a better job.

People suffering from chronic physical pain have 60–90 percent less pain-reducing endorphin than others. Fortunately, dozens of pain studies show complete or significant relief of arthritis, migraines, and even cancer pain using two endorphin-boosting amino acids that I'll be telling you lots more about soon.

Whether endorphin depletion is caused by physical or emotional pain, or both, these aminos can usually relieve the problem very quickly.

Is it your gender? Endorphin levels rise during puberty in both boys and girls, but in adulthood, men have higher endorphin levels than women do. Female endorphin levels reach male levels only if women do regular, *vigorous* exercise (or suffer chronic stresses—remember, stress triggers a compensatory endorphin surge).[15] But too much of this ill-gotten endorphin can interfere with normal menstruation. Using a drug that reduces endorphin can induce ovulation in women who have lost their normal menstrual rhythm because of too much exercise.[16]

Ideally, in women, endorphin levels should peak at ovulation (midcycle), but in women who have PMS they don't peak and, in fact, tend to be low throughout the menstrual cycle.[17,18,19] Endorphin levels predictably sag in menopause along with feelings of well-being. Estrogen, the mood queen, rules the release of endorphin (as well as serotonin) in the brain.[20] If estrogen or the adrenal hormone DHEA (some of which converts to estrogen) is low, which often happens in menopause, taking estrogen and/or DHEA supplements can raise endorphin levels substantially, among other benefits.[21]

Note: Be sure to test your sex hormone levels before you experiment with hormone replacement to see if your levels really are drooping. Find details on testing and balancing sex hormones in the "Sex Hormone Tool Kit."

Emotional vulnerability is typically associated with being female. In fact, women are often proud of being the more sensitive of the two sexes. They often feel superior to "insensitive men," who in turn typically feel superior to "overly emotional women." As I mentioned, it turns out that endorphins really do have a gender bias: men tend to have higher levels than women.[22,23] Because of this, women really are more sensitive than men and are more inclined to become too emotional if their naturally lower endorphin levels drop even further. This can exaggerate the essential endorphin differences between men and women and make it even harder for them to understand each other's built-in emotional styles. However, men can also become endorphin depleted and often learn early to cover their ultrasensitive feelings so that only *they* know how hard life can be for them. Knowing the real biochemical factors affecting each other's moods and behavior can make a big difference for couples trying to work things out; and raising endorphin levels with amino acids can be even more helpful, as you're about to discover.

ENDING ENDORPHIN DEFICIENCY

The Endorphin-Boosting Amino Acids

If your pleasure chemistry is deficient, there really is a simple and direct way to build it up in a single day. The winning formula? Twin amino acids, backed up by high-protein foods three times a day and a few other nutritional armaments. This nutritional strategy can almost certainly restore the pleasure in life that you're missing and help you to more easily survive times of emotional stress and grief. The twin formula is DLPA, a combination of the D- and L- forms of the amino acid phenylalanine. The two aminos work well together, because each offers a different but synergistic benefit in the pain prevention department. This comforting combo can be found in any health food store and really can start taking effect in minutes.

One of the two aminos, L-phenylalanine, helps amplify pleasure sensations only indirectly. It's one of the fifteen or more base aminos needed to form endorphin and one of the five needed to form enkephalin—one of the most powerful of the painkilling subgroups in the endorphin family. This remarkable amino directly raises energy and decreases depression by increasing the brain's stimulating neurotransmitters, the catecholamines. Additionally, it forms PEA (phenylethylamine), another energizing brain chemical (also found in chocolate) that may be the chemical most responsible for feelings of euphoria. Just as low endorphin is associated with pain, low PEA is routinely associated with depression, and LPA helps increase both![24]

The second component of the twin formulation DLPA is D-phenylalanine. DPA is the mirror image of L-phenylalanine, but it's a much more potent endorphin booster.[25] DPA is a rare substance known to effectively and safely neutralize the enzymes in the brain that destroy endorphins. Each of your brain's big four mood enhancers has an enzyme nemesis that destroys it, regardless of how desperately you might still need it. This natural process is designed to prevent an excess of endorphin production, but you need protection against it when the problem is deficiency, not excess. In the case of your endorphins, it's enzymes called "endorphinase" and "enkephalinase" that you're up against, and their terminator is DPA. DPA quickly disarms these enzymes, thus protecting your supply of endorphin and allowing it to build and expand.

In one study reported in the richly researched book *DLPA*,[26] endorphin levels tripled ninety minutes after one dose of DPA was taken and stayed that high for six days! Author Arnold Fox, M.D., past president of the American Academy of Pain Management, has been using DPA and DLPA in his clinical practice for over twenty years, and he's even more enthusiastic now about their benefits than he was when he published his best-selling book on the subject in 1985.

Many studies have confirmed that DPA and LPA even significantly relieve the physical pain of arthritis, migraines, and cancer.[27] In one study, ten chronic pain patients were given both aminos for three to seven days. Good to excellent results were noted in *every* case![28] In a French study, nine patients in severe pain from a variety of causes were given low levels of DPA only, for twenty months. Seven *never* needed any other pain relievers *ever* again.[29] In several studies, DPA and LPA together (DLPA) were very successfully combined with either acupuncture or pain medication.[30] Adding DLPA lowered the need for pain medication and reduced pain more effectively than acupuncture used alone.

DLPA in Action

Holly came to us because her husband had died six months earlier and she could not function, her grief was still so deep. She had just had to quit her high-level civil service job and her teaching position at the local college, and she was turning, for comfort, to chocolate and wine too often. She was in constant emotional pain and could not muster any of her former cheerful optimism. Bouncy, spirited, and resourceful most of her life, she had rarely had serious mood problems until her tragic loss.

Holly took 2 capsules of DLPA in a formula called Comfort Zone in our office. In fifteen minutes she said, "I haven't felt this good since before my husband died." She went home with her "comfort pills," as she called them, and reported back two weeks later: Her grief was ebbing to tolerable levels, but she still needed her supplements every day to keep it that way. Four weeks later, Holly reported needing fewer of her aminos. She was skipping days with no relapses. After another month, she was using her Comfort Zone formula (see page 117) only occasionally. By the end of four months, she didn't need it at all anymore. She was able to manage a new job and was back to feeling more like herself again. She was moving normally through the stages of her grieving.

DLPA as an Antidepressant

Studies confirm that some forms of depression respond very well to DLPA—better, in fact, than to some antidepressant drugs.[31] In one study, DLPA was twice as effective as imipramine, with 60 percent of the depressed patients improved on it, compared to 30 percent on the drug.[32] In another study, 85–95 percent of depressed patients showed complete or significant improvement on DLPA.[33] Finally, in a study using very low doses of DLPA for just twenty days, two-thirds of the patients were discharged symptom-free![34]

Why? L-phenylalanine (and to a lesser degree D-phenylalanine) can be converted into the stimulating brain chemicals PEA and norepinephrine, which are known to be deficient in many depressed people. I think it's obvious, too, that low-endorphin feelings of sadness and hurt can often be part of the complex state of mind we call depression. When D- and L-phenylalanine raise pain-relieving endorphin *and* energizing norepinephrine and PEA levels, several possible aspects of depression can fall away, sometimes leaving no other negative feelings behind at all![35]

You'll love DLPA, especially if your energy as well as your pain tolerance is a bit lower than you'd like. If you need coffee to get going or caffeinated sodas to keep going, you'll do very well on DLPA, since it combines the painkilling D- with the energizing L- forms of phenylalanine. You may find yourself free of caffeine and depression as well as pain before long on DLPA.

When DPA Alone Works Best

Not everyone who needs comfort and a stronger sense of well-being needs both the D- and L- forms of phenylalanine supplements. Some people do better with the D- form alone. We learned this from a man who had all the low-endorphin symptoms in spades. Dan was an emergency room nurse. Very sensitive to emotional pain, he was apt to tear up easily and "loved" chocolate and pot for comfort and numbing, especially after a stressful night at the ER. Part of the problem was that Dan was hyperenergetic both mentally and physically and had trouble "shutting it off" to get to sleep. He did not need more stimulation, so DLPA had an overamping effect on him. He could see that it eliminated his pain sensitivity and his taste for chocolate and pot, but it also made him jumpy and interfered with his sleep.

About the same time that Dan was having this mixed reaction to DLPA, we learned that the D-phenylalanine portion of DLPA, by itself, was available. We immediately sent for some and asked Dan to try it.

He reported being very happy on his DPA right away. He still had no interest in chocolate and pot, and had lost his tendency to be oversensitive, but he no longer felt wired or sleepless.

If you have sleep problems at night but need energy in the morning, you'll probably be fine taking 1 or 2 DLPA capsules first thing in the morning and in the midmorning, but you shouldn't take DLPA in the afternoon, certainly not after three P.M. Many of our clients are in this boat. If they need an endorphin boost in the afternoon—for example, if they're three P.M. chocolate nibblers—we suggest they try DPA just at that time. *Note:* Rarely, even DPA, some of which can convert into energizing LPA and PEA, can also be too energizing in the afternoon. Usually, though, it's well tolerated.

What Other Supplements Can You Use to Raise Your Endorphins?

More aminos: As you know by now, there are twenty-two different amino acids altogether in protein-containing foods. Your body can use all twenty-two aminos if it has plenty of at least the nine "essential" amino acids: histadine, isoleucine, leucine, lysine, methionine, phenylalanine, threonine, tryptophan, and valine. Taking a supplemental blend of at least these nine aminos (freeform) for a few months, in addition to your DLPA and your protein-rich meals and snacks, can help get your endorphin building off to a strong start.

Please note that it's very important to get an amino acid blend that contains *all* nine of the essential aminos. Many blends contain only a few of the nine essential aminos. The one most often left out is tryptophan. Since tryptophan indirectly helps to boost your endorphin levels and directly boosts levels of antidepressant serotonin, it can be mood damaging to take amino blends that lack it. In fact, giving test subjects an amino blend lacking tryptophan is a common way of studying depression, panic, and insomnia. (If you're taking tryptophan or 5-HTP separately as a supplement, as per chapter 3, you can safely take amino blends that don't contain it.)

The serotonin-endorphin connection: There's another factor to think about—your serotonin levels. Did you have a high score in part 1 of the

Mood-Type Questionnaire? If you did, but you skipped reading chapter 3, you might want to take a closer look at "Lifting the Dark Cloud" when you're finished with this chapter. Here's why: Serotonin and its precursors, 5-HTP and L-tryptophan, have been shown to stimulate endorphin levels, thereby improving mood and pain tolerance dramatically.[36] But it can take up to a month to raise endorphin levels indirectly this way. Combining serotonin-boosting supplements like 5-HTP or tryptophan with DLPA can create the same effect more powerfully and in less time.

We've had several clients with only a few low-endorphin symptoms, but with quite a few low-serotonin symptoms like worry and irritability, who had been put on Prozac or a similar serotonin-boosting drug before they came in to see us. They reported that Prozac had stopped their tendency to "cry all the time." (In fact, several of them said that they couldn't cry at all, even after the death of a loved one.) I found it fascinating that the drug had eliminated their low-endorphin symptoms (perhaps *too* completely) but had not done as thorough a job on their low-serotonin symptoms. More than half of our low-endorphin clients also show clear signs of being low in serotonin and respond beautifully to the combination of DLPA in the morning and midmorning and 5-HTP or tryptophan in the afternoon and evening. Be sure to look into chapter 3 for a sense of whether you'll need to add serotonin boosters to your endorphin-building protocol.

How your basic vitamin and mineral supplements can help boost your endorphins: Your basic supplements are vital for mood (and health) maintenance. Some of them are also dazzlingly effective painkillers in their own right, and most of them help your brain convert aminos into neurotransmitters like the endorphins.

A multi-vitamin/mineral containing the basics can have a real impact on your overall sense of well-being. A British study of men and women taking a potent multi for twelve months confirmed this. The results were reported with typical British understatement: Both the men and the women felt significantly "more agreeable" by the third month. The nutrients given the most credit for the mood boost here were B vitamins, whose levels had increased most significantly.[37]

All of the basic *B vitamins* have been shown to help eliminate every kind of emotional discomfort and significantly relieve physical discomfort as well. One of our clinic's early clients, Larry, had been in emotional and physical pain for many years since the Vietnam War, when he had been shot and seriously injured. Larry had tried many painkillers but hated their side effects. Finally, and reluctantly, he'd settled into regular alcohol use instead and found himself using far too much alcohol whenever his pain got too bad or his love life took a nosedive. We didn't know about endorphin-building DLPA then, but we did know about a local pain expert who had developed a simple and effective pain-relieving nutritional protocol using B vitamins.

We referred Larry to physician Michael Margoles, M.D., author of *Chronic Pain*, who had found that the B vitamins helped restore endorphin function and regenerate damaged nerves. After a week on his B complex, Larry found himself in much less pain and much less inclined to reach for a drink. Over the next months, he began to feel better and better. By using DLPA as well as B vitamins, our clients get faster results now, but we know that taking the basic Bs is essential for long-term pain relief.

The mineral *magnesium* can also accomplish marvels with pain by neutralizing some of the body's most pain-provoking chemicals.[38] Postoperative patients, for example, are able to cut their painkilling medications significantly when magnesium is provided before surgery.[39,40] Migraine pain and PMS discomfort, too, can respond dramatically to magnesium supplementation.[41,42] In one study, *all* subjects on magnesium got major relief from severe migraine headaches.[43] Pain and stress increase your need for magnesium, too. Even a loud noise can cause magnesium levels to surge and then drop for two days, so it's all too easy to get depleted in this soothing mineral.[44]

Vitamin D plus calcium can stop the pain of osteoporosis, PMS, and bone cancer, since the pain of these conditions is caused by a calcium and vitamin D deficiency.[45]

Vitamin C has a definite effect on our endorphin levels. It can even reduce the severe discomfort of withdrawal from painkillers like heroin all by itself.[46]

The *omega-3 fats* block inflammatory pain directly. These fabulous fats also promote the effective production and protection of all your mood-enhancing brain chemicals, including endorphin. So do vitamins D and E, the B complex, and zinc.

THE BEST FOODS FOR ENDORPHIN BUILDING

Fill Your Plate
with Endorphin-Boosting "Joy Foods"

Have you been getting enough protein and the other foods that help with pain coping? Endorphin building requires a big, consistent supply of high-protein foods like fish, eggs, cottage cheese, and chicken. Unlike the other neurotransmitters that regulate your feelings of well-being, your endorphins are composed of not one but at least fifteen amino acids. As you've probably gathered by now, amino acids can be found only in protein-containing foods. You'll need plenty of protein, at least 20 to 30 grams three times a day, to start and keep the process going. Only animal sources of protein contain all twenty-two possible aminos. Have you been avoiding animal products? Unless you are a very careful vegetarian, you can easily become deficient in the proteins you need to make your endorphins on typically low-protein vegetarian fare.

Lots of fresh vegetables and good fats are also vital. Vegetables are loaded with the vitamins and minerals that your brain needs to convert protein into the endorphins.

Fats and oils also encourage endorphin release, making you satisfied with your meals. Fats are naturally combined with protein in most high-protein foods (like fish, eggs, and meats), so if you're on a low-fat diet, you may not be getting enough fat or protein to allow your brain to produce endorphin at optimal levels. For example, have you been throwing out the fat-rich egg yolks and eating only egg whites or removing the fatty skin from chicken? If so, you're reducing your endorphin levels, too.

Low-fat, low-calorie, and high-carb diets can definitely deplete your endorphin stores by reducing both protein and fat. The two teary clients I described at the beginning of this chapter, Paula and her daughter, Amy, had both been chronic dieters for years.

So what do you need to eat to keep your endorphins at optimal levels? Take a look at the following sample menu. The word that comes to mind is *satisfying!*

A Sample Endorphin-Building Menu

Breakfast: A three-egg omelette with vegetables and potatoes in the morning; or a protein powder and fresh fruit shake with coconut milk.

Lunch: Plenty of turkey or other meat and cheese on a whole-grain sandwich or in a big salad with plenty of olive oil and balsamic vinegar salad dressing.

Dinner: A substantial piece of fish, chicken, or lamb, with asparagus in lemon butter and a buttered baked potato; or, if you are vegetarian, rice and beans with cheese, cashews, and vegetables stir-fried in ghee or coconut oil.

Why *Not* Use Exercise, Sweets, or Other Comforts to Raise Your Endorphins?

It's true that you should be able to stay high on your own endorphins, since things like sunlight, music, romance, exercise, and nature can all raise endorphin levels. But they can't help you if your basic levels are so low that you have nothing to work with. That's when a sunset does nothing much for you, and that's where your protein and DLPA come in. Without them you're stuck with addictive needs for exercise, sex, sugar, or alcohol and drugs that *force* a brief release of endorphin at a very high price. Sex, for example, raises endorphin levels 200 percent.[47] But, if your natural levels are low, a temporary boost from sex, chocolate, or pot won't take you very far for very long.

Regarding exercise, the short answer is this: If you've exercised hard enough to get an endorphin "high," you've exercised too long. Runners' "highs" typically kick in *after* they have hit the wall of exertion that should have been their signal to stop running. Please don't push yourself with exercise past pain. Forget about that kind of gain. You can be fit and feel great using moderate exercise and smart nutrition instead. If you're addicted to the exercise high, use your DLPA and taper back to more moderate levels.

If you've stopped feeling the high after intense exercise, your endorphin levels have definitely bottomed out. This was discovered by measuring endorphin levels in endurance athletes after their events. Even if they'd done well in the events, if they didn't feel that triumphant euphoria afterward, their endorphin levels were considerably lower than those of their happier counterparts (probably depleted by the stress of overexercise).

Again, the solution is DLPA, the basic nutrients, and plenty of protein. But please reconsider the extent of your exercise.

Certain foods can have druglike effects on your brain's pleasure sites. Chocolate and other sweets, baked goods (anything made from wheat or white flour), and dairy products can all raise endorphin levels dramatically.[48] In fact, these three foods can have a uniquely pleasurable, druglike effect. Think about how many sweet "treats" are triple endorphin boosters made from flour and milk products as well as sweeteners: chocolate cheesecake, chocolate-chip cookies, or the ultimate triple hitter: cookie dough ice cream. So why *not* rely on these foods to keep your endorphin levels soaring? No matter how good they may make you feel, that feeling doesn't last! These foods are also unhealthy, highly addictive, and likely to put on unneeded pounds.

Chocolate contains not only plenty of sugar, but at least five druglike substances: theobromine, caffeine, salsolinol, PEA, magnesium, and amandamide (a marijuana-like brain chemical). All are either stimulating or opiatelike. This extraordinary collection of psychoactive ingredients explains a great deal about chocolate's superaddicting allure.

Sugar, especially combined with chocolate, forces a rise in endorphin levels. It is the ultimate "pleasure" drug food, but many people can attest to the addictive pleasure of bread and cheese as well. When we ask our clients what foods they "love," pizza is often high on the list, right after chocolate. As we know, wheat flour and milk products (even low-fat ones) can both trigger the production of false endorphins, or "exorphins,"[49,50] that fit like keys into endorphin slots and force them to "turn on." That makes for food addiction as the brain becomes dependent on those foods for the druglike pleasure they release, however briefly.

Another thing that can make flour and dairy products so pleasurable and addictive, ironically, is their ability to cause more uncomfortable allergy reactions than just about any other foods. Both can cause major inflammation of both the digestive and respiratory tracts. You may not be aware of pain while digesting these foods because there are few nerves in your digestive tract, but if you feel bloated, gassy, or constipated on a regular basis, or are tired or sleepy regularly after your meals, you're getting the message that something is wrong in your digestive system. You may also have become resigned to other allergic symptoms such as sneezing, wheezing, postnasal drip, and sore throats. And that is where the endorphins come in. They can comfort us from both digestive and/or respiratory distress. Remember how endorphins are released when we've had an injury? Same principle here.

Allergic reactions to certain grains and milk products usually kick in during childhood, when we're typically fed so much milk, wheat-based cereals, noodles, and bread. Allergy symptoms like earaches, stomachaches, constipation, asthma, and other respiratory problems are typically ignored or misdiagnosed, so the body begins to increase endorphin activity to comfort us from this chronic allergic irritation and damage. Ironically, this makes these foods irresistible. More on these two foods and how to decide if you're allergic to them in chapter 7.

Breaking an Addiction to Comfort Foods, Drugs, or Alcohol

If you've tried to stop eating endorphin-boosting foods, you may have faced formidable withdrawal reactions that made quitting almost impossible. Have you felt so deprived and moody that you just *had* to have some sweets, bread, or cheese? Sound familiar? This is why so few people can stay away from their comfort foods. If your brain's endorphin production is weak, it can easily come to rely on external stimulation, because without it, there really may not be enough endorphin being activated naturally to keep you comfortable. Unfortunately, if you're overeating sugar, wheat, and/or dairy products, diabetes is a real danger, along with a host of other potential health problems.

The good news is that by using DLPA or DPA and the other nutritional tools described in this chapter to raise your endorphin level, you'll be much less attracted to these foods and can stop using them without much regret. If you follow the Action Steps listed next and still find that your addiction to comfort foods is a problem, turn to the "Food Craving Tool Kit" for more information on how to understand and eliminate biochemically based emotional eating. If alcohol, drugs, or pleasurable activities have you hooked, see chapter 13.

Saying Good-bye to Your Oversensitivity

When you combine the special supplements I've recommended in this chapter with your basic supplements and good-mood foods, you should feel relief right away. You'll stop working so hard to avoid pain, and you'll stop overreacting to it when you inevitably do get hit with some. To start assembling your endorphin-building gear, move on to the Action Steps. You're almost there.

ACTION STEPS

Before you focus your attention on the details of the endorphin-building strategy that follows, remember that you'll need to use the special repair supplements described in this chapter *in conjunction* with the basic supplements and good-mood foods described in the chapter on creating your nutritherapy master plan. If you don't, you'll be disappointed in the results.

Read chapter 10, "Your Master Supplement Plan," for complete directions on taking your supplements. The basic supplements are described there and listed in a daily master supplement schedule. This is followed by a list of all the special repair supplements recommended in every chapter of the book, including this one. Study the Action Steps below to decide which special supplements you'll need, the best doses, and the appropriate times to take them. Insert this information into your master supplement schedule (pages 202–205) and you're ready to go. Be sure to check the "Caution Box" on pages 199–200 for any contraindications before you add any amino acids or other special supplements to your master supplement schedule.

	AM	B	MM	L	MA	D	BT*
DLPA 500 mg	1–2	—	1–2	—	1–2	—	—
(250 mg D-, 250 mg L-)							
Comfort Zone	1–3	—	1–3	—	1–2	—	—

If you tend to crave sweets or alcohol for comfort, you might consider trying the Comfort Zone formula, which combines DLPA with L-glutamine, an amino acid that helps reduce cravings for sweets, starches, and alcohol by normalizing blood sugar levels, is great for your digestion, and can also convert to calming GABA.

continued

Or DPA 500 mg (if you need to avoid more stimulating DLPA)†

	AM	B	MM	L	MA	D	BT
Or DPA 500 mg	1	—	1	—	1	—	—
Freeform amino acid blend 700–800 mg	1–2	—	1–2	—	—	—	—

You probably won't need the complete amino blend after the first month if you're eating plenty of protein three times a day.

---

*AM=on arising; B=with breakfast; MM=midmorning; L=with lunch; MA=midafternoon; D=with dinner; BT=at bedtime.
†Why you might want to take DPA rather than DLPA: you are jittery, hyper; headache prone; have high blood pressure; have insomnia; or have a personal or family history of melanoma.

To order DPA or Comfort Zone, which are hard to find, call our clinic's order line (800-733-9293) or order from our Web site: www.moodcure.com. For DPA only, contact Montiff (310-820-4883) or Bios Biochemicals: www.biochemicals.com

See chapter 10 for all the details on taking your supplements and when to stop taking them.

RECOMMENDED READING

Fox, Arnold, M.D. *DLPA to End Chronic Pain and Depression* (New York: Pocket Books, 1985). Now out of print, but available used.

Braverman, Eric R., M.D. *The Healing Nutrients Within* (North Bergen, N.J.: Basic Health Publications, 2002).

Ehrenpreis, Seymour, Ph.D. *Degradation of Endogenous Opioids: Its Relevance in Human Pathology and Therapy* (New York: Raven, 1983).

Step 3

Creating Your Nutritherapy Master Plan

CHAPTER 7

Out with the Bad-Mood Foods

Ridding Your Diet of Emotionally Hazardous Edibles

Now that you've identified your own mood type (or types) in step one and learned how to use special nutritional repair strategies to restore your true emotional self in step two, it's time for the basics. In step three you'll discover which foods to avoid and which foods and supplements to pursue in order to build and maintain a nutritional foundation that will keep false moods permanently at bay.

I've been making ominous allusions to bad-mood foods throughout the book, and now I'm going to get down to the possibly unwelcome but definitely fascinating details. Most of us in the West eat nutrient-poor food most of the time and frequently skip meals, particularly breakfast, altogether. As a result, our levels of many of the nutrients that create good moods have been subnormal for years. We're low in key vitamins and minerals, and many of us eat too little protein. You may be surprised to know that most of us don't consume enough healthy fat, either. On the other hand, we're eating too many nutritionally void sweets, starches, and fatty junk foods. Between the good-mood food that we *don't* eat and the bad-mood food that we *do* eat, we have come up with the perfect recipe for an emotional hash.

Is your daily menu a minefield? Certain foods—brace yourself, they might be your favorites—can be mood monsters. Four of the most frequently eaten foods in the United States are so mood toxic that I can't recommend them to anyone. In addition to eating lots of these top bad-mood foods, you're probably relying on coffee or diet soda, sweets, and snack foods to get you through. Fast food and diet food provide skimpy, low-quality fuel and fast loss of mood quality. The current epidemic of bad moods is definitely linked to an epidemic of deteriorating food quality and quantity: junk moods come from junk foods. Junk foods are addictive and lead to overeating. Overeating leads to overweight. Overweight leads to dieting. The only thing harder on your mood than junk food is diet food—that is, *no* food.

This is the law of malnutrition: When your food quality or quantity deteriorates, your mood is the first casualty, even before your physical health begins to deteriorate.

AND NOW, FOR THE FOUR TOP BAD-MOOD FOOD AWARDS

Bad-Mood Food Numbers One and Two: A Tie Between Sweets and White-Flour Starches

I call them the "gruesome twosome": first, the refined granules, powders, and syrups we call sugar; and second, the refined white-flour starches. Since these foods are so often teamed together and have almost identical effects, they are tied for first place in the bad-mood category. Many of our clinic's clients have been freed from the moodiness they've endured for years, simply by dropping these two items from their menus. No supplements, no other changes, dietary or otherwise, required.

Let's begin with sugar, one of the most addicting substances on the planet. Brought to Europe from the East in the 1100s as a precious drug, along with other rare substances like frankincense, myrrh, and opium, sugar was kept under lock and key by apothecaries and worth its weight in silver. Called "crack" in France, it was destined to become a prized and popular delicacy by the sixteenth century, well-known for its tremendous addictive potential. For quicker and cheaper access to this potential bonanza, European merchants developed the slave trade, with all the cruelty and displacement that still causes so much suffering.

Addiction, greed, slavery—that is the origin and legacy of sugar's "sweetness." Added to most processed foods, from cereal to ketchup to frozen entrées, sugar guarantees sales through its highly addictive effects.

As it does with all addictive substances, our vulnerability varies. Some of us may develop only a mild dependency, with few negative consequences. If push came to shove, we could even live without sweets. If you're in that category, you're a rare bird who should feel free to skip this first section entirely. Most of us have been more seriously hooked, either caught up in the perpetual yo-yo of dieting and overeating or in the epidemic of full-scale eating disorders. My first book, *The Diet Cure*, deals extensively with sugar addiction, its devastating effects on both mood and health, and how it can be overcome.

Sugar is bad enough all by itself, but it's often teamed with the other top bad-mood food—refined white-flour starch. In fact, high-starch foods like breads and cereals are more of a problem for some people than sweets. They can actually be almost as shocking to our sugar-regulating system, because, like sweets, they are converted into glucose—blood sugar—so massively and so quickly.[1] For reasons I'll reveal in the section coming up, some people are drawn more to floury products than to sweetened ones, but usually these mood-toxic twins are inseparable. You'll find them together in cookies, crackers, breads, cakes, and cereals. Why? Because the sugar-and-starch combo can make foods doubly addicting.

In a way, it's unfair to categorize sweets and white-flour products as foods. They're really more like drugs. That's why they have such mood-altering power. The sugarcane and sugar beets that sugar is extracted from, and the grains that flour is extracted from, contain fiber, vitamins, and minerals. But after the extraction process, most of those beneficial nutrients are gone. What's left is a potent crystallized concentrate, not unlike other plant concentrates we're familiar with, like cocaine or opium, also extracted from lovely plants full of vitamins, minerals, and fiber. These two refined white carbs can force a release of your brain's natural feel-good neurotransmitters, serotonin and endorphin. This brain chemistry disruption and depletion leads to the need for another cookie for another brief mood boost . . . then another . . . and another.

American consumption of sweetened foods has increased from 25 pounds a year to 125 pounds a year in the past one hundred years and increased 30 percent just in the past twenty years, according to the USDA. This increase in our intake of sweets along with our high intake of refined starchy carbohydrates (both sweets and starches are carbohydrates) really is the primary cause of the fastest-growing disease in the world, diabetes, with its doubled incidence of depression.[2]

The first chapter of this book begins by comparing our current rates of depression (high) with those of one hundred years ago (low). What I didn't mention was that the same time period has seen a similar increase in sugar consumption and diabetes. The Pimas, native people living just south of the Mexican border, eat close to the way they did one hundred years ago and have no diabetes. Yet their relatives just north of the border have one of the highest rates of diabetes in the world, fueled by the bad-mood twins.

The twins specifically contribute to two other emotional and physical scourges: stress and sex hormone imbalance. The adrenal glands get so enormously overworked processing sweets and refined starches that they can't keep up with the demand when a stressful life is added to a stressful diet. Since the adrenals are also responsible for making half of our sex hormones before the "pause" and *all* of them afterward, diet can make all the difference to both men and women. Our clients *routinely* lose their PMS and menopausal or andropausal depression as soon as they drop these carbs.

The sugar-starch combo, along with bad-mood fats, also produces a type of blood-congesting fat called "triglyceride" that greatly increases the risk of heart disease (another illness associated with very high rates of depression). On top of that, they sabotage your mood and health in yet

---

Let's see what a typical high-carb breakfast can do:

Orange juice—Even without added sugar, this, like all fruit juices, is so concentrated in fruit sugar and devoid of the vitamins, minerals, and fiber that should dilute the sugar content that it qualifies as a junk carb. (Most vitamins can't survive *any* processing, and most fruit juice is highly processed.)

Cereal—The milk on top helps if it's full-fat milk, but it's typically low-fat, which means high (milk) sugar. When they take the fat out of milk, what's left is sugar, water, and protein, which we pour on top of sugar-and-flour concoctions that have been refined beyond recognition.

Toast or bagel—All or mostly refined starch (white flour) and usually heavy on the sweeteners. Even "whole wheat" bread usually has white "enriched" flour as the number one ingredient and some kind of sweetener added.

another way. They steal your appetite for the good-mood foods. You just don't feel like a shrimp salad when there's soda, pasta, or ice cream around. The result, according to the USDA: significantly less protein and other key mood-enhancing nutrients, like calcium, magnesium, zinc, vitamin C, and B vitamins, especially in the diets of our children.[3]

What's the problem with high-carb "meals"? If you consume these food bombs *with* plenty of real foods like eggs, they land more softly. If not, within seconds your body is highly stressed trying to neutralize their destructive impact. First, it sends out precious adrenaline, intended to cope with real stresses like a mugging or a divorce. That sends your endorphin levels up (which is what makes you feel so good). Then your insulin levels go up (that's what puts you at risk of becoming diabetic). Most of the sugar and starch, after almost instantly converting into a system-shocking mass of glucose, is moved hastily out of your bloodstream and into your muscles by insulin, where it's converted into fat for storage (that's when you gain unneeded weight). Then your blood sugar drops to an alarmingly *low* level (that's when you become hypoglycemic and get grouchy, headachy, or weepy). Finally, your most vital stress-coping chemical, cortisol, is rushed in to release emergency blood sugar stores to keep you from going into a coma. This blood sugar–regulating maneuver is extremely costly. It's a procedure that should be performed infrequently, in emergencies. It's like having a five-alarm fire drill three or four times a day. Your stress-coping equipment gets used up dealing with the high-carb twins and can't help you out with all your other stressors (that's when you become less and less able to cope).

Have you had enough? How about this: Sugar is the preferred food of cancer cells! I do have three more words left to say about sugary, starchy so-called foods—*Don't eat them.* But if you still can't imagine life without these junk foods, see the "Food Craving Tool Kit" for the eight secrets of how to break a carbohydrate addiction.

Bad-Mood Food Number Three: Wheat (and Its Cousins Rye, Oats, and Barley)

Most people never suspect that among the most ordinary food they eat every day lurks a potential mood disaster. The items that tend to have this upsetting effect are (I'm sorry) bread, pasta, bagels, and cookies made out of flour ground from the grain wheat and its cousins rye, oats, and barley. You may be immune. Not everyone is affected by these grains, but a surprising number of people are. I've seen it in over a thousand clients and have experienced it myself.

These unhappy grains, whether "whole" or refined, all harbor a peculiar protein called "gluten" (think glue), which can irritate, inflame, and rupture the lining of the digestive tract, to the point that nutrients from food don't get absorbed well (or sometimes at all). Food can't be properly broken down and digested, so malnutrition sets in. In addition to digestive distress, bowel problems, headaches, and high rates of colon cancer and diabetes, depression and manic-depression can result because the nutrients responsible for regulating our moods can't be absorbed. Dozens of studies confirm that depression is a common symptom of gluten intolerance (also called "celiac disease"), one that usually disappears when wheat and the similar grains are withdrawn.[4] People with gluten intolerance have low levels of the antidepressant, antianxiety brain chemical serotonin,[5] and gluten has been implicated in mental illness since at least 1979, which is when I first noticed psychiatric journals reporting tremendous improvement in the symptoms of patients with depression and manic-depression in mental hospitals who had been experimentally taken off gluten-containing foods. More recently, anxiety, Tourette's, ADD, epilepsy, and other neurological problems have been associated with these grains.[6]

Wheat grown in the United States is a hybrid developed specifically to increase the gluten content so that baked goods will have more puff. But the hybridization has made it the most indigestible flour in the world. Fluffy biscuits and bread turn to a gluey, irritating mass in the small intestine. Pastry recipes from other countries don't work well in the United States, because our wheat has been so altered (and vice versa). Rye, barley, and oats contain less gluten than wheat does, which is why we don't make Wonder Bread out of them. All four grains were originally grasses. (If you are allergic to grass, you might think about crossing all these grains off your grocery list.) The gluten they contain is one of the few comestibles that can affect the brain like a drug. It's called a "brain allergen" by experts on diet and mood like author Doris Rapp,[7] a pediatric allergist, and psychiatrist/author Dwight Kalita.[8] The gluten in these grains affects the brain like an opiate, stimulating the production of exorphins. That's why you may "love" and feel comforted by your bread or pasta—your brain gets a druglike rush every time you eat those foods. As a result, gluten is one of the few food substances that can actually create a full-scale addiction. Allergic clients who go off it can actually feel a tired and headachy withdrawal reaction for a few days. If your cravings for baked goods, pasta, and the like won't allow you to go without them, turn to the "Food Craving Tool Kit" for information about how to turn off those cravings.

Among the first things that the gluten-containing grains, particularly wheat, can eliminate are your vim and vigor. If you start keeping a food/mood log, you may find that you routinely get lethargic and unfocused after a meal that contains these grains.[9] (Rice and corn are usually fine. They contain no gluten.) How do you feel after a plate of pasta? a bowl of cereal? a sandwich? a burrito? . . . Sleepy? Feel as if you swallowed a brick? One of our clients went off the flour gluten–containing grains for ten days, then brought a piece of bread to work to try at her break. Her other co-workers came looking for her half an hour later and had to shake her awake. Chronic exhaustion caused by gluten intolerance has been the secret behind the mystery of why some of our clients have become addicted to stimulants like diet pills, cocaine, and "speed." These people no longer feel the need for their drugs when they quit eating wheat and experience their own energy surging back.

Gluten intolerance is also associated with thyroid disease.[10] An Italian study found that those with a significant allergy to gluten also developed a significant allergy to their own thyroids (thyroiditis), which disappeared when the gluten was removed for three to six months.[11] Thyroiditis is quite common and has many negative symptoms, including depression, anxiety, and low energy. We've seen this condition many times, and you can read about it in the "Thyroid Tool Kit."

Gluten can not only sedate us, it can produce agitated moods in some people. One of our clients, a social worker of 45, had suffered from severe anxiety for years. She was unable to use calming amino acid supplements because of a liver problem, but she found that just removing wheat, rye, barley, and oats from her diet eliminated her anxiety and panic in a week. When she tried them again, her anxiety came right back. Another client, a psychiatrist, discovered that frequent feelings of anguish, hurt, and rage disappeared when she stopped eating these grains.

One other thing: Bowel problems (including an increased incidence of colon cancer) are common symptoms of gluten intolerance. Think for a minute about what chronic constipation can do to your mood.

If you suspect that you might be gluten intolerant, do the two-week home test described on page 140 to be certain. If you test positive, I suggest you explore the gluten-free resources in the "Resource Tool Kit" and get *The Diet Cure,* which contains more information on living gluten-free than I can include here. I know it's a major inconvenience, but please get serious about this. If gluten is the cause of your bad moods and low energy, you'll feel better within two weeks once you stop eating it. But it will all eventually come back if you start eating these grains again.

Bad-Mood Food Number Four: Bad-Mood Fat

The award for bad-mood food number four goes to vegetable oil and the margarine and shortening made from it. I don't mean extra-virgin olive oil, which is a good-mood fat. I am referring to—surprise!—corn oil, soy oil, canola oil, safflower oil, sunflower oil, peanut oil, sesame oil, wheat-germ oil, cottonseed oil, walnut oil, and the like. The reason we didn't use these oils much before 1930 was that we preferred traditional fats like butter and cream. And not so coincidentally, our rates of depression, heart disease, and cancer were much *lower* then.

All that changed in the 1950s, however, when the medical establishment told us that saturated fat in butter and other dairy products could cause heart attacks and that the polyunsaturated fat in vegetable oil and margarine was beneficial for your heart. By the 1960s, vegetable oil and margarine had become staples in the American kitchen, at what now appears to be the cost of a substantial measure of both our health and our happiness.

Here are the reasons I fear these fats. First, they are very unstable—that is, they can become dangerously rancid very quickly. Rancid means oxidized, and in your body, oxidized means damage to your cells and tissues, especially to the areas rich in fat like your brain. You know what happens when an apple is exposed to the air? Oxidation is the process that turns it brown and makes it go bad. If you eat vegetable oils that are already oxidized from heat and light in processing, you are exposing your own healthy tissues to a volatile substance that will damage them. Here's where butter is truly better. You can keep it on the table for days at a time and it won't spoil. Why? It's not damaged by light and heat, and it's packed with natural substances called "antioxidants" that prevent oxidation. In contrast vegetable oils have had their antioxidants removed and destroyed in processing. The reason they don't *smell* rancid is that they've been *deodorized* by being exposed to high heat. Unfortunately, all this processing seriously damages these oils by the time we pour them onto our salads and skillets or add them to our recipes. Oxidation, or rancidity, is a major contributor to most degenerative diseases, and we consume, on average, fifty-seven pounds a year[12] of rancid vegetable oils, 400 percent more than we did in 1920.

Vegetable oils are pressed out of seeds, nuts, and beans that are high in a fat that has a special name and very particular qualities. Its name is "omega-6." We need a little of it on a regular basis. In fact, it's considered essential. We need it to clot our blood, shed the lining of the uterus when we menstruate, and constrict our blood vessels, for example. Producing inflammation, though, is the thing that most of the omega-6 fats are best known for, and inflammation is useful, up to a point. It can kill things like viruses and bacteria. But overconsuming omega-6 can result in overkill of healthy tissues all over the body, including the brain. Chronic inflammation of the brain can interfere with neurotransmitter functions in any number of brain cells. For example, omega-6 interference with the neurotransmitter dopamine can lead to Parkinson's disease, bipolar moods (manic depression),[13] schizophrenia, and obsessive-compulsive disorder.[14]

It's the combination of rancidity, excess intake, and inflammation that makes the omega-6s such a serious modern health hazard. We used to get the small amounts of omega-6 we needed from eating whole grains and beans and from seeds and nuts that we'd keep in the freshness-maintaining shell till we were ready to eat them. Now these are the only oils many people *ever* eat or cook with. They're also the oils used in almost all prepared foods like baked goods, salad dressings, and mayonnaise.

These fats have even crept into important foods that used to be almost totally omega-6 free. Fish, meats, and poultry are now raised on high-omega-6 grains instead of low-omega-6 algae, grass, and bugs. There is no question that ever increasing rates of depression, heart disease, and cancer have been direct results. The Japanese and Israeli scientific communities have concluded, after several decades of consuming these "Western" oils and suffering epidemic increases in "Western" diseases as a consequence, that the high-omega-6 vegetable oils have been a disaster for their people. A grim report to the National Institutes of Health by the top Japanese experts concluded that omega-6 vegetable oils "are inappropriate for human use as foods."[15]

Okay, so vegetable oils are killing us, but do they really have that much to do with our moods? Yes! For the first time in history, we have been using these rancid oils in huge quantities. Even if the omega-6 vegetable oils were not rancid, they should be consumed only in very small quantities. When we eat too much omega-6, it takes over. Most notably in terms of our moods, it takes over our brains. In addition to provoking the damaging brain inflammation I've just mentioned, there's another kind of brain malfunction that it sets in motion. Omega-6 molecules are similar in form (long and slinky) to that of another fat—the omega-3s that we're *supposed* to use to make our brain's cell walls. When we don't get enough of the right stuff and pinch-hitter omega-6 steps in, our brain cells quit sending and receiving signals properly. This is a disaster for our moods. It's very clearly an issue in depression, with rates of depression over the past one hundred years rising right along with our consumption of omega-6 fats.[16]

Putting aside its terminal rancidity for the moment, let's move on to the final nail in the omega-6 coffin (and our coffins, if we eat it). Let's look at what is done to these rancid oils, so liquid by nature, to make them harden into the margarine and shortening that we find in most prepared food and use at home to "protect" our hearts.

The fragile, already damaged vegetable oils, so ultrasensitive to heat, are boiled again for many hours with hydrogen and bits of nickel until their essential molecular structure is entirely changed into a "hydrogenated" or "trans" (think *trans*-formed) fat. The toxicity of this "trans" fat *far* outstrips any dangers attributed to saturated fats (except for saturated fat that is hydrogenated). Hydrogenation (*trans*-forming) turns any fat into something that a biochemist friend calls "one step away from a plastic." The process not only keeps liquid fats firm, it keeps them firm forever. Shelf life versus your life.

The evidence, building for decades, exploded in the 1990s with dozens of studies describing the fatal effects of the hydrogenation of our arteries and hearts. One of many similar studies found ". . . a significant association between the intake of trans-fatty acids and the risk of coronary death."[17]

What's the brain and mood impact of these "partially hydrogenated" fats that still crisp up nearly every packaged food on the market shelf, *though many manufacturers don't list them among their ingredients?* Transfats prevent your brain from using brain-protective omega-3 fats, thus contributing to the takeover by omega-6 fats that leads to depression and other mood disruption.

Avoiding the bad-mood fats. One of the reasons that lithium and similar drugs help with bipolar, or manic-depressive, mood swings is that they protect the brain against the effects of the omega-6 fats.[18] But most of us don't need drugs to clear out our brain passages. We need to stop using the bad-mood omega-6 vegetable oils, hydrogenated or not, and start using lots more of the good-mood fats. (More about them in the next chapter.)

This is a tough order, since it involves avoiding processed foods like mayonnaise and prepared salad dressings, in addition to all those "baked goods" (baked bads), like crackers, cereal, crisps, and cookies. It will take a while for you to identify the culprits at the store and dodge what you can when you eat out. But it will be worth your life as well as your mood!

Bad-Mood Food Number Five: Soy

Much to the dismay of all of us who have come to regard soy as a wonder food, soy turns out to have a number of mood- and health-deflating effects. Here are some of the findings that I think you should know about: my main concern is to let you know how soy can adversely affect mood-regulating sex and thyroid hormones, but I'd also like you to know how soy can adversely affect the brain and digestion.

Soy and babies. Soy milk–based infant formula poses such a risk that the health ministers of the United Kingdom and New Zealand have formally advised parents not to use soy formula.[19] There is no question that soy-fed infants have estrogen levels an average of seventeen thousand times higher than infants fed human or cow's milk. This equates to the estrogen in 5 birth control pills a day! The epidemic rise in premature sexual development in 15 percent of Caucasian girls and 50 percent of African American girls, reported in the cover article of the October 30, 2000, issue of *Time* magazine, may be directly attributable to the effect of soy formula. This is exactly the conclusion reached by a study of girls with premature breast and pubic hair growth in Puerto Rico.[20]

Among infants fed soy milk, diabetes rates are twice as high as among those who are breast-fed,[21] and no one questions the fact that soy milk inhibits thyroid function in infants.[22] The ratio of available tryptophan in soy milk is lower than that in breast milk, setting infants up for the misery of low-serotonin moods and sleeplessness,[23] along with diabetes and thyroid disease, both strongly associated with depression.

Soy and digestion. Soy contains an unusual kind of protein, which, though high in most amino acids, is so hard to digest (except perhaps in the case of fermented miso or tempeh) that its constituent mood-protective amino acids are not easily absorbed. This protein can also damage the digestive tract, and that can result in generally impaired digestion and further decreased protein absorption.

The soy industry has a very helpful Web site aimed at the piglet farmer. On it is a warning about the amount of soy feed that has been found to be safe for piglets: *1 percent.* Next to this warning is a ghastly photograph of a baby pig's damaged intestine, as evidence of the harm that can befall overly soyed swine.[24] Unfortunately, the soy industry, in its pursuit of human consumers, has not been so forthcoming regarding soy's negative effects on the digestive apparatus of *Homo sapiens.*

The thyroid factor. A local physician had been encouraging her patients to use soy isoflavones in menopause until she began to observe an odd thing: Many of them were developing low-thyroid symptoms. Actually, soy's depressing effect on thyroid function has been well documented for forty years.[25] Soy contains mineral-blocking phytates, acknowledged even by the soy industry as interfering with the absorption of antidepressant thyroid hormones as well as the thyroid- and brain-crucial minerals iodine, iron, and zinc. We know that soy eaters have a high incidence of autoimmune thyroiditis,[26] which you can read about in the "Thyroid Tool Kit."

The hormone factor. Recently, soy has been promoted as an "anticancer" food that could protect against breast cancer and prostate cancer. Proponents of soy often point to the remarkably low levels of these cancers in Asian countries, where soy is widely consumed, as evidence of its cancer-fighting power. What they fail to say, however, is that the average amount of tofu consumed in a day in Japan is *less than 2 teaspoons.* In China, even less is eaten. In Japan and elsewhere in the Orient, the use of soy milk has been virtually unknown. In the United States, we're eating much more soy than has ever been used by humans anywhere: big tofu burgers and high-potency soy protein shakes, big glasses of soy milk, and highly concentrated soy-derived supplements. When you eat soy in such high quantities, it's the equivalent of taking unmonitored hormone replacement therapy.

Several menopausal women with low estrogen have told me that as little as half a cup of soy milk has stopped their hot flushes in minutes. Research confirms that soy raises estrogen levels, but is this always good? Raised estrogen levels may be fine for women who definitely have low estrogen levels (though the other adverse effects of soy can still impact them), but few menopausal women are ever tested to see what their estrogen levels are, and many of them have perfectly normal or high levels that should not be tampered with. Males and females who have normal or high levels of estrogen already (that is, most men and women under 40) should be neither raising nor lowering their levels of powerful estrogen, certainly not without testing. (See the "Sex Hormone Tool Kit" for how to test your own sex hormone levels.)

For one thing, over 80 percent of U.S. breast cancers are associated with estrogen supplementation. Not surprisingly, in many studies soy is associated with increasing risks for breast cancer.[27] In one study, women who already had breast tumors were given a soy drink for fourteen days. Their breast tumor growth increased significantly. Breast tissue cell growth was activated in another study using 45 milligrams of isoflavones. (This is double the Japanese daily intake from soy foods of this potent phytoestrogen).[28] Yet a typical recommended daily dose of soy isoflavone in U.S. supplements is 40 to 80 milligrams.

Disturbed menstruation, so common in young vegetarians, is also thought to be a soy-related phenomenon.[29] Predictably, males on soy lose testosterone, and their estrogen levels may rise to abnormal heights or fall too low.[30]

Soy and premature brain aging. A thirty-five-year Hawaiian study of 8,900 Japanese men and 500 of their wives, all of Japanese descent, showed tofu intake to be the only factor that correlated with brain aging and shrinking and Alzheimer's disease.[31] The more tofu consumed, the more impaired the brain. My mentally sharp father, on his own for the first time at age 75, began eating tofu twice a day, almost every day, and developed an unusual late-onset form of Alzheimer's that his doctors couldn't explain. Like many of us, he was just trying to be healthy, but his mood and his mind were never the same, even after he stopped eating tofu.

The soy story, initially so promising, appears to be headed for an unhappy ending. If you've never liked it much anyway, you won't be too upset by this development, but I know that this news will be a real blow to vegetarians and other health-oriented people. I was shocked and skeptical myself, until I looked closely at the ever increasing research.

THE SPECIAL NONFOOD AWARD FOR DIET FOODS

Not eating *enough* food may be even harder on your mood than eating too much bad-mood food. A large Johns Hopkins study found that dieting was the number one cause of depression among overweight people and concluded that food restriction was an unsafe means of weight loss. Low-calorie dieting is also well-known to be the primary cause of all eating disorders and the terrible moods associated with them. The short-term nutrient losses sustained in a diet can easily add up to long-term mood deficits.[32] Dieting, fasting, restricting—all have indelible effects on your brain. There is no such thing as a "successful" low-calorie diet: dieting starves and literally shrinks your brain. Skipping meals is starvation, too. Your body doesn't keep all its mood-maintaining nutrients in a tidy cupboard somewhere. If you don't swallow them, they won't arrive. We know from the concentration camps, from famine, from anorexia, that people can go on living without sufficient nutrients, but are they *happy*? *No!* Here's a snapshot of what's really going on when you don't eat:

1. Skipping meals automatically throws off your blood sugar levels for the entire day. Lots of credit can be given to the nonfood *coffee* here, as it can kill your morning appetite, in particular, leading to the most common bad-mood eating practice: the skipped breakfast syndrome (SBS). SBS is famous for promoting high stress and low energy, and making you ready for chocolate by ten A.M. Caffeine is profiled as a food additive in the next section.

2. Low-calorie dieting can be like skipping meals all day, plus it almost immediately inhibits the levels of two of your biggest mood enhancers—serotonin and thyroid hormone.

3. Fat really is jolly. Low-fat diets are firmly associated with depression and irritability. Low-fat typically means high-carb and, therefore, low blood sugar, leading to mood swings, hypoglycemia, and diabetes. Blood sugar levels can drop even lower with no fat to provide an alternative fuel that actually burns more steadily than carb fuel. Without certain fats, your brain functions poorly, and your sex hormones and stress-coping hormones can't be properly made.

4. Low-protein diets (for instance, a typical vegetarian diet) usually mean low energy and low mood, because your brain and body are low in the amino acids that they need for making their natural antidepressants and stimulants serotonin and norepinephrine and their naturally relaxing GABA (not to mention muscle building and the thousands of other body functions that require protein). That means protein at least *three* times a day. You'll notice the difference on the first day.

5. Prepackaged diet foods are deficient not only in calories, they're deficient in nutrients as well, being highly processed and loaded with chemicals.

Regarding aspartame (NutraSweet): This queen of the diet world is one of the most complained-about substances on the market. The FDA received 4,800 complaints in one year alone. Huge quantities can be ingested by a single person, because aspartame is found in so many different diet foods. Yet, like real sugar, this synthetic sugar can raise insulin levels and has actually been linked to diabetes.[33] Our clients often complain about adverse physical symptoms, such as headache and bloat, but the *top mood complaints* are depression, irritability, confusion, anxiety attacks, insomnia, and phobia.[34] Sound like the list of low-serotonin symptoms? It should, because aspartame can definitely inhibit serotonin. Aspartame can also be highly addictive, as it forces a rise in our natural stimulants and painkillers norepinephrine and endorphin. A psychiatric study researching the effects of aspartame on people who already had problems with depression had to be halted because the effects were so severe: 63 percent experienced memory loss, 25 percent became irritable, 37 percent became more depressed, and 40 percent experienced nightmares![35] Combined in ubiquitous diet sodas with caffeine (which you'll read about next), aspartame can be particularly mood toxic.

DISHONORABLE MENTIONS: AWARDS FOR BAD-MOOD FOOD ADDITIVES

Caffeine. The average person is ingesting lots more caffeine than ever before, in coffee, diet sodas, chocolate, and the increasingly popular iced tea. Besides the predictably negative effects on the quantity and quality of your sleep, making you tired and irritable, you can count on caffeine to contribute to feelings of anxiety. Studies show that the individuals who drink the most coffee often suffer chronic depression as well.[36] The mood seesaw that caffeine sets up is part of what gets you hooked. When you crash, you pick up more caffeine. In the process, your own natural "uppers" are getting depleted as they do when any stimulant drug is used, making you more dependent on caffeine.

Among this drug's worst mood offenses is its inhibiting of the brain's levels of antidepressant serotonin and sleep-inducing melatonin. Caffeine also depletes some of our most mood-vital nutrients: the B vitamins, vitamin C, potassium, calcium, and zinc. It also overstimulates and weakens the kidneys, pancreas, liver, stomach, intestines, heart, nervous system, and adrenal glands and overacidifies the pH (causing premature aging). Coffee is laced with pesticides and free-radical-producing hydrocarbons that weaken cell membranes. What's more, it takes only a small amount of coffee to set off these negative effects—as little as two small cups or one mugful a day. (Decaf, unless it's organic, still contains some caffeine as well as all the pesticides and hydrocarbons.)

Colorings, preservatives, and other chemical additives. The chemicals used to color and preserve food are known to have effects on mood. These effects, particularly on children, have been studied extensively since the 1970s.[37] They are irritability, distractibility, and hyperactivity. Some artificial colors are more apt to upset than others, with yellow the most upsetting of the lot. (Ironically, antidepressants are often coated with a yellow dye that has caused significant problems.[38]) Dr. Benjamin Feingold alerted us to this problem originally, and his work has been confirmed internationally, see www.feingold.org and *Helping Your ADD Child* by John Taylor, Ph.D.,[39] for important details.

Since artificial flavors, colorings, and other chemical additives are in every processed item from cheese to Tylenol, you may have been affected but not known that it was these brain irritants that were the culprits. There's one standout, though: the "flavor enhancer" MSG, notorious for its adverse effects on the brain and its ability to trigger depression in particular.[40] Found in many common foods like flavored crisps and crackers, it is also a component of "hydrolyzed vegetable protein" (HVP), one of the most common additives of all in processed foods.

To avoid additives, try health store foods, which are usually free of most of them—and check labels.

Pesticides. Another mystery ingredient, present in both fresh and processed foods, pesticides can definitely affect your mood as well as your health.[41] Choose organic produce, packaged food, and dairy products and organic or range-fed eggs, poultry, and meat whenever you can.

THE ALLERGY FOOD AWARDS

Allow me to list the foods that have been found to be the most common irritants, in order of annoyance. You may already be having adverse reactions to these (or other) foods and already be avoiding them. Does any food give you the runs, hives, or trouble breathing? Surprisingly, most allergy symptoms are much more subtle, constant, and familiar—like being tired or constipated every day. Certainly not everyone is troubled by allergic reactions to foods, but there's an easy way to find out if *you* are. It's a home test that I describe at the end of this chapter.

Are Certain Foods Giving You Allergic Moods or Other Symptoms?

Most common allergic mood reactions: Irritability, angry outbursts, glum lethargy, teariness, hyperactivity, stress, depression. Allergic moods could hit within minutes or any time in the twenty-four to forty-eight hours after exposure.

Most common allergic physical reactions: (1) Respiratory problems, including asthma, sore throats, earaches, stuffy nose, and postnasal drip. We've found that food allergies often aggravate other allergy reactions to inhalant pollens or grasses, and research bears this out. In a study of allergic individuals eating anything they wanted, 25 percent reacted to inhalants, while those on an allergy-food-restricted diet had half as many reactions.[42] (2) Digestive problems such as constipation, diarrhea, stomachache, bloat, gas, reflux, and heartburn.

Other common allergic reactions: Low energy and sleepiness (especially right after meals), joint pain, achiness, poor concentration, addictive cravings for the allergy food or for sweets.

First Place: wheat (and its cousins rye, barley, and oats). I've already pronounced these grains bad-mood food number three, but I just thought I'd mention them again here.

Second Place: cow's milk products.

Runners-up: soy and the nightshade family (tomatoes, peppers, white potatoes, aubergine, and tobacco).

Runners-up especially for children: chocolate, peanuts, eggs, and high-salicylate food like apples and oranges, as per Dr. Feingold.

Second Place: Dairy Products

Milk, cheese, or anything else made from the modern cow: Whether it's the antibiotics, the feed, or the processing, more of us than ever are finding dairy products a problem. At our clinic we hear almost as many complaints about cow's milk products as we do about first-place wheat and the other gluten-containing grains. There's lots of evidence that these can adversely affect mood in both children and adults. Anger and even violence are particularly associated with allergic reactions to milk products.[43] The first time I heard about the negative effects of food on mood and behavior was in a report given by a juvenile probation officer about a "hopeless" repeat offender delinquent who had had a complete change of "character" when he was diagnosed with a milk allergy and taken off milk and cheese.

If you have any of the emotional or physical traits listed in the "Allergy Symptom Box," please test this food and see if it's a problem for you or not. Even if your mood isn't improved by avoiding it, you may still discover a priceless health secret—like the secret behind your chronic asthma, earaches, sore throats, or diarrhea. Be aware that the milk protein called "casein" can be as addictive as gluten, the grain protein. It's one of the reasons for the enormous popularity of milk-based foods. Consult the "Food Craving Tool Kit" if you find you need help in freeing yourself from stubborn cravings for these foods. First, try lactose-free milk to see if you lose your symptoms. If not, it's probably the casein or whey that your body can't tolerate. In that case, even lactose-free milk and low-lactose yogurt or butter won't work, and you'll have to go entirely dairy-free. If you do, try clarified butter (ghee), which has all the lactose and protein removed from it and is great for cooking. Most dairy-intolerant people do well with goat's and sheep's milk products. Also, try raw cow's milk products that have been neither homogenized nor pasteurized. They affect some people much differently from processed milk products. If none of this works, you can still enjoy coconut milk and oil (more on this yummy alternative soon). Do avoid rice milk, soy milk, and almond milk, all overly sweetened or otherwise objectionable.

Runners-up: Soy, Chocolate, Peanuts, Eggs, and the Nightshades

In our experience, these foods are far less likely to cause mood symptoms in adults than the gluten-containing grains or milk products. Among them, soy and the nightshades are the most common allergy-provoking foods. In children, chocolate, peanuts, and eggs are the foods in this category found to be most likely to trigger reactions like tantrums, hyperactivity, tears, and/or apathy. Adults with allergic symptoms, especially if they have extreme trouble concentrating (or ADD), should also consider eliminating and challenging all these foods if they don't get significant benefit from eliminating just wheat, rye, oats, barley, and dairy products.

HOOKED ON BAD-MOOD FOODS?

Have you known for a while that your mood improved a lot when you ate more protein, vegetables, or fresh fruit and less bread, cereal, pasta, and sweets? Many of our clients tell us they never felt a more solid sense of well-being than when they were on the Atkins or Paleolithic diet. The trouble was that they never *stayed* on the good-mood foods in those diets. They *couldn't*. Why? Because they'd gotten really hooked on sweets and starchy carbs, dairy products, and fatty junk food. Are you food addicted? Most Americans are, to some degree. Detaching from food addiction so that you can easily choose foods that you *know* make you feel better is what the "Food Craving Tool Kit" is all about. Please read it.

How do you know if you're addicted to junk food? It's simple. Even with all your good reasons not to, you keep eating it. "Continuing use despite adverse consequences" is the formal definition of addiction. Your mood is bad, but you keep on eating bad-mood food. If you're stuck on junk food, like so many of us are, taking the amino acids and other supplements recommended for your particular mood imbalances may well relieve those cravings by eliminating the moods that trigger them. But if for any reason your junk food or carb cravings persist, turn to the "Food Craving Tool Kit" for more help.

HOME TESTING FOR FOODS YOU MAY BE ALLERGIC TO

Any suspect foods should be subjected to the following simple and effective home test. No other kind of testing, in our experience and that of other food allergy experts, is as accurate.[44] Food allergies are more common than any other allergies, but they are harder to diagnose. The traditional "scratch" testing doesn't work nearly as well for foods as it does for inhalants, for example, and blood-testing results have also been disappointing. We rarely do these kinds of testing because the home test is so effective and convincing. (There are a few testing methods that we do use occasionally when allergy symptoms persist even after the most common allergens have been tested or eliminated. See the "Resource Tool Kit" for a list.)

Keep a food/mood log to monitor your testing process. Write down what you eat at what time on the left side of a sheet of paper and how you feel *in detail* (mood, energy, sleep, digestion, congestion, bowels, and so on) on the right.

➤ Stay off suspect foods for fourteen days.
➤ Reintroduce only one food or food group at a time.
➤ Wait two full days before reintroducing or "testing" a new food. If you are intolerant to a food or food group, your body will react negatively. For example, if you react to reintroducing wheat, stop the wheat and wait two days before you try rye. The reason for this is that sometimes you can get allergic symptoms hours or days after your test. If that delayed reaction hits on the day that you try the next food, you won't know which food is the problem. Some people have problems only with wheat, not with all gluten-containing grains. If wheat was not a problem, the other three gluten-containing grains— rye, oats, and barley—are not likely to be troublemakers, either, and you probably don't need to test them.
➤ Women should test *after* their period and *before* the onset of PMS symptoms.

Here's how to do the actual testing:

Days One to Fourteen: Making the Break. Do not consume any of the foods that you have decided to test. Be very careful to examine contents of packaged foods, and cross-examine waiters about the possible presence of test foods. Wheat, dairy, soy, and corn are everywhere. If you aren't sure, don't eat it during the testing period! (For instance, hydrolyzed vegetable protein could be wheat or soy, modified food starch could be wheat or corn.) The supplements you'll be taking will assure that your withdrawal reactions (if any) from these foods is fairly short and mild, so don't dread this testing period. You won't miss the foods you eliminate, and by day 5 (if not before), you should be feeling better than you have in a long time. You may notice quick weight loss in this first week, too.

Day Fifteen: The Challenge. On this "testing" day, notice whether any of your originally bothersome symptoms have gone away. Then eat a good-size serving of one test food for breakfast and the same test food again at lunch. For example, if you're testing for a milk allergy, have a glass of milk at breakfast and a glass of milk with lunch. Make a note of how you feel. Also note any food cravings, your mood, energy, digestion, respiratory symptoms, bowel function, appetite, skin changes, headaches, and sleep patterns—any and all information that your body imparts. You may have a very strong reaction, such as a migraine if you're prone to them. If you get even a little tired, bloated, or headachy after your challenge meals, don't ignore it. If you gain weight or start craving the tested foods again, don't be surprised. It's not a coincidence.

When testing the gluten-containing grains, test first with wheat (bread, pasta, or another very plain form of wheat), because it is the grain highest in gluten and will therefore give you the clearest results. Do not eat any more of the food or food group for the next two days (after waiting two days, you can test another gluten-containing grain, like rye).

Allergic reactions to milk products and gluten-containing foods can be very similar, so you'll get a clearer response to your testing if you eliminate both, then reintroduce one at a time to see which is the problem or whether both are problematic. If it feels too overwhelming to let go of milk products and the gluten-containing grains all at once, test the grains first.

Do not eat any more of your convicted allergy foods as you go on to test other foods (or ever).

If you have no leftover adverse symptoms from your first challenge, you can test another food a few days later. If, after you reintroduce wheat, milk, or any other food, you determine that you need to avoid it permanently, you can expect to feel better for as long as you stay away from it. If you suddenly feel irritable, depressed, anxious, bloated, tired, achy, or distracted again, you'll know that you've inadvertently (or advertently!) consumed your allergen.

Perhaps you'll eat a little of it because of convenience or pressure when there's nothing else available on the menu or everyone's indulging in a traditional holiday treat—and you'll experience some of your old symptoms for a while. But they'll fade, or you can use two tablets of Alka-Seltzer Gold to get rid of them quickly. Just don't do it often or you'll be back to allergy square one.

RECOMMENDED READING

Bernstein, Richard K., M.D. *Dr. Bernstein's Diabetes Solution* (Boston: Little, Brown, 1997).

Taylor, John, Ph.D. *Helping Your ADD Child* (Roseville, Calif.: Prima Publishing, 2001).

Rapp, Doris J. *Is This Your Child? Discovering and Treating Unrecognized Allergies* (New York: William Morrow, 1992).

Philpott, William H., M.D., Dwight Kalita, Ph.D., and Linus Pauling. *Brain Allergies: The Psychonutrient and Magnetic Connections* (New York: McGraw-Hill, 2000).

DesMaisons, Kathleen. *Potatoes, Not Prozac* (New York: Simon & Schuster, 1999).

Simontacchi, Carol. *The Crazy Makers: How the Food Industry Is Destroying Our Brains and Harming Our Children* (New York: J. P. Tarcher, 2001).

Schlosser, Eric. *Fast Food Nation: The Dark Side of the All-American Meal* (New York: HarperCollins, 2002).

Carper, Jean. *Your Miracle Brain: Maximize Your Brainpower, Boost Your Memory, Lift Your Mood, Improve Your IQ and Creativity, Prevent and Reverse Mental Aging* (New York: Quill, 2002).

Hagman, Bette. *The Gluten-Free Gourmet: Living Well Without Wheat* (New York: Henry Holt/Owl, rev. ed. 2000). Recipes concentrate on breads and other normally gluten-containing foods. Good general info on celiac disease and other gluten-intolerance problems in introduction.

Sully's Living Without (magazine). A lifestyle guide for people with food and chemical sensitivities (www.livingwithout.com).

Soy Alert! (www.westonaprice.org/soy/soy_alert.html) for info on negative effects of soy.

ADD, ADHD and other conditions, and additives and salicylates: see www.feingold.org

CHAPTER 8

Your Good-Mood Food Master Plan

Choosing the Best Foods for You

A nd now for the happy news about foods that will please both your palate *and* your disposition. Let's start with the specific foods that are guaranteed to improve your mood: protein, vegetables, healthy fats, and fruit. Then we'll move into general guidelines for how to get enough of the right foods for your particular needs.

THE FOUR TOP GOOD-MOOD FOODS

Good-Mood Food Number One: Protein

There's no question about this one. I've seen hundreds and hundreds of people add more protein to their lives and report great changes in their moods within days as a result. The word *protein* actually means "of primary importance" in Greek. As I've said in every chapter of this book, without protein you cannot feel optimistic, enthusiastic, calm, or comforted. The neurotransmitters that send out all of these positive feelings can be made only by using certain of the twenty-two types of protein called "amino acids." The more protein, the better you're able to feel. Most people seem to need 20 to 30 grams of protein per meal. That means at least a palm-of-your-hand-size portion of protein *three* times a day!

Our office had a visit recently from a tall, handsome vegetarian of 43 who had been so anxious and depressed most of his life that he actually threw up every morning, because he was so nervous about facing the coming day. A month before his appointment with us, he had joined a gym and been told to cut his carbs and increase his protein and vegetables, which he'd done. By the time he got to us, he was almost entirely relieved of his panic. We simply suggested a trial of tryptophan and GABA to take the remaining edge off and told him to call in with a progress report. He called in with positive reports four times before we told him to stop and just call if he had any problems. We never heard from him again.

The following foods provide the highest concentrations of protein:

Fish
Poultry—chicken, turkey, and, especially, Cornish game hens
Eggs
Lamb, beef, pork, and venison (including liver!)
Dairy products from cows, goats, and sheep (as tolerated)
Shellfish

Fish

Please try to eat fish at *least* twice a week. Why is fish first on my list of high-protein foods? Because it's so quick to prepare, so easy to digest, and contains, along with *plenty* of all twenty-two aminos, the unique omega-3 fat that your brain needs to correctly form the cells in your brain, your eyes, and the lining of your arteries, among other things. More about this wonder fat soon. Fish even contains vitamins as well as minerals like calcium, magnesium, and potassium, and we can safely eat up to 2.2 pounds of it a week, despite mercury warnings, according to the FDA. (Serve your fish with a delicious garnish of coriander, an effective mercury detoxifier.) Fish and shellfish definitely qualify as fast food in the best sense of the word. Most cuts of fish cook in less than ten minutes. Ditto for shellfish like shrimp and scallops. Canned sardines and salmon are the fastest fish. Always keep a can or two on hand for emergencies. A word of encouragement: the rate of depression worldwide corresponds to the amount of fish consumed. The Japanese eat ten times *more* fish than we do, and they have ten times less depression![1] A word of caution: farmed fish are low in omega-3 and high in omega-6.

Poultry

In terms of their protein content, all birds are created equal; but of all the kinds of poultry, succulent game hens, so quickly roasted in the oven, contain more of the invaluable omega-3 fat. All poultry contains all twenty-two aminos, but because poultry is grain fed, its fat content tends to be higher in the omega-6 bad-mood fats. Somehow game hens are able to produce a slightly better ratio of omega-3 to omega-6.

Ode to Eggs

In 2001, the American Heart Association exonerated eggs, announcing that these high-protein foods don't contain much saturated fat and don't significantly contribute to LDL (bad) cholesterol.[2] So eggs are back to being the perfect food. First of all, they're perfectly nutritious: loaded with protein, vitamins, minerals, and the lecithin that helps us digest fat easily. The yolks contain as much protein as the whites and *much* more additional nutrition. I have witnessed what cardiologist Robert Atkins has been claiming for years, that most people *reduce* their cholesterol levels and their weight eating lots of eggs, *if* they drop sweets and overly starchy foods.

Eggs are also *perfectly fast:* scramble, boil, poach, or bake as a frittata in minutes. As crepes you can wrap them around anything—ricotta and fresh fruit or sautéed veggies. They're *perfectly portable,* too: keep hard-boiled eggs ready in your fridge for instant protein in an emergency, in the delicious deviled version, sliced in a salad, or blended with olive oil, vinegar, and seasoning for a salad dressing. The only trouble with eggs is that we aren't eating enough of them. Two gives only 13 grams of protein, and we need over 20 grams per meal—so have three at a time! And look for the higher-omega-3 eggs at health food stores. Unless you have a genetically high-cholesterol problem, you don't need to limit the eggs you eat.

Beef, Lamb, Pork, and Venison

All these foods are loaded with protein, including the rare amino acids carnitine and taurine and the best-absorbed forms of zinc and iron. I learned how important red meat could be from working with young vegetarian female athletes whose injuries did not heal quickly, who'd lost their endurance and their periods, and who tended to develop eating disorders at a phenomenal rate. All of these problems turned out to be directly attributable to deficiencies of iron, zinc, and protein. Those girls who were willing to resume eating red meat saw a quick reversal of these symptoms.

Note: For better protein digestion, people with type A blood seem to do best adding supplements of hydrochloric acid when eating animal protein, as they are known to be weak in this protein- (and mineral-) digesting acid. More on this in chapter 10.

Dairy Protein

Cottage cheese is a super source of protein, with 28 grams in every cup. Hard cheeses are protein rich, too, though often so fatty and strong in flavor that it's hard to eat a palm-size portion (though mothers in Italy do feed their meat-hating children big hunks of Parmesan cheese, one of the cheeses highest in protein and calcium).

Many people find that cow's milk and cheese are hard to digest, though for some, lactose-free milk or raw milk and cheese are more digestible. Cheese is a more concentrated source of protein than milk, since most of the liquid (and milk sugar, or lactose) has been removed. Yogurt is easier to digest, too, but, like milk, it has more water and less protein—8 to 10 grams per cup.

Eating goat's and sheep's milk products helps many dairy-intolerant people, and these foods are delicious. Not only is traditional sheep's or goat's milk feta available now, but almost any kind of cheese, from cheddar and ricotta to a Parmesan-like cheese to a Brie-like cheese made from sheep's or goat's milk, can be found. Goat's milk yogurt is readily available in health food stores, and goat's milk is available even in supermarkets.

Vegetarian Protein

Since we've thrust soy firmly into the bad-mood category, what's left for a vegetarian in the high-protein department? Many vegetarians eat dairy products, eggs, and fish. Some also eat chicken. If you're in that group, you're okay. If you are vegan (no eggs or dairy), you'll need to eat *lots* of carefully selected food to get enough protein. Beans are only 5–10 percent protein. Compare that to canned salmon at 20 percent and roast beef at 28 percent protein! And vegetable protein sources do not contain all twenty-two amino acids. They're particularly low in antidepressant tryptophan, the serotonin precursor.

The vegetarian morality, though powerfully convincing, has tended to lead us toward the same high-carbohydrate, low-protein, low-tryptophan, low-serotonin morass as the low-fat, high-carb diets have done. Where can we get L-tryptophan now? Since it's an amino acid—in other words, a building block of protein—it's found only in foods that contain protein. Some protein-containing foods have more tryptophan than others; generally, the more protein a food has, the more tryptophan it contains. Take turkey. It's a high-protein food with about seven times more protein than rice (which has only 6 percent protein, like most grains). The same is true of most other high-protein foods like eggs, fish, pork, beef, and cottage cheese. Vegetarians will really need to supplement with tryptophan or 5-HTP. For a complete amino acid supplement blend that includes 5-HTP balanced with vegetarians in mind, see the "Resource Tool Kit."

By mixing vegetable protein sources, you can get all twenty-two aminos. For example, hummus, a spread made of chick peas and sesame paste found in most stores, combines all the amino acids. But it has only about 14 grams of protein in a 7-ounce container. If you eat the whole container over grain, you can bring the protein content up to 20 grams. The trouble is, this puts the proportion of protein to carbs at twice what is ideal, unless you're a fast metabolizer or an athlete. Too many carbs can overwork insulin and the stress hormones and store as unneeded fat. If they're carbs from whole foods, though, you're safer.

A cup of any cooked beans will give you about 15 grams of protein. The other most concentrated vegetarian protein source is nuts and seeds, with black walnuts (which have almost twice the protein of English walnuts and only two-thirds the carbs), peanuts, and sunflower and pumpkin seeds being highest (all about 7 grams of protein per ounce). But then your total omega-6 fats, already present in your beans and grains, can run too high because most nuts and seeds are high in omega-6 fat. But there are some exceptions. Flaxseeds are known for their lower omega-6 and higher omega-3 fats. Other nuts, lower in both omega-3 and omega-6, are considered neutral, and, like olive oil, all are high in safe omega-9 fats; they are cashews, macadamias, hickory nuts, filberts, almonds, pecans, and pistachios.

You can also use protein powder made from rice or whey (for instance, with fresh fruit in a smoothie) to supplement your food, 20 to 30 grams in 2 to 3 tablespoons. Mix it into a morning smoothie or hot cereal; add it to a pureed bean soup (it comes plain as well as vanilla flavored) or a vegetarian burger recipe. But watch your mood. You'll still need to take amino acid supplements additionally to protect your serotonin and melatonin stores, especially if you're a vegan. If you're blood type A, vegetable protein sources should agree with you better than with the O blood types, who don't seem able to thrive without animal protein in plenty.

Protein in Common Foods

Food	Quantity	Protein in Grams
Beans	1 cup	15
Bread	1 slice	2–3
Buttermilk	1 cup	8
Cheese, firm	1 ounce	6–10
Cheese, soft	1 ounce	2–4
Corn	1 cup	4
Cottage cheese	1 cup	30
Eggs	1	6
Fruits	1 (apple, banana, orange, etc.)	1
Meat, poultry, fish	3–3½ ounces (not including fat, skin, or bones)	17–27
Milk	1 cup	8–10
Nutritional yeast	1 tablespoon	8
Nuts	¼ cup	2–7
Oatmeal, cooked	1 cup	6
Rice, cooked	1 cup	6
Seeds	1 ounce	6
Yogurt	1 cup	8–10

Good-Mood Food Number Two: Fats

Your body is supposed to be full of fat, about 18 percent if you're a man and 28 percent if you're a woman. Your brain must be particularly fatty. Up to 60 percent of it should be composed of specialized fatty substances that have to be replaced constantly and have very complex mood-related duties that can't be performed by French fries or corn chips. To feel your best, you need to feed your brain regularly with only the best fatty foods. If you're wondering how *any* fatty foods could actually be good for *anything*, you're about to get a nutritional villain adjustment, so hold on to your hat.

Think of the positive words associated with fat: rich, soft, moist, shining, good-natured . . . In ancient times, fat was associated with joy, wealth, and even sanctity. We *need* fats! In 2001, even the fat-phobic American Heart Association became so convinced about our need for more fat that it raised our fat allowance from 30 to 40 percent![3] It also recommended more eggs and shellfish and urged us to eat more fatty fish. Why? It caved under the overwhelming evidence. It recognized that happier and healthier cultures all over the world have a higher intake of certain fats than we do in the West and that low fat has not led to low heart disease. It also recognized that the "low fat" sweet and starchy carbohydrates that we've been eating in our efforts to cut fat have led to record rates of a new health and mood scourge—diabetes. Indeed, the incidence of diabetes has *doubled* in the past thirty years.

Omega-3 Fats

Let's start out with the most spectacular good-mood fat. It's called "omega-3," and its first home is your brain. Every time you consume this extraordinary oil, your brain gets first dibs, because no other fats can do as good a job. In fact, the "other" omega-6 fats may be your brain's worst problem and the cause of some of your worst moods. The rate of depression among individuals correlates precisely with the ratio of omega-3 fats to omega-6 fats in the brain. The more omega-3, the better your mood; the more omega-6, the worse your mood. In the West, we are very low in omega-3. If we add more omega-3, we can quickly raise a potent natural antidepressant brain chemical called "dopamine" by 40 percent![4] That translates to mental and physical alertness, focus, and excitement.

A depressed, sedentary, achy, mentally confused woman of 80 was brought to us by her daughters. We decided to give her high doses of omega-3 when her basic supplements and a better diet did not help much. Not only did she begin daily exercise with pleasure in two days, but her aches decamped, her head cleared, and her emotional outlook improved. She began to arrange flowers again for the first time in years. She also quit "needing" her evening martinis and lost her taste for overly rich food.

Our clients generally love the way they can come alive on their omega-3 foods and supplements. It turns out that, among other things, omega-3 is an MAO inhibitor, meaning it slows down the MAO enzymes that destroy mood-boosting brain neurotransmitters like dopamine and serotonin.[5] Believe it or not, these fats can even be *over*stimulating to some people. If you find yourself waking up bright and early at four A.M. after too much omega-3-rich fish or fish oil supplementation, you'll have to cut back a bit.

Severe depression and manic-depression are being treated successfully now with this fat,[6] and ADD and alcoholism are also showing preliminary clinical response.[7,8] (We successfully treat addiction to fatty foods with it, too.) Alzheimer's and schizophrenia are clearly affected by altered fatty acid function,[9,10] and omega-3 fat may help.[11] And, as if all this weren't enough, after you've been eating more omega-3s for a few months and your brain's needs are met, the omega-3s will move into the linings of your arteries and remove any plaque that has built up in your body's botched efforts to repair its linings *without* enough of its preferred omega-3! (The studies on omega-3's positive impact on artery health and heart disease are heartening!)[12,13,14]

Where can you get this wonder food? Omega-3 fat comes in two forms: a ready-for-brain-use form found only in fish and a cruder form found in flaxseeds and some other seeds and nuts. The latter is a shorter form of omega-3, alpha linolenic acid (ALA), which has to be worked over by certain enzymes that two-thirds of us don't have and that decline with age. For all of us, ALA helps the body expel excessive omega-6 fat but can't be used reliably to form the long chains that our brains need. These brain chains should wrap around in our brain cells, forming very special membranes that can transmit billions of molecular messages instantly and accurately. These fatty chains are called "DHA" and "EPA."

Fish fat is full of EPA and DHA. Fish like sole contain some, and there's a little bit of the shorter ALA (flaxlike) version in almost all fatty foods, both animal and vegetable. But by far the best sources of the omega-3 fats are wild salmon, sardines, herring, anchovies, and mackerel. They have about *three times more omega-3* than other fish and five times more than flaxseed oil. Their good-mood fat is concentrated in and under the skin.

To get enough of the vital omega-3 fats, you'll need to eat fish more often, as your ancestors did. For example, the Japanese still eat two and a half pounds of fish weekly, and their depression rates have historically been nil, as have their heart disease rates. But when was the last time *you* ate fish five times a week? That's how much they eat, and you might need to eat, to get enough omega-3s to elevate your mood and energy and counterbalance the omega-6s.

Recommendations about the ideal ratio between the two fats range from one to one (omega-6 to omega-3) up to seven to one, but in the United States the actual ratio is now over twenty-five to one.[15] The vital ratio has begun to change in Japan now, too. As I mentioned in chapter 7, the Japanese have been eating too much of the omega-6 vegetable oils and trans fats, and depression, heart disease, and cancer rates are increasing alarmingly as a result.

In the United States people used to get quite a bit of omega-3 from meat and chicken as well as fish, but now most of these animals are fed grain high in omega-6 rather than grass, hay, or bugs with high omega-3 content. Grass-fed beef is coming back, though, and it's *fourteen times* lower in omega-6 fats. (See the "Resource Tool Kit" to locate sources.)

According to the FDA, we can safely eat 2.2 pounds of fish a week (preferably not higher-omega-6 farmed fish). That's about five or six servings weekly (otherwise the mercury and other pollutants will get us). *Note:* Don't cook that fish in high-omega-6 oil, and don't dress it with mayo or tartar sauce, unless made yourself with olive oil. (See recipes in chapter 9.) If you're unlikely to eat that much fish, don't worry, you can take fish oil supplements to help fill your omega-3 quota. Your basic supplement schedule (page 202) includes about 2 grams a day of fish oil (combined DHA and EPA). That's the equivalent of one-quarter pound of salmon or sardines a day (without the mercury, which is stored in the fish muscle). If you also eat fish at least twice a week, you'll make your omega-3 quota nicely. So eat as much fish as you can, take your supplements, and enjoy more energy, more focus, and healthier arteries!

Note: Flax oil is helpful *in the brain* only for one-third of us, at best. The rest of us can't convert its ALA omega-3 fat into DHA and EPA. We'd need to use five times more of it than of the fish oil to get equivalent effects, but flax also contains significant amounts of omega-6 fats.

The SAT (for Satisfying) Fats

Now for the real fun. Think of the fatty foods you'd love to eat if you thought they wouldn't kill you or make you fat. When I tell my clients that butter and sour cream are safe and healthful, they beam incredulously as if a loved one were being returned from the dead. Little do they know that they may be the loved one in question. We have been "good" for sixty years. We've cut down hard on what we thought were "bad" fats, meanwhile stocking up on "safe" vegetable oils and hydrogenated fats, but the results have been terrible. Heart disease has escalated, and cancer and diabetes have become epidemic.

So are you ready now for some good news about cream cheese, whole-fat yogurt, chicken skin, and coconut milk? I know that this is going to be hard for you to swallow. Part of it is the term *saturated fats.* Let me give it a new spin. Let's call it *SAT,* short for *SATISFIED.* All saturated fats are complete in their molecular structure, unlike the omega-6 or even the omega-3 fat molecules, which look like combs with broken teeth. This density gives SATs their undisputed stability and strength. It's also why they don't easily get rancid, something no one disputes.

The study I mentioned in chapter 7 that convicted the trans fats in margarine and shortening of murder by heart disease also pardoned the saturated fats. "There was no association between intake of saturated fat and the risk of coronary death."[16] The scientific literature is loaded with this exonerating evidence. In fact, SATs are the *preferred* energy source for your heart because they burn at such a reliable pace, much steadier and longer than carbs do. Many studies confirm that saturated fats can also protect you from stroke.[17]

One mood benefit provided by these creamy fats we've been avoiding all these years is that they support the function of the omega-3s in our brains, reducing the negative effects of the excess omega-6s. They actually lower levels of the most potentially damaging omega-6 fat, arachidonic acid.[18,19]

Four recent studies, three on Type II diabetics (with their doubled rates of depression) and one on mildly obese men and women, used a high-saturated-fat, low-carb diet. Their results: All showed improvement in cholesterol levels, weight, and insulin levels.[20,21] But these studies are really just confirming common sense. Many peoples all over the world have consumed lots of these full-fat foods and thrived physically and emotionally. We did, too, before 1910. In 1909, we ate about twenty-six pounds of saturated fat per year and nine pounds of omega-6 fats (on top of what was in our eggs, meat, and so forth). In 1998, we consumed less than *nine* pounds of saturated fat and sixty-six pounds of omega-6 fat![22] SATs are *not* our problem. The high omega-6s—margarine and vegetable oils—are (as I hope I made clear in chapter 7).[23]

You can safely cook with SATs, because at a heat that would toxify any vegetable oil, the sturdy SATs hold up. In your brain and body the SATs build protective cell walls. In your skin they keep damaging UV rays from penetrating and keep moisture in. Many SATs are also great for energy.

They slow the entry time of refined carbohydrates, protecting you from diabetes. They keep your blood sugar levels rock solid, which keeps your mood solid, too. The medium-chain saturated fats are wonderful, steady, stress-relieving energy fuels that athletes use to perform better.

The crucial fat-soluble vitamins A, D, and E cannot be absorbed into our bodies without their carrier, saturated fats. Nor can calcium! For example, spinach has lots of calcium, which is not absorbed well unless it's eaten with butter (or olive oil, which also contains some SAT). Same principle with collard greens and bacon fat.

Speaking of butter, let's take a look at my personal favorite SAT. *Butter* is so packed nutritionally, with its ten vitamins, ten minerals, eighteen amino acids, and eleven kinds of fat that it's hard to know where to begin. It's tremendously high in vitamin A, which it helps deliver to your eyes (night vision is absolutely dependent on an adequate vitamin A supply). Vitamin A regulates the female sex hormone progesterone, too, providing many mood as well as fertility and other benefits. (While saturated fats like butter assist vital vitamin A absorption and uptake, too many omega-6 fats can prevent it.[24]) Then there's butter's butyrate, the fastest burning of all fats. This very special fatty acid is used extensively in your brain. For one thing, it serves as a base for making GABA, your natural Valium (GABA stands for gamma-amino*butyric* acid). It can also protect you from colon cancer and is used as a medicine in precancerous colon problems to do just that.

How did I lose my own fear of SAT fats? Through twenty years of working with people who had eating disorders. The overeaters and bulimics in our program often avoided both protein and fat to save their calories for carb binges. At first we asked them to increase protein, which helped stop their moodiness, overeating, and obsessiveness. They added lots of vegetables as the only carbohydrates allowed and tried to keep fat levels low. At the same time, we expected them to exercise regularly, but this low-fat, low-carb diet didn't give them enough energy to do so. It didn't always lower their high cholesterol levels, either, and it kept them feeling deprived. They didn't enjoy eating. Because nuts and seeds were often binge foods and too high in omega-6 fats, we couldn't recommend them, so we tried a new food plan that ended up working like a charm. It was very simple: high protein, high vegetables, and more, mostly saturated, fat. No sweets (even fruit) or high-starch foods at all. The results: no cravings, high energy, *satisfied* with the food, mood fine, weight normalizing, and cholesterol *lowering!*

What About Cholesterol?

Cholesterol is not a fat, but I could go on at the same length about the health and mood benefits of cholesterol as I just have about the benefits of saturated fat. An impressive review of 195 international studies showed that a cholesterol level between 160 and 260 seems to be ideal.[25] With levels above or below that range, we can have more health troubles, but more of the trouble than you think comes with cholesterol levels that are too *low* rather than too high. A forty-year study of four thousand people in Hawaii found that "the earlier that patients start to have lower cholesterol concentrations, the greater the risk of death."[26] Many other studies concur.

Surprisingly, cholesterol is one of the most valuable nutrients there is for mood, particularly for stress coping, since it is the substance that we use to make our stress-coping hormones and our mood-regulating sex hormones. If you've been avoiding it stringently, you may have innocently compounded your mood problems.

Low cholesterol is firmly associated with depression, anxiety, irritability, violence, suicide, and insomnia. Cholesterol in the brain is essential for natural antidepressant serotonin production.[27] A huge amount of the brain, about 25 percent of it, is cholesterol. Cholesterol is (surprise!) an antioxidant that actually protects our tissues, including our brain tissues, and is the base from which we make all the stress and sex hormones that direct our brain's whole mood show. Cholesterol is not a fat; it's an alcohol that can be made from many foods. Cows can obviously make it from grass. I recommend several books in the Action Steps that will tell you much more of the fascinating true cholesterol story.

Now let's talk about my second favorite SAT, the delectable one that makes so many of my clients smile when I recommend it: *coconut milk*. Do you enjoy this food in Thai cooking? I defy you to find more beautiful or cheery people than the Thai. They, like so many equally healthy and cheerful peoples in southern climates, eat lots of this saturated fat. Coconut fat contains powerful antiviral and antifungal fat and is probably a bit more stable even than butter, as it is a little more saturated (think satisfying, satiating, and rancidity resistant). That's why the milk and oil of coconut is so safe as well as yummy to cook with.

The omega-9 fats are the final good-mood fats. The oil most endowed with this fat is *olive oil*. Just being the *only* oil that you can still safely use on your salads, now that I've demoted most of the competition, should qualify olive oil (extra-virgin olive oil, to be precise) as a major mood enhancer. Olive oil contains very little of anything but omega-9 fats, which are almost as stable as saturated fats. It has a little saturated fat and almost no omega-6 fatty acids, so it doesn't get rancid easily. It keeps well in cool, dark places, even after it's been opened. Although it's low in the omega-3s, the omega-9s in olive oil are very supportive of the omega-3s, and they specifically help promote serotonin's antidepressant activities in your brain.[28,29]

The nuts highest in omega-9 (but low in omega-6) are cashews and macadamias. Peanuts, almonds, filberts, hickory nuts, and pistachios are high in omega-9, too, and lower in omega-6 than all other nuts and seeds except cashews and macadamias. Eat them in moderation, though, because they do still contain considerable omega-6.

Happy omega-3 fats from fish, saturated fats from foods like chicken skin and butter, and olive oil are primary fat sources for some of the healthiest people on earth. In the Mediterranean, for example, the people of Crete and Italy are certified with world-class health. A 93-year-old woman from the Mediterranean coast of Syria, in perfect health and mood, told me recently that she still uses only olive oil for her salads and vegetable sautés and eats fish four times a week, plus lots of lamb, poultry, and butter.

Good-Mood Food Number Three: Vegetables

They're bright, they're colorful, they're energizing and calming. They come in interesting shapes, sizes, and textures. Some of them are among the only *healthy* fast foods on the planet. They're loaded with the vitamins, minerals, and other nutrients that make good moods possible. They're the indispensable partners to the good-mood proteins and fats in providing the nutrients your brain needs most. They're the only carbs guaranteed not to cause blood sugar shocks. (Yes, vegetables contain carbohydrate as well as fiber and water.) Some of them are outstanding cancer preventives. Several large studies have found that increasing the intake of fresh vegetables can cut stroke risk by as much as 50 percent.[30] A few specific examples of vegetable power: Tomatoes and peas protect against prostate cancer, while brussels sprouts, broccoli, and cabbage protect against colon cancer.

The antidepression diet of the traditional Japanese contains not only almost half a pound of fish per day, per person, it also contains generous amounts of vegetables from both land and sea.[31] "How many vegetables fill my mood requirements every day?" you ask. Answer: From 4 to 5 cups *a day,* the amount of veggies that would overflow if you put them into a quart container like a milk carton. Think a good-size salad plus 2 cups cooked or raw vegetables. Or a big salad (8 cups) containing lots of veggies. Think a large Caesar at lunch and a stir-fry with snow peas, cabbage, and broccoli florets at dinner. (It takes 2 cups of leafy greens like lettuce or raw spinach to make a cup, because it's so fluffy and insubstantial.)

Do You Hate Your Veggies?

Some people don't like to eat vegetables. They're usually people who are zinc deficient and don't enjoy much of anything unless it has a strong sweet or spicy flavor. If you're in this category, take a 50-milligram zinc capsule every day for a month and see if you don't start to enjoy your 4 cups of vegetables a day (okay, start with 2 cups a day). You'll also be boosting your immune, thyroid, reproductive, and neurotransmitter systems, which all depend on zinc. You might buy a bottle of liquid Zinc Status by Ethical Nutrients and see if you can taste it. By the end of your month on zinc supplements, it should taste awful, indicating your zinc levels are now fine.

Whenever you eat vegetables, you're eating next year's exciting scientific health discovery. Science is only very gradually testing vegetables for their hundreds of specific mood- and health-promoting contents. Every month, new and exciting study results get published, and the most praise goes to dark green leafy vegetables. Sautéed with fresh garlic in olive oil, or snipped into a soup, they will provide you with lots of absorbable mood-boosting B vitamins like folic acid. Folic acid deficiency is consistently found to be a factor in depression as well as in schizophrenia. My favorite B vitamin study found that folic acid supplements "significantly improved clinical and social recovery" in both depressed and schizophrenic patients![32] Reams of research like this attest to the antidepressant powers of folic acid alone, but, truthfully, all the B vitamins are known to effectively reduce stress and promote a sense of well-being.

Dark green leafy vegetables get their color from the mineral magnesium. Spinach, chard, beet greens, and kale are all loaded with this relaxing, soothing mineral as well as lots of B vitamins plus vitamin K, which enhances bone density and preserves omega-3 fat stores. I could go on and on. Popeye wasn't kidding.

Note: Spinach is high in magnesium and B vitamins all right, but it needs to be cooked to eliminate phytates (chemicals that block iron, calcium, and other minerals from being used in your body). (Look for New Zealand spinach, which contains no phytates.)

For pure vitality, it's the potassium in most vegetables that is so precious. Lettuces are loaded with potassium. So are tomatoes, even cooked in sauces. All raw or cooked vegetables and vegetable juices are full of potassium. Cooking veggies in a soup or sautéing or roasting them with a protective coating of olive oil preserves the potassium. And it's in the peels—so don't peel, just scrub. If you steam veggies or boil them, you lose quite a bit of potassium in the water (so drink it!). We need 4,000 milligrams of potassium a day for protection against stroke, and vegetables are our best source, though beans and fruit also contain good amounts.

The *only* problem with vegetables is that they take time to wash, chop, and cook. Even salads require the first two steps. If this is a problem for you, turn to page 165 for helpful tips on time, food, and mood. The short, brutal version is "Get over it"—but actually, raw carrots, celery, cherry tomatoes, and snap peas are instant veggies, and you can eat raw red bell peppers and cucumbers like apples.

The more organic and fresher the veggies you eat, the more vitamins and minerals you'll get. Go to farmers' markets or get a home delivery of equivalent produce. This produce typically lasts twice as long as what's available in markets because it's fresher when you buy it. Cooking destroys some of the vitamins and minerals and most of the enzymes in veggies, so have some *raw veggies*—either in a salad or as nibbles—every day. When you can, stir-fry quickly or simmer (heat a vegetable soup, for example, just *below* the boiling point) to retain maximum nutrients in your cooked food.

Good-Mood Carbs: Fruits, Vegetables, Legumes, and Grains

We need good-quality carbohydrates, especially for fueling our brains. The brain is particularly dependent on a constant supply of glucose from carbs for quick energy, which it burns to keep its millions of cellular engines running at all times (a goodly percentage of which are generating our moods). High-carb foods are absorbed instantly *in our mouths* as well as farther along.

I explained in the bad-mood food section that processed sweet and starchy white flour products give us too much energy (glucose), too fast, and no nutrients. Unprocessed carbs fuel us more gradually and give us nutrients at the same time. Green vegetables contain some starch, but not much. We can get whatever additional quick energy we need from fruit, starchier vegetables, legumes, and whole grains, all nutrient rich. All are *whole* foods that break down gradually. *Fruits* are the easiest to digest. Raw fruit contains all the enzymes and vitamins that are destroyed by cooking. It also contains lots of the fiber that keeps our bowels working well (constipation is not conducive to a good mood!). We need several servings daily.

Bananas, for example, contain not only lots of energizing potassium, but some antidepressant serotonin and lots of sleep-promoting melatonin, too. Fruit also tends to be rich in vitamin B_6, the vitamin that your brain must have in order to make serotonin. (Most of us are deficient in B_6.)[33] They are also full of the antioxidants that protect all our brain's cell membranes, promoting *all* neurotransmitter activity.

Many of the long-term studies showing the cancer protective effects of vegetables also credit fruit. Those who ate the most of both vegetables *and* fruit had the best results. Fructose, the primary sugar in fruit, is slower to convert to glucose than table sugar or white flour. So for most people it doesn't cause blood sugar and mood to start swinging, especially if it's eaten when it's best digested, *before* meals or as a between-meal snack. If diabetes is not a problem for you, eat two to four raw fruits, or their equivalent, per day (1 apple equals 1 cup of berries). Most fruit is very high in Vitamin C, and ninety percent of the vitamin C we consume is used by the adrenals for stress fighting. Vitamin C is easily destroyed by heat, so raw fruits (and veggies) are by far our best sources.

All foods *except* fruits and vegetables acidify your body. These two foods alkalinize, the opposite of acidify. Even citrus fruit becomes alkaline in the digestive process. The body works best when its pH (acid/alkaline) level is balanced. This balance can't be kept without fruit and vegetables.

What about starchy veggies? Do baked potatoes count? They're certainly nutritious and energizing, especially with their potassium-loaded skins left on. You need the energy of higher-carbohydrate vegetables like potatoes, corn, winter squashes, and yams *in addition* to your low-starch veggies. In relation to other high-carb foods, like grains or beans, starchy veggies are lower in protein, but they're easier to digest, and they contain neither the omega 6s nor the digestion-blocking lectins which grains and beans always contain. Serve some on the side, next to your mixed greens salad and your steamed asparagus if they sound good to you.

Higher-carbohydrate vegetables are alkaline and contain lots of potassium and vitamin A (beta-carotene). Beans are high in potassium, too, but are more difficult for some people to digest and are more acidic than high-carbohydrate vegetables, as are grains. Beans and grains like corn contain good fiber and other nutrients, but they are more allergy-provoking than most vegetables or fruits and must be soaked and cooked for a long time to be edible; this destroys many nutrients. Watch for allergy symptoms, especially with the grains wheat, rye, oats, and barley. Especially if you're an O blood type, these grains will definitely tend not to work well for you.

GENERAL GOOD-MOOD FOOD GUIDELINES

Put your first emphasis at all three meals on *protein, fat,* and *vegetables.* Eat *20 to 30 grams of protein* at every meal, *about the size of the palm of your hand.* Eat lots of green and some red, orange, purple, and yellow vegetables every day. Your goal is *at least 4 or 5 cups of vegetables* a day.

The menus, recipes, and suggestions in the next chapter will give you a detailed idea of what your new meals will look like: lots of colorful cooked veggies on your plate or a big bowl of salad next to it (not a bitsy salad plateful); a good (at least palm-size) portion of protein; and glistenings of butter or olive oil everywhere. Plus nourishing carbs like fruit, potatoes, yams, squash, or grains and beans, as needed.

Now that you have an idea of *what* to eat, here are some guidelines for *how* to eat:

Eat Regularly

Don't let more than five hours go by without eating good-mood foods.

1. Eat three good meals plus snacks to create a *stone* foundation that your moods just *can't* sink below.
2. Skipping meals destroys your mood foundation.
3. Breakfast: Skip it at your peril. Without it, your mood will swing all day.
4. Supplements are great, but only food can keep you stable all day, every day.

Eat Enough

Especially for weight-conscious women and men, it's easy to undereat as a regular habit, and undereating is mood starvation.

Colleen had a tendency to be easily stressed and anxious and overate sweets and starches. A bright, talented woman, she was always looking for answers. After reading *The Diet Cure,* she started taking aminos and the basic supplements, increased her protein, and cut out refined carbs. She lost thirty-five pounds, and she became energized, calm, and focused. She began exercising and stretching daily with great pleasure. So far, so good. There were some essential foods, though, that she was not eating enough of. Eventually it began to cause problems: she became a bit too thin, even gaunt, and became more easily stressed again. She was eating more than 4 cups of low-carbohydrate vegetables and 90 grams of protein a day (including lots of fish). But she wasn't eating enough fat or higher-carbohydrate food for *her* body's needs, especially considering the amount of exercise she was doing (one and a half hours of walking almost daily). We suggested she eat more butter, avocado, coconut milk, and olive oil, as well as high-carb potatoes, taro (she lived in Hawaii), and fruit. She did, and the resulting increase in body fat made her look lovely and feel stress-resistant again.

I'm telling you this story to remind you that there is no "diet" that is right for everyone at all times. Though Colleen intellectually appreciated the need for fat, her years of training in the religion of low-fat/low-cal still unconsciously led her into trouble, and her new low-carb zeal led her into undereating the healthy higher-starch foods that she needed, too.

Eat According to Your Genetic Heritage

Knowing what foods your ancestors traditionally ate could save your life as well as your mood. Recent immigrants to the United States are healthier physically and have one-fifth as many psychiatric disorders as the U.S.-born; but after ten years, they begin to lose that edge. Why? Largely because their "poor third world" diets were so much healthier than the "rich" U.S. ones.[34]

A Nicaraguan woman with a significant weight problem, low energy, mood swings, and borderline diabetes told me in our assessment session that she always lost weight and felt great when she visited Nicaragua. U.S. food had literally made her moody, sick, and overweight. When she stopped eating fast food and began to eat more fresh vegetables and fruit, beans, corn, chicken, and fish—Nicaraguan style—she felt fine.

The Japanese, who develop heart disease and mood problems in the United States, are well protected in Japan by their high-protein, high-vegetable, high-omega-3 diet. A typical breakfast is eggs, fish, spinach, rice, and seaweed soup. (Greens are served in Thailand for breakfast, too!)

Blood type can be a helpful guide in choosing the most beneficial foods. We have found that type Os tend to do best with diets that emphasize animal protein (but not dairy products) and most vegetables and fruits. Type As can usually tolerate beans, rice, and corn well, in addition to protein (though dairy can be a problem for them, too) and vegetables. (They need to add hydrochloric acid to digest animal protein well.) Perhaps because Bs and ABs are so rare, we have not noticed clear-cut nutritional needs unique to them. The Peter D'Adamo books (*Eat Right for*

What Is *Enough* Concentrated Protein in One Meal?

- ➤ 3 eggs (24 grams of protein)
- ➤ ½ of a 6-ounce can of tuna (22 grams of protein)
- ➤ at least ⅓ of a 16-ounce carton (⅔ cup or 5.3 ounces) of cottage cheese (20 grams of protein)
- ➤ 1½ cups of beans (20 grams of protein)
- ➤ 3–4 ounces of meat, fish, or poultry, approximately the size of the palm of your hand (20 grams of protein)

YOUR GOOD-MOOD FOOD GUIDE

I. Protein

20–30 grams *per meal* from fish, meat, chicken, turkey, eggs, cottage cheese, beans, grains, nuts, or seeds.

II. Low-Carbohydrate Vegetables

4–5 cups (cooked or equivalent) per day of courgettes, asparagus, broccoli, green beans, cabbage, and the like (1 cup = 3 celery stalks, 2 medium tomatoes, or 2 cups uncooked leafies such as spinach or lettuce).

III. Fat

There's no quota here for *added* fats. If you eat full-fat protein sources in the required amounts, you'll get plenty of essential and saturated fat. But please use only extra-virgin olive oil for salads; coconut oil, butter, ghee (clarified butter), or extra-virgin olive oil for cooking; plus avocados, coconut milk, and so on as desired.

IV. Liquids

Eight or more 8-ounce portions from filtered water, herb tea, or vegetable juice (not carrot alone).

V. High-Carbohydrate Foods

The following carbs can be added as metabolism, weight, and energy require, in the order given (unless you're a vegetarian and require more legumes and grains for protein). If you cut back on high-carb foods, be sure to compensate by eating more protein, fat, and low-carbohydrate vegetables.

A. *Fruit:* 2–4 servings per day (1 serving = ½ banana, 1 apple or peach, 1 cup berries, and so on).
B. *High-Carb Vegetables:* carrots, winter squash, potatoes, yams, sweet potatoes, and the like.
C. *Legumes* (⅔ carbs, ⅓ protein): beans, lentils, split peas, and so on.
D. *Whole Grains:* rice, corn, or other grains (including products like tortillas or bread). Be sure to check whether or not you tolerate wheat, rye, oats, and barley well, as per the allergy food section in chapter 7.

Your Type) can provide you with some suggestions, but don't take them too literally. See what actually works best for you.

Eat Organic and Range-Fed Whenever Possible

Ideally, the eggs, fish, poultry, meat, and dairy products you eat at home will come from wild, grass-fed, or organically raised sources. Otherwise your system will have to contend with hormones, antibiotics, pesticides, genetically engineered feed, and other unnatural "additives," none of it conducive to good health or mood—though even this is better than *no* protein! The same is obviously true of vegetables, fruits, oils, grains, beans, nuts, and seeds. Use farmers markets, health stores, and the organic produce sections in some supermarkets to find organic foods. Whenever you can, grow your own! See the "Resource Tool Kit" for shopping ideas.

RECOMMENDED READING

Fallon, Sally. *Nourishing Traditions,* 2nd ed. (Washington, D.C.: New Trends Publishing, 1999).

Ravnskov, Uffe. *The Cholesterol Myths: Exposing the Fallacy That Saturated Fats and Cholesterol Cause Heart Disease* (Washington, D.C.: New Trends Publishing, 2000).

Eades, Michael R., and Mary Dan Eades. *Protein Power* (New York: Bantam Books, 1997).

Schmidt, Michael A. *Smart Fats: How Dietary Fats and Oils Affect Mental, Physical and Emotional Intelligence* (Berkeley, Calif.: Frog Ltd., 1997).

Enig, Mary. *Know Your Fats: The Complete Primer for Understanding the Nutrition of Fats, Oils, and Cholesterol* (Silver Spring, Md.: Bethesda Press, 2000).

Byrnes, Stephen, Ph.D. *Diet and Heart Disease* (Warsaw, Ind.: Whitman Publishing, 2001).

Stoll, Andrew L., M.D. *The Omega-3 Connection: The Groundbreaking Antidepression Diet and Brain Program* (New York: Simon & Schuster, 2001).

Gittleman, Ann Louise, M.A. *Your Body Knows Best* (New York: Simon & Schuster, 1997).

Cordain, Loren, Ph.D. *The Paleo Diet* (New York: John Wiley & Sons, 2001). Ignore his low-fat prejudice.

Geary, Amanda, *Food and Mood Handbook: Find Relief at last from Depression, Anxiety, PMS, Cravings and Mood Swings* (London: Thorsons, 2001).

CHAPTER 9

Good-Mood Menus

Recipes and Ideas for Everyday Eating

N ow it's time to eat.

Eating at Home

The very best meals and snacks for your mood are usually the ones you prepare at home, where you have the most control over the ingredients and cooking methods. My cooking consultants and I have created good-mood menus and recipes for you with three things in mind:

1. The food should be tasty.
2. The food should be easy to prepare.
3. The food should be stretchable, so that you can make extra to use in other meals to minimize the work and time involved in feeding yourself well.

Both the menus and the recipes concentrate on getting you used to cooking and eating more fish and greens and to using only the best oils for salads and cooking. To make your preparations as easy as possible, we've included a list of helpful kitchen implements after the menu section.

Eating at Home, Without Cooking

Is your energy too low to cook? Or do you need extra help with preparing meals to de-stress your lifestyle? Whether on a temporary or permanent basis, you might want to try a *personal chef*. Usually your chef comes to your home once a week and prepares a number of meals that you can heat up during the week. Some personal chefs cook in their own kitchen and deliver food to your home. For more information, check the web for companies and individuals providing this service. But make sure that they can and will cook *good-mood* foods for you.

Take-out from restaurants or delis is another possibility. Some markets have counters with cooked prepared foods, and many meat and fish counters now also have seasoned or marinated meats ready for you to cook or heat up at home (like cracked crab). See the eating-out tips that follow, as they apply to take-out food, too. The main thing to watch for here is the oils they use.

Eating Out, but Well

You are probably going to be eating out at least once a day. Today, half of our meals are eaten out, as compared with one-third ten years ago. If you work in the same location every day, you'll quickly discover which local food places serve good-mood meals and which don't. If you strike out entirely or can't stand the same restaurant's food every day, take a small cooler bag filled with your own delicious leftovers or other creations. If you travel and have to eat out three meals a day, here are some eating-out tips that will help you survive the worst fast food joints in town. (Just read *Fast Food Nation: The Dark Side of the All-American Meal*, by Eric Schlosser, if you're reluctant to change your eating-out habits):

➤ Order a sandwich without the bread (or open faced on whole-grain bread, if you can tolerate wheat). Add side orders of soup, salad, and vegetables to complete your good-mood meal.

➤ Get a baked potato and top it with whatever protein and vegetable choices are available. Add a salad for more vegetables.

➤ Order several side salads if they don't have a large vegetable salad. Side orders of salads or vegetables with cottage cheese, a hamburger patty, or a chicken breast (throw out the bun) will make a decent salad meal. Most restaurants have olive oil and vinegar to bring to the table. Avoid their dressings, unless they make them in-house with olive oil (unlikely except in nicer Italian places).

➤ You can get a hamburger patty or chicken breast or two almost anywhere, and even fast food places often have salads or salad bars now. Cut pieces of your hamburger or chicken into as much salad as you can get and have at it.

➤ Eggs—order three—are available everywhere for breakfast. Some places offer fresh fruit or tomato juice (if you can, get it with fresh lemon to squeeze into it). You'll probably need to fill up on potatoes or whole-wheat toast (if you're okay with wheat). Lots of butter is fine. Keep fried foods to a minimum because of the excessive heat and bad vegetable oils used.

➤ Chinese food is good, except for the oil (ask for no MSG). Avoid any deep-fried and breaded food like egg rolls, shrimp, and crispy noodle dishes. Japanese restaurant food can work, especially if you ask for plain, not sushi (sugar-sweetened), rice and avoid deep-fried tempura. Thai foods, especially curries and the coconut soup, are great choices. Try to avoid the sweetened dishes in all these restaurants—sweet and sour sauce and the like.

➤ Mexican food—eat anything but fried taco shells. Ask for soft corn tortillas to go with your lettuce, meat or chicken, beans, and salsa (and guacamole, if available) or get extra and just eat the filling. Burrito fillings are usually fine, but many people find the white-flour wrap too heavy, like digesting limp cement. Get two, unless they're huge, and just eat the fillings with a fork; or ask for the filling in a container with soft corn tortillas on the side.

GOOD-MOOD MENUS
FOR TWO WEEKS

When a menu item is starred (*), it means that a recipe for that item is included in the recipe section that follows the menus. If a menu item sports an (M) after it, that means "make more," you're going to use it for another meal later in the week. Whenever a menu item is decorated with an (L), it means it contains leftovers from a previous day.

Sat. I	B	*Cottage Cheese Pancakes with fresh fruit (M).
	L	*Complete meal salad (skip cheese, since you ate cheese at breakfast).
	D	*Roasted Cornish game hens (M).
		*Roasted veggies (include potatoes and/or yams) (M) and cherry tomatoes.
Sun. I	B	Grapefruit half or 2 (best to eat fruit before a meal); turkey or chicken sausage (no nitrates); sautéed veggies scrambled with 2–3 eggs per person; warmed and buttered corn tortilla (or wheat toast, if you can tolerate wheat gluten).
	L	1 cup or more of cottage cheese on a large bowl of chopped fresh fruit, with a sprinkling of fresh almonds.
	D	*Fish-spinach roll-ups; *steamed basmati and/or wild rice (M); raw finger veggies (carrots, celery, cherry tomatoes).
Mon. I	B	*Fresh orange–coconut milk Protein Blender Smoothie.
	L	*Complete meal salad with leftover Cornish hen (L).
	D	*Lamb chops (M), roasted veggies (L), and sliced cucumber with finely chopped mint, yogurt, and lemon juice.
Tues. I	B	*Cottage Cheese Pancakes (L), warmed up, with fresh fruit.
	L	Tuna-stuffed avocado (prepare tuna with *Perfect Blender Mayonnaise or *olive oil vinaigrette) on a thick bed of salad greens. Add leftover rice for a more filling meal.
	D	*Thai Coconut Milk Soup, including greens and potatoes, for a one-dish meal (M).
Wed. I	B	*Fresh or frozen strawberry-yogurt Protein Blender Smoothie.
	L	*Complete meal salad with cheese, beans, and pan-toasted seeds.

continued

	D	Cut-up meat (L) and heat in marinara sauce from a jar. Serve over fresh polenta (or sliced packaged precooked polenta rolls) with crumbled goat's or sheep's milk feta cheese on top. Thinly slice purple and/or green cabbage for slaw (2 cups per person), toss to coat with olive oil, then add balsamic or apple cider vinegar, salt, and pepper to taste.
Thurs. 1	B	*Oven Pancake topped with fresh fruit, and turkey, chicken, or pork sausage or bacon without nitrates.
	L	Thai Coconut Milk Soup (L)—reheat and take in a wide-mouth thermos.
	D	Pan-browned dinner sausages (no nitrates), *One-Step Baked Ratatouille.
Fri. 1	B	*Blueberry-banana Protein Blender Smoothie.
	L	*Complete meal salad.
	D	*Oven-Roasted Fish (M); whole-wheat or rice fettucini with butter and grated Pecorino Romano or Parmesan cheese *and olive oil–sautéed greens with vinegar.
Sat. 2	B	*Quick Rice Pancakes (L)(M) with fresh fruit.
	L	Stir-fry (L).
	D	*Beef or lamb roast with carrots and potatoes in drippings. Big green salad with *Balsamic Salad Dressing.
Sun. 2	B	Orange slices (or peaches and berries in summer). Sautéed spinach, onions, and other veggies scrambled with three eggs. Leftover baked potatoes or yams, sliced and cooked in butter or ghee
	L	*Fish (L) tostadas (reheat fish in oven on a corn tortilla), with avocado slices, shredded cabbage, cheese, green onion, and tomato.
	D	*Crispy Chicken Tenders, steamed broccoli with butter and lemon, and baked potatoes.

continued

Mon. 2	B	*Tropical Protein Blender Smoothie (fresh or frozen pineapple and banana with coconut milk).
	L	*Tuna and Bean Salad.
	D	*Chicken breasts and/or thighs (M), served with *sautéed greens, baked butternut squash (M) with butter, and cherry tomatoes.
Tues. 2	B	Warmed-up Quick Rice Pancakes (L) with butter or yogurt and sliced bananas.
	L	*Chunky Salad (M) with Creamy Lemon Salad Dressing.
	D	*Steak (M), baked potato with butter and/or sour cream, sautéed summer squash, and raw pea pods and baby carrots.
Wed. 2	B	*Peach or apricot Protein Blender Smoothie with sunflower or almond milk.
	L	*Complete meal salad.
	D	Grilled brochettes: prawns and/or scallops skewered with slices of onion, courgette, bell pepper, and cherry tomatoes, marinated in extra-virgin olive oil, freshly pressed garlic, lots of lemon juice, and salt, cooked on barbecue grill or grill. Serve with buttered corn on the cob or polenta (M).
Thurs. 2	B	Chopped tomato and cucumber with lemon or yoghurt. 3 eggs with polenta slices (L), all sautéed in butter in the same pan.
	L	Tostada: oven-crisped corn tortilla topped with steak (L) strips, cheese, green lettuce, onion, avocado, and salsa.
	D	Chicken breasts/thighs (M) with mashed-buttered butternut squash (L), *sautéed chard, and cherry tomatoes.
Fri. 2	B	1 cup or more cottage cheese with 2–3 pieces fresh fruit.
	L	*Complete meal salad.

continued

D	*Dredged and pan-seared fish with fresh lemon juice. Serve with buttered green beans and mixed green salad with *Creamy Lemon Salad Dressing.

Snacks	Deviled, pickled, or plain hard-boiled eggs and raw vegetables.
	Raw veggies or chips (baked, not fried—see "Resource Tool Kit") with or without dips.
	Dip suggestions: salsa; salad dressings (see recipes, page 186); cottage cheese (or hard-boiled egg) blended with avocado, garlic (fresh or powder), salt, and lemon juice; bean dip; refried beans (no oil) mixed with salsa; hummus; plain cottage cheese.
	Apple or pear with or without a chunk of cheddar.
	Fruit with cottage cheese.
	Fruit with a handful of lower-omega-6 nuts (cashews, macadamias, hickory nuts, filberts, almonds, pecans, or pistachios).
	Buttered popcorn with cheese or lower-omega-6 nuts.
	Rolled slices of meat or poultry (if you go to a deli for lunch, bring back a couple of slices of meat for a midafternoon snack) and carrot sticks.
	A mixture of chopped black olives and cream cheese spread on slices of ham and rolled up.
	Leftovers, such as high-protein pancakes or smoothie.
	A small fresh smoothie.

HELPFUL KITCHEN IMPLEMENTS

➤ Large skillet or sauté pan (about 12 inches in diameter), with a metal handle so that it can be put in oven.

➤ Blender or food processor.

➤ Steamer basket that fits in a large cooking pot for reheating leftovers or steaming vegetables.

- Large bowl.
- Large roasting/baking pan.
- 2–4-quart pot (for vegetables and grains).
- Large 6–8-quart pot (for soups).
- Kitchen scissors and chef's knife.
- Wooden spoon.
- "Salsa" chopper (a round plastic container with a blade that rotates and chops when you turn the handle by hand—for quickly chopping onions, pepper, celery, garlic, tomatoes, and so on for recipes).
- A 10 × 10-inch (approximate) baking dish, either glass or metal.

Skip the microwave—our experience is that eating food nuked in the microwave can cause fatigue, not suprising when you consider the violent cellular friction applied to the food by this method.

RECIPES

Breakfast

PROTEIN BLENDER SMOOTHIE

As a base, put any of the following into a blender:
2 tablespoons to ⅓ cup full fat coconut milk (add water
     if necessary to this smoothie), or I cup goat's milk,
     plain kefir, plain whole-milk yogurt, buttermilk, or
     organic cow's milk (if you can tolerate them)

Add:
A banana and/or other fresh fruit—½ cup berries,
     I peach, I pineapple wedge (mix and match); or
     ½ cup pumpkin or sweet potato (with a dash
     of cinnamon) for a change
2 tablespoons protein powder from rice, egg, or whey
     sources (totaling over 20 grams of protein)

Plus any or all of the following options:
1 tablespoon (or to taste) powdered green foods
1 teaspoon to 1 tablespoon nutritional yeast
2 tablespoons flaxseeds or meal
Fresh ginger or mint to taste

Blend all together. Add water (or ice in hot weather) if you'd like it thinner.

Makes 1 serving.

COCONUT MILK

Delicious in smoothies, or with chicken or vegetable broth or water for a soup base. Great in hot spicy herb teas or with fruit instead of whipped cream (it solidifies in fridge) or diluted in any recipe that calls for milk or cream. Look for first-press (full-fat) canned milk without preservatives (see "Resource Tool Kit").

From scratch:
(Method 1) Break open a fresh coconut and pour the clear milk into a blender. Remove the coconut meat, chop, and place in the blender. Add enough hot water to bring the level to 4 cups. Blend at high speed for 3 minutes. Strain, pressing pulp to get out all liquid (this can be done in cheesecloth). Return pulp to the blender, just cover with hot water, and blend on high speed for 2 minutes. Strain, press again to remove all liquid from pulp, and discard. Refrigerate or freeze.

(Method 2) Soak dehydrated coconut (unsweetened) overnight. Strain and press as above.

OVEN PANCAKE

4 tablespoons butter
½ cup whole-grain flour
½ cup milk or substitute
½ teaspoon salt
4 eggs

Place butter in a large (10- or 12-inch) ovenproof skillet and put into oven heated to 400°F. Place flour, milk, and salt in a blender. Blend to mix thoroughly, scraping sides with a spatula. Add eggs one at a time, blending after each addition. Pour egg mixture into hot skillet and return to oven. Bake until puffed and golden brown, 10–12 minutes.

Serves 2.

QUICK RICE CREPES OR PANCAKES

For each person, combine in blender:
**½ cup cooked rice, or ⅔ cup for more substantial
    pancakes (Use leftover basmati and/or wild rice.
    Always keep some around.)**
3 eggs
Salt to taste

*Blend all together until it forms a batter. On a griddle or in a
    skillet, melt:*
1 tablespoon butter, ghee, or coconut oil

Heat skillet until a drop of water sizzles. Using about ¼ cup batter for each pancake, cook until set and lightly brown on both sides. (Believe it or not, this recipe is tender and tasty made with plain canned beans if you're out of rice.)

COTTAGE CHEESE PANCAKES WITH
FRESH FRUIT TOPPING

3 eggs
1 cup cottage cheese
2 tablespoons melted butter or coconut oil
¼ cup wholegrain flour
¼ teaspoon salt
1 cup fresh fruit
Ground cinnamon

Whirl eggs and cottage cheese in a blender or food processor until blended. Add melted butter or coconut oil, flour, and salt; whirl until smooth.

Lightly grease a griddle or large frying pan and preheat over low-medium heat. When pan is hot, pour ¼ cup batter into pan for each pancake. Cook until tops are bubbly, turn, and cook other sides until lightly browned.

To serve, spoon 2 tablespoons fresh fruit onto each pancake and sprinkle lightly with cinnamon.

Makes 8 pancakes.

Lunch and Dinner: Fish, Poultry, and Meat Entrées

Cooking Fish and Seafood

Fish and other seafood are fast; fish cooks in less than half the time it takes to cook most meats and poultry. These fish are hearty, taste good, and don't fall apart or overcook too fast:

Salmon (preferably wild—not farmed)
Bluefish
Tuna
Sea bass
Halibut
Red snapper
Mahi-mahi
Swordfish
Blue marlin
Calamari steaks
Or any rich white fish, like flounder or haddock

These fish are more delicate and cook much faster:

Sole filet
Trout filet

Cooking methods for fish:
1. Pan searing with herbs.
2. Marinating and baking in the oven.
3. Dredging and pan searing for a crisp texture.

4. Stuffing with spinach and baking (only for delicate, thin fish like trout and sole).

Pan Searing Fish with Herbs

This is an excellent way to cook, because it seals in the flavor and allows the fish to remain very moist inside.

> **You will need:**
> Preheated 375°F. oven
> 2 tablespoons spice blend of your choice. These can
>   be bought in most stores. Health food stores often
>   carry them in bulk, and grocery stores usually have
>   a brand name, such as McCormick-Schilling, Spice
>   Islands, or Dean & DeLuca, or a generic brand
>   they produce. Avoid MSG and hydrolyzed vegetable
>   protein. Some suggestions:
> Italian seasonings
> Curry powder
> Mexican seasonings
> Spike (or other brand "healthy" seasoning)
> Lemon-pepper blend
> Mediterranean blend
> Thai seasonings
> 8–10 ounces fish (serves 2, or 1 with planned leftovers for
>   another meal)
> About 2 tablespoons olive oil

How to do it:

Simply take the dry ingredients and rub all over the surface of the fish. For more flavor, allow the seasoning to soak into the fish for about 10 minutes.

Once you have done this, heat the olive oil in a skillet or sauté pan over medium flame or coil until oil begins to ripple a little. Place the fish in the pan and sear for 2 minutes until it is brown, then flip it over for another 2 minutes to brown the other side.

When fish is browned, place your sauté pan with the fish in it in the preheated 375°F. oven until it is cooked (about 5–10 minutes). Make sure it is cooked through by testing with a fork.

Marinating and Baking Fish in the Oven

You can use bottled salad dressings to make a liquid marinade (use a fat-free type—with no oil added—so you can add your own extra-virgin olive oil). The marinade will result in a sauce to go along with your fish. You can make your own marinade, using one of the following combinations:

> 4 tablespoons olive oil and 2 tablespoons balsamic vinegar, with 1 tablespoon fresh basil and 2 tablespoons minced onion
>
> 4 tablespoons olive oil, a squeeze of lemon juice, and 3 tablespoons chopped tomato (either canned or fresh), with 1 tablespoon basil or thyme and 1 tablespoon capers
>
> 2 tablespoons garlic (either chopped fine or pressed), 2 tablespoons ginger (chopped fine or garlic pressed), 1 tablespoon chopped lemongrass, and ½–1 cup coconut milk
>
> 2 tablespoons tamari, 5 tablespoons sesame oil, and 2 tablespoons ginger (chopped fine or garlic pressed)

> *You will need:*
> **Preheated 375°F. oven**
> **8–10 ounces fish (serves 2, or 1 with leftovers for another meal)**
> **Any of the above marinades; or ½ cup of bottled fat-free salad dressing with 2 tablespoons of extra-virgin olive oil added**

How to do it:

Lay the fish out so it's flat in a 10 × 10-inch baking dish. If you're cooking more than one piece, make sure that they don't overlap. You may need to use a large roasting pan if you are making extra for later meals.

Pour the marinade over the fish and let sit about 10 minutes.

Place in the preheated (375°F.) oven and roast until fish is done (when it is still moist but flakes easily when pulled away with a fork), about 15 minutes for hearty, thick fish and 10 minutes for the thinner fillets, such as sole and trout.

Dredging and Pan Searing Fish for a Crisp Texture

You will need:
Preheated 375°F. oven
½ cup rice flour (or wheat flour,
   if you tolerate it)
2 tablespoons herb blend (choose one):
   Italian seasonings
   Curry powder
   Mexican seasonings
   Lemon-pepper blend
   Mediterranean blend
   Thai seasonings
Salt and pepper
8–10 ounces fish (serves 2, or 1 with leftovers for another
   meal)
2 eggs, beaten (or a little milk or water) and placed in a
   shallow dish
2 tablespoons olive oil, ghee, or coconut oil

How to do it:
In a shallow bowl big enough to lay the fish out flat, mix flour and dry herb mixture together, and season with a little salt and pepper.

Dip the fish in the egg to moisten. (Or you can use a little water or milk to moisten the fish so flour will adhere, if you'd rather not use egg.) Then dredge the fish pieces in the corn or rice flour coating. Set aside on a plate.

In your skillet or sauté pan, preheat oil for about 1 minute, then place the fish in it. Let it crisp on both sides (about 2–4 minutes on each side).

If you are cooking sole or a similar thin fish or fillet, it will cook through on the stovetop (about 4 minutes on each side).

If you are cooking hearty, thick fish, place the pan (with the fish still in it) in the preheated 375°F. oven and cook until done (about 10–15 minutes).

Stuffing Sole or Trout Fillets with Sautéed Spinach and Lemon Butter

You will need:
Preheated 375°F. oven
1 tablespoon olive oil
4 cups cleaned and chopped fresh spinach
1 teaspoon minced garlic (optional)
Two 4-ounce pieces fillet of sole or trout
Salt and pepper, for seasoning
1–2 tablespoons butter
4 long toothpicks (2 for each fillet)
Lemon wedges or juice

How to do it:

Heat 1 tablespoon of olive oil in a skillet or sauté pan. Add the spinach and toss until it's wilted. (If using garlic, add and let it open up in the pan until it's light golden.) Season with salt and pepper, and remove from the heat. Cool a few minutes until you can comfortably touch the spinach.

Lay the fillets out flat. Salt and pepper to taste. Place half the spinach at the top of each fillet. Roll up each fillet and place 2 pats of butter on each. Secure with toothpicks, sticking them through the butter pats.

Put the rolls in the sauté pan and place in the oven for about 8 minutes until done (when the fish is still moist but flakes easily when pulled away with a fork).

Squeeze lemon juice on fish and serve.

Cooking Poultry

Roasting Poultry

You will need:

Preheated 350°F. oven

1 whole chicken, 2 Cornish hens, 4 chicken breasts,
6 chicken thighs, or 1 turkey breast to serve 2–3

Salt and pepper

Seasoning mixture (choose from the following):

1 tablespoon fresh or 1 teaspoon dry each of
rosemary and sage

1 tablespoon each of thyme and lemon zest

½ cup yogurt mixed with 1 tablespoon lemon zest or
1 tablespoon curry powder or any combination of
herbs we've mentioned in other recipes

Homemade or store-bought pesto, either with dairy
or dairy-free

Fresh lemons for stuffing in the cavity of whole birds
along with 1 tablespoon fresh or 1 teaspoon
dry herbs

How to do it:

Take whatever poultry you have chosen, salt and pepper to taste, and coat with dry herbs or with wet mixture and place in a roasting pan. If using a whole bird, rub a little herb mixture inside the cavity and add halved lemons, if desired. Place poultry in the refrigerator for 1 hour to overnight.

Take the marinated poultry from the fridge and roast it in the oven until golden brown and the juices run clear. For whole birds, when you jiggle the leg it should come away easily and juices should run clear. About 35–45 minutes for cut pieces and for game hens. Larger whole birds should be cooked by weight—20 minutes per pound or to 170°F. on a meat thermometer.

CRISPY CHICKEN TENDERS

½ cup whole-grain or gluten-free bread crumbs (see
  gluten-free food sources in the "Resource Tool Kit")
½ teaspoon granulated garlic or garlic powder
¼ teaspoon celery salt
Pepper to taste
1 pound chicken breast strips
Melted butter

Mix bread crumbs with garlic, celery salt, and pepper.

Coat each strip with melted butter, then with seasoned crumbs.

Put on lightly oiled cookie sheet or in large roasting pan and bake at 325°F. for 10–12 minutes or until lightly browned and done through.

Serves 2: ¼ pound per person, plus planned leftovers.

Cooking Pork, Beef, and Lamb

Pork Loin, Rack of Lamb, or Leg of Lamb with Bone

You will need:
Preheated 375°–380°F. oven
1 cup basil leaves
1 tablespoon rosemary
3 cloves garlic
Approx. ¼ cup olive oil (drizzle in until it forms a paste)
Pork loin, rack of lamb, or leg of lamb with bone in

How to do it:

Puree the basil, rosemary, garlic, and olive oil together until it forms a loose paste.

Coat the meat and roast in a roasting pan for 15–20 minutes per pound, until done.

Pork or Lamb Chops or Beefsteak

> *You will need:*
> **Preheated 375°–380°F. oven**
> **2 pork chops or 2–4 lamb chops or 1–2 beefsteaks (serves**
>   **2, or 1 with leftovers for another meal)**
> **Salt and pepper**
> **1 tablespoon olive oil**

How to do it:

Season the chops or steak with salt and pepper. Heat 1 tablespoon oil in a large skillet or sauté pan. Place meat in hot oil and sear until light brown on one side. Turn and sear the other side. Finish cooking in the oven until done the way you like, following these guidelines:

Pork chops—A minimum of 10 minutes for each inch of thickness.

Lamb chops—5 minutes for rare, 8 minutes for medium-rare, 10 minutes for medium, and 15–20 minutes for well done.

Beefsteak (1 inch thick)—No oven time for rare, 5–7minutes for medium, 7–10 minutes for medium-well, and 10–15 minutes for well done. Increase the time approximately 5 minutes for each additional inch of thickness.

THAI COCONUT MILK SOUP

Coconut milk is delicious and great for you. The curry in this soup makes it even more delicious, and it's easier than you'd think. This one-dish meal will make about 3 quarts—enough for 6 servings. It keeps well in the fridge or can be frozen and reheated at another time for succulent leftovers.

> *You will need:*
> **3 tablespoons ghee or olive or coconut oil**
> **1 tablespoon chopped garlic**
> **3–4 tablespoons curry powder (according to your taste,**
>   **as these vary in heat)**
> **1 cup chopped onion (½ very large onion)**
> **2 tablespoons chopped fresh ginger**
> **6 cups of a variety from the following:**

Broccoli florets

Carrots, cut in ½-inch slices

Celery, cut in 1-inch slices

Cabbage, cut in approx. 2-inch chunks

Green beans, cut in 2-inch pieces

Potatoes, cubed with skin (include up to 2 cups, but only if this soup is a complete meal with no other high-carb foods)

Greens, chopped or snipped with scissors, if large (add in last 10 minutes)

Pea pods or snow peas (add in last 10 minutes)

Green onions, tops and all, cut in 1-inch pieces (add in last 10 minutes)

About 1½ pounds protein. Examples of different proteins you can add to this soup:

Fish, cubed

Shrimp (add frozen, works fine)

Scallops, cut into bite-size pieces, if large (add frozen, works fine)

Turkey, cubed

Chicken, cubed

Pork loin, cubed

5 cans coconut milk, *full-fat* and with no preservatives (substitute chicken or vegetable broth for some of the coconut milk, if you'd like)

¼ cup fresh basil, minced, or 1 tablespoon dried

In a large pot, heat the ghee or oil. Add the garlic, curry powder, onions, and ginger. Sauté about 5 minutes, then add the veggies (except greens, pea pods, and green onions), and the protein choice. Stir until coated with the spice mixture.

Sauté another couple minutes, then add the coconut milk. Stir until all the flavors are incorporated, then let simmer until the protein is cooked through (about 20 minutes for thawed seafood, 30 minutes for meat, poultry, and frozen seafood), stirring now and then. During the last 10 minutes, add greens, pea pods, and green onions, if you are using them.

When it's all cooked, add the basil and let it open up a few minutes. It's ready to serve.

Salads and Dressings

Select-a-Salad

Salads are a great way to enjoy all your food groups and get the nutrients you need. They're also easy to make, lovely to look at, and delicious when made fresh. Use the following chart, which was developed for *The Diet Cure*, for hundreds of salad variations.

For a complete meal salad: Select items from lists 1, 2, 3, 4, and 5 and combine for a salad that is a satisfying meal.

For a side salad: For a salad to go along with a protein entrée, select from lists 1, 2, 5, and, if there's no other starchy carb in the meal, 3.

1. 2 cups or more from this list	2. 1 cup or more from this list	3. Total of ½ cup from this list	4. ¾ cup or more from this list	5. 2 tablespoons from this this list
· green- or red-leaf lettuce	· raw broccoli or cauliflower	· green peas	· roast beef, chicken, or turkey	· vinaigrette
· spinach leaves	· steamed broccoli, asparagus, green beans, or cauliflower	· black-eyed peas, lima, kidney, chick peas, cannellini, black, or pinto beans	· ¼ cup nuts and/or seeds	· Creamy Lemon Salad Dressing (see recipe on page 186)
· romaine lettuce			· cottage cheese	
· arugula				
· mesclun	· tomatoes	· rice or other cooked grains	· ¼ cup feta cheese	· other salad dressing with good oils and no sugar
· other mixed greens	· cucumber		· ½ cup beans or peas	
· cabbage	· bell peppers	· cooked potatoes or sweet potatoes		
or omit this list and use 1 more cup from list 2	· avocado			
	· carrot, sliced or grated			

CHUNKY SHRIMP AND FETA SALAD

2 tomatoes
4 stalks celery
½ red onion
1 cucumber
2 carrots
4 ounces crumbled feta cheese
12 ounces cooked salad shrimp

Cut all vegetables into large (½-inch to ¾-inch) chunks. Mix with feta and shrimp. Use your favorite dressing.

Makes 4 servings.

TUNA AND BEAN SALAD

1 (14.5-ounce) can chick peas, drained and rinsed
½ medium red onion, thinly sliced
Salt to taste
1 (6-ounce) can tuna
4 tablespoons extra-virgin olive oil
2 tablespoons red wine vinegar, or balsamic vinegar
Cracked pepper to taste
¼ cup chopped fresh parsley

Place the beans and onion in a serving bowl, sprinkle with salt, and toss. Drain tuna, break into large chunks, and add to serving bowl. Coat well with oil. Add vinegar, pepper, and chopped parsley. Toss thoroughly. Adjust seasoning to taste. Serve on a bed of salad greens, sliced avocado, and sliced tomato.

Makes 2–3 servings.

PERFECT BLENDER MAYONNAISE

1 large egg
1 tablespoon vinegar
½ teaspoon salt

¼ teaspoon dry mustard
½ cup extra-virgin olive oil, plus ½ cup more
1 tablespoon lemon juice

Combine in a blender the egg, vinegar, salt, and dry mustard; cover and blend about 5 seconds. With blender running *on the slowest speed*, add ½ cup olive oil in the thinnest stream you can, still making a stream. For best results, the stream of oil should hit the combination in the container halfway between the side of the container and the vortex in the middle.

Add lemon juice; running the blender on the slowest speed, gradually add ½ cup more olive oil. If the oil quits moving into the vortex, stop the blender and break the surface tension of the mayonnaise, using a spatula to scrape the sides (sometimes just turning the blender off and on again will do this). Store for up to 4 weeks in a tightly covered jar in the refrigerator.
Makes about 1¼ cups.

CREAMY LEMON SALAD DRESSING

½ cup olive oil
¼ cup lemon juice
3 tablespoons nutritional yeast
1 teaspoon salt
1 teaspoon mustard

Shake until blended in glass jar or whisk in bowl.
Makes about 1 cup.

BALSAMIC SALAD DRESSING

¼ cup balsamic vinegar
¾ cup extra-virgin olive oil
1 teaspoon salt
1 tablespoon mustard
1 teaspoon minced garlic

Whisk in bowl or shake in jar.
Makes about 1 cup.

RANCH OR BLUE CHEESE SALAD DRESSING

½ cup Perfect Blender Mayonnaise
¼ cup lemon juice
¼ cup buttermilk
2 teaspoons salt
I teaspoon pepper
I teaspoon chopped garlic
I tablespoon minced green onion
¼ cup water to thin
I teaspoon garlic salt
I teaspoon onion powder

Blend or whisk all ingredients until well mixed.
Makes about 1 cup of dressing or dip. Optional: *Add ¼ cup crumbled blue cheese to make Blue Cheese Salad Dressing.*

DILL TAHINI SALAD DRESSING

¼ cup sesame tahini
¼ cup lemon juice
I cup yogurt
I teaspoon garlic (pressed or chopped)
I teaspoon dill
I teaspoon salt
I teaspoon pepper
½ cup water

Blend or whisk all ingredients until well mixed.
Makes about 2 cups of non-dairy salad dressing or dip.

Vegetables

Roasting Vegetables

Roasting vegetables and potatoes is so easy. It requires only a little prep and some oven time.

Types of veggies you can roast:

Turnips

Carrots

Asparagus (need only 15 minutes of roasting)

Green beans (need only 15 minutes of roasting)

Courgette or summer squash (need only 15 minutes of roasting)

Sweet potatoes

Potatoes—all types

Kohlrabi

Onions

Swede

Brussels sprouts

Cabbage (cut in 2-inch cubes)

Broccoli

Fennel (especially good with balsamic vinegar and olive oil)

Aubergine (Japanese in halves or quarters or large in cubes)

Bell pepper strips

These are only examples—you can roast most veggies, except greens, which are better sautéed.

You will need:

Preheated 350°F. oven

2 tablespoons olive oil per every 2 cups of vegetables

1 tablespoon chopped garlic

1 tablespoon chopped savory herbs such as rosemary or thyme

How to do it:

Cut your veggies into 1- or 2-inch pieces, or, for broccoli and cauliflower, separate into florets. Place in a big bowl and toss with olive oil.

Lay out a single layer on the roasting/baking pan and cook in oven until almost done (15–30 minutes).

Remove the vegetables and put them back into the bowl. Add the garlic and herbs, toss around with a wooden spoon, then put them back on the baking pan and return to the oven for about 3–5 minutes, until the garlic and herbs open up. The reason for waiting until the end to add them is that the flavors will open on the veggies without burning the garlic and herbs. (You can save this last step if you'd prefer the veggies without garlic and herbs. In that case, just salt them before or after roasting.)

Sautéed Greens

Here are some of the many types of tasty greens—they're easy and quick to cook:

Kale
Swiss chard
Spinach
Arugula
Curly endive
Mustard or turnip greens

You will need:
1 tablespoon olive oil or ghee for each 4 cups of chopped
    greens
Your choice of seasoning for greens—per each 4 cups
    raw, chopped greens:
    1 tablespoon chopped garlic and pinch chili flakes
      (add late in cooking)
    1 tablespoon chopped onion and bits of bell pepper
    Juice of ½ lemon and salt (add late in cooking)
    Salt and pepper (add late in cooking)
    1 tablespoon chopped ginger and a squeeze of lime
      juice (add late in cooking)
    A dash of cumin and a small dash cayenne pepper,
      then more to taste

How to do it:
Chop the greens you've chosen with a knife, or snip them with kitchen scissors. Heat olive oil or ghee in a large sauté pan or skillet (add onion and pepper, if using), then sauté the greens quickly, and just when they wilt, add the seasonings. Allow the heat to open up the flavors a little (for 1–2 minutes), then turn off the heat. Tougher greens, like some kale, turnip, and mustard, can be steamed until tender by adding a little liquid (2 tablespoons water or broth) and cooking covered till tender.

ONE-STEP RATATOUILLE

This tastes even better when it is made ahead and reheated, and it even tastes good served at room temperature. Vary the vegetables according to what you like and what's available.

> 1 medium aubergine, cubed
> 6 small courgette and/or crookneck squash, cut in
>   ½-inch slices
> 1 large red or yellow onion, sliced
> 4 cloves garlic, minced
> 6 plum tomatoes, cut in quarters
> 1 medium red bell pepper, seeded and cut in 1-inch
>   squares
> ½ teaspoon oregano or marjoram and ¼ teaspoon
>   thyme (optional), or 1 teaspoon Italian herb blend
> 1–1½ teaspoons salt, to taste
> ½ cup extra-virgin olive oil

Place all ingredients except olive oil in a 3-quart ovenproof pot or casserole dish. Drizzle olive oil over all and mix. Bake uncovered for 1½ hours in a 325°F. oven. The vegetables will cook down considerably.

Makes 6–8 servings.

Cooking Whole Grains Simply

There are many interesting kinds of grains. Cooking them is pretty simple; there are instructions on the packages, if you buy them in the grocery store. However, if you buy them in bulk, here are the basics.

Grain	Liquid Needed per Each Cup of Grain	Approximate Cooking Time
Basmati rice	2¼ cups water or stock	30 minutes
Brown basmati	2¼ cups water or stock	40 minutes
Wild rice	2 cups water or stock	1 hour
Black rice	2 cups water or stock	45 minutes
Buckwheat groats	2 cups water or stock	45 minutes
Amaranth	3 cups water or stock	25 minutes

You will need:
Water, or vegetable or chicken stock
Measuring cup
Pinch of salt, or if you want more flavor:
For each cup of uncooked grain, add 2 tablespoons of any
of the following to the water:
Italian seasoning
Curry powder
Mexican seasoning
Lemon-pepper blend
Thai seasonings
Or add
2 chopped cloves of garlic and chili flakes to taste
2 tablespoons chopped onion and 2 tablespoons bell
pepper
1 tablespoon chopped zest of lemon

How to do it:
Bring your measured water and herbs to a boil. Add the grain, cover,
turn down to a simmer, and cook until done.

RECOMMENDED COOKBOOKS

Ross, Julia. *The Diet Cure* (New York: Penguin, 2000).

Audette, Ray, Troy Gilchrist and Raymond V. Audette. *Neanderthin: Eat Like a Caveman to Achieve a Lean, Strong, Healthy Body* (New York: St. Martin's, 2000).

Doyen, Barbara. *Back to Protein* (New York: M. Evans, 2000).

Hagman, Bette. *More from the Gluten-Free Gourmet: Delicious Dining Without Wheat* (New York: Henry Holt/Owl, rev. ed. 2000). This is a more complete cookbook than *The Gluten-Free Gourmet,* since it contains vegetable and meat recipes.

Okamoto, Sam. *Incredible Vegetables* (Gretna, La.: Pelican, 1994).

Katzen, Mollie. *New Moosewood Cookbook* (Berkeley, Calif.: Ten Speed Press, 2000).

Katzen, Mollie. *Vegetable Heaven* (New York: Hyperion, 2000).

Also see the recommended reading list for chapter 8.

CHAPTER 10

Your Master
Supplement Plan

Putting Your Mood Repair Program Together

Your master plan is almost complete. Now that you have your good-mood food guide and recipes in hand, it's time to assemble the final component: your master supplement plan. This will be laid out in two parts. *First,* I'll describe and list the basic supplements that I recommend for everyone, long-term, regardless of which particular mood repair needs they have. *Second,* I'll list *all* the special repair supplements recommended in the book, so that, once you've scanned the "Caution Box" for any contraindications, you can check off just the supplements best suited to your particular mood repair needs.

Your basic supplement list will include suggested supplement amounts and the best times to take them. The special repair supplements will be listed by name as they appear in the book, chapter by chapter, but the dose and time schedule will be left blank. That way you can fill in the specific amounts and times that seem most appropriate *for you.* Before you fill it in, though, make copies of this master supplement list (pages 202–205) so that you can change it as time goes on.

The combined master supplement list will be followed by some important general information and guidelines for you to use in taking and gradually eliminating your special repair supplements.

The supplements I recommended are usually elements that occur naturally in foods and are generally recognized as safe. They're supplements that you'll be able to find easily in health food stores, through mail-order sources, and in some drugstores. I have suggested less accessible supplements only when I knew of no other supplement that worked as well for the particular purpose. This doesn't mean that good options don't exist, merely that at our clinic we have not yet discovered them. *Any* of the exact supplements we use for our clients can be ordered from our clinic's supplement order line or from other mail-order sources that I list in the "Resource Tool Kit" on page 289, if you have trouble finding local sources.

YOUR BASIC SUPPLEMENTS

I have been alluding to the basic supplement plan throughout the book because it really is the basis for your Mood Cure, along with the good-mood foods. The nutrients included in this basic supplement plan are intended to restore any depletions that have eroded your mood and to keep your nutrient levels and mood permanently strong.

One of our nutritional consultants has been doing very detailed diet analyses for years. She has never found any diet, including the *best* diets of superathletes, that contains 100 percent of the essential nutrients at even the most minimal, outdated, RDA (Recommended Daily Allowance) levels. There are just too many obstacles—among them heat, light, age, processing, and inadequate soil—blocking you from obtaining enough nutrients from food itself.

For many years, the RDA was the standard for how many nutrients we needed to prevent severe deficiency problems like scurvy. More recently, the U.S. government has developed the DRI (Dietary Reference Intake) to help us more adequately support optimal nutrition, not just prevent deficiency. But the higher DRI levels are still very low for many, perhaps most of us. That's partly because they're based on the assumption that we're eating fairly well, which we aren't; and even if we were, the needs for nutrients can vary tremendously from person to person. Genetics, stress, illness, and exercise are just a few of the things that can cause us to need extra nutrients, even if we are eating well and often.[1]

The following basic collection of vital nutrients is intended to be safe enough to take permanently, yet potent enough, in combination with your good-mood foods, to prevent your relapsing into false moods after you stop taking your aminos and other special repair supplements.

Are Supplements Safe?

The U.S. deaths due to prescription and over-the-counter medications: 106,000 per year (290 deaths per day), according to a study published in the *Journal of the American Medical Association* in April 1998.[2]

Deaths due to nonherbal supplements: one in 1995–1996, according to the most recent report by the American Association of Poison Control Centers (and even that one death is still being hotly contested).

Poison control and the FDA lump amino acids, vitamins, minerals, and herbs under the one term *supplements*. In fact, the herb ephedra, which has been used for weight loss and has been very much in the news, has caused fatalities but will certainly not be part of your program!

In the "Caution Box" on pages 199–200, you'll find information to help you avoid any adverse reactions to supplements. Be sure to read the labels on any supplements you buy, to note any similar cautions.

Your Basic Multivitamin

A good-quality multivitamin is the crown jewel of your basic supplement program. In numerous studies, vitamin and mineral deficiencies have been associated with mood and depressive disorders,[3] and taking vitamins and minerals has proved to correct these same disorders.[4] People who take multivitamins tend not only to be healthier, they tend to be happier. Look at the results of just two of many studies on multis like the one you'll be taking (for the rest of your life, I hope).

➤ In the first study, over a hundred healthy young men were tested for vitamin deficiency. Even mild vitamin deficiencies were clearly correlated with a decreased sense of well-being and increased irritability, fear, nervousness, and depression. The group that was given a moderate-potency multivitamin supplement for eight weeks became less nervous and depressed, had greater self-confidence and concentration, were more active and social, and had a "markedly improved mood."[5]

➤ In a second study of nine hundred people over ten years, those who took a multi daily lowered their risk of colon cancer by half.[6]

True Balance Multiple by NOW Foods is our clinic's favorite multiple, because it is unusually high in both B vitamins and the mineral chromium. For blood sugar stability, coping with stress, and brain function, these are key nutrients. When we have been unable to get this multi and our clients have had to purchase other multis instead, they have really noticed the difference. Health food stores and supplement mail-order houses can get it for you if they don't actually carry it in stock. In case you need an alternative to True Balance, I will also recommend two other easily found multis that our nutritionists have determined to be high in quality—My Favorite Multiple Original Formula by Natrol and Allergy Multi by TwinLabs.*

Unfortunately, it is impossible to get enough of the nutrients you need without taking 4 to 6 multis per day, and even the best multivitamins will still be lacking in some key ingredients. That is why I recommend taking the following supplements *in addition to* your multivitamin.

Your Basic Magnesium, Calcium, and Vitamin D

The minerals calcium and magnesium, along with vitamin D, are inseparable mates (or should be). But their levels are suboptimal in all sex and age groups, except adolescent males.[7] They can not only reverse osteoporosis, they can sometimes improve sleep and stabilize mood all by themselves.[8,9,10,11] Unfortunately, even very good multis, such as the three I've suggested here, never contain enough of these three nutrients. Recommendations for *calcium*—best known for its bone-building importance but intimately involved in many crucial functions, including brain neurotransmitter function—have risen from 800 milligrams daily to 1,300 milligrams (and as high as 1,500 milligrams when osteoporosis is present).

Many people need as much *magnesium* as calcium, or even more, though most supplements provide only half as much. Magnesium protects us from many conditions associated with insomnia, depression, stress, anxiety, and anger, as well as heart attack, Alzheimer's disease, constipation, low blood sugar, diabetes, chronic fatigue, low thyroid, PMS, and osteoporosis.[12,13]

Vitamin D is actually a hormone that regulates the adrenals, the thyroid, and calcium, among other things. We recently learned that our need

---

*Both these multis have higher calcium and lower magnesium. If you tend to be constipated, or develop constipation, take extra magnesium.

for D is *much* higher than we had thought, with recommendations varying from 400 IU (international units) to at least 2,000 IU.[14] (The successful U.K. prison study included 800 IU of vitamin D per day.) Raising levels can result in a "sunny" mood, increased energy and bone health, and decreased feelings of stress, especially in those suffering from depression, SAD, and PMS. The trouble is that excessive levels of vitamin D can be toxic, so do not exceed 400 IU daily *without testing for your levels first.* Good blood tests for vitamin D are listed in the "Resource Tool Kit," page 289. Particularly if your levels are below 35, take 2000 to 4000 IU extra. (Be sure to retest in three to six months.)

Calcium, magnesium, and vitamin D are listed right underneath your multi on your basic supplement plan. Take them together with dinner. Alter your levels as needed for your unique biochemical needs—for instance, too much magnesium can cause loose bowels, while too much calcium can lead to constipation (or depression in rare cases).

Basic Vitamin B Complex

B vitamins are some of the most important factors in mental health. Low levels of folic acid, B_{12}, thiamin, riboflavin, and B_6 have all been associated with mood disorders, and supplements of all these nutrients have been used successfully to correct them.[15,16,17,18,19] The brain requires lots of the B vitamins for repair and permanent maintenance of proper brain neurotransmitter and adrenal function. Stress causes the B vitamins to be quickly depleted. The vitamin B content of your multi probably won't be high enough to do the job without extra B complex, at least for your first few months, if stress has been a significant fact of your life.

We like the coenzymate form of the vitamin B complex, which is rapidly and efficiently utilized by your body and won't upset your stomach. If this form is not available, just use an ordinary low-potency B complex with no more than 10 to 25 milligrams of each B vitamin. (Higher B complex can have side effects, such as nausea and insomnia, *especially when not taken with food.*) After your first three months, take this extra B complex only as needed during high-stress periods.

Basic Vitamin C and Bioflavonoids

In nature, vitamin C, minerals, and bioflavonoids are always combined; they work best together as antioxidants to help prevent stress burnout, cancer, heart disease, and asthma, among other things. Our nutritionists generally recommend 2,000 to 3,000 milligrams per day—what you'd get if you added two 1,000-milligram doses to the vitamin C in your multi. Make sure the bioflavonoids total 300 milligrams or more per 1,000 milligrams of C.[20,21] NOW Foods' Ascorbate Mineral C is a good example of the complete "C complex."

Basic Vitamin E

This extraordinary antioxidant can cut your risk of stroke and cataracts by 40 percent! All of us need vitamin E to help protect our entire brain and body from the serious dangers of free radicals caused by rancid (oxidized) fats. Vegetable oils (except olive oil) and trans fats in margarine and shortening are particular problems and have had their natural vitamin E content removed or destroyed during their processing. Stress reduces our vitamin E reserves, making supplementation vital for most of us.[22]

Basic Fish Oil

These are the super omega-3 fats that enhance and protect your brain, your arteries, and your digestive lining. Look for 300 to 600 milligrams of combined DHA/EPA in a single gel capsule. (Add up the total in *1 capsule* of just the DHA and EPA noted on the back of the bottle; don't judge by how much general fish oil is claimed on the front of the bottle.) Avoid supplements that combine fish oil with any other oils. These combinations actually reduce the ability of the omega-3s to do their job. A study of manic-depressives found that 9,600 milligrams per day of DHA/EPA was remarkably effective as an antidepressant, but we've found that 1,800 to 3,600 per day is enough for most of our clients. (If you go over your own ideal dose, you may get too energized and even have trouble sleeping.)

Safety and Effectiveness of Flax Oil and Algae Oil

Up to 80 percent of Americans cannot convert flax oil to DHA/EPA,[23] and there is reason to fear its association, confirmed by several studies, with prostate cancer (while fish oil is associated with lowered incidences of this cancer).[24] Flax is great for skin and hair for everyone, and up to one-third of us can effectively convert it to DHA/EPA. Algae oil (e.g. by Nature's Way) contains DHA and can be used with or without flax oil. (See page 199.)

Fish Oil, Blood Coagulation, and Vitamin K

Fish oil supplements, like any added fats, increase your need for vitamin K, which keeps your blood from getting too thin. Consult your medical practitioner about whether to take fish oil, if you're taking any blood thinners, even aspirin or ibuprofen, on a regular basis (note that vitamin E thins blood, too). If you take more than 1,800 milligrams of DHA/EPA a day, you'll need to take 1 milligram (1,000 micrograms) of vitamin K to counteract blood-thinning effects. Vitamin K is found in its most concentrated form only in leafy greens and seaweed. The astronauts use it in space, where, without gravity, their bones otherwise become too thin. It also helps prevent plaque buildup in the arteries. Take 10 tablets (100 micrograms each) daily. (And eat your dark green leafies!)

Note for People with Blood Type A

You are typically deficient in hydrochloric acid, which diminishes your ability to absorb minerals and protein (and to burn up hostile invaders like germs and parasites). Taking 1 to 8 capsules of HCl (600–700 milligrams) along with your multi with meals can help. Start with one and go up until you feel a mild acidic burning, then go down one capsule lower.

Suggestions for Vegetarians and Vegans

If you eat no animal products, neither fish, chicken, milk products, nor eggs, your multi won't give you all the extra nutrients you need. Check your multi's contents against the following suggested amounts of key nutrients, and get any additional supplements you'll need to reach the following levels:

Vitamin B_{12}	100–400 mcg daily
Vitamin D	800 IU daily (more should be avoided unless you test your levels first)
L-carnitine	500 mg daily
Zinc	25–50 mg daily (upper limit of safety is 100 mg, except during illness)
Selenium	100–200 mcg daily (upper limit of safety is 400 mcg)

continued

Iron	27 mg daily; NOW Iron Complex (with Ferrochel) in nongelatin tabs is the only vegan nonsweetened source I know of
Omega-3 fatty acids	Algae Oil by Nature's Way or Martek Biosciences at 410-740-0081, but be aware that they use gelatin caps; you can purchase them and squirt the oil out, if you don't want to swallow these caps
HCl	These come in tablets or gel caps by Freeda for A blood types (and for all to use on exotic travels to protect from parasites)

Caution Box: When Amino Acids and Other Nutrients Should <u>Not</u> Be Taken

Important: Read this information about contraindications to amino acids and other supplements before you decide which nutrients to try.

➤ You should consult a physician before taking any amino acids, if you have a serious physical illness, including high or low blood pressure, lupus, migraine, liver impairment, severe kidney damage, an inborn error of amino acid metabolism, an overactive thyroid, or ulcers; are pregnant, nursing, taking methadone, or taking any medications, especially antidepressants or MAO inhibitors; or have severe mental or emotional problems, such as schizophrenia or bipolar disorder.

➤ If you are taking a selective serotonin reuptake inhibitor such as Prozac (or any other mood-altering medication), you should consult with your doctor before taking 5-HTP, L-tryptophan, Saint-John's wort, or SAM-e.

➤ If you are taking an MAO inhibitor (including phentermine) for depression, you should ask your doctor if it would be appropriate for you to take 5-HTP, L-tryptophan, L-tyrosine, D-phenylalanine or L-phenylalanine (*probably only after discontinuing* your MAO inhibitors).

continued

➤ If you have manic-depression (bipolar disorder), do not use L-glutamine, L-tyrosine, SAM-e, or Saint-John's wort, high doses of fish or flax oil, or chromium without consulting with a psychiatrist or psychopharmacologist. All can trigger mania in some people. Even with an expert's okay, watch your reactions very carefully. Even 5-HTP and tryptophan might cause problems at higher doses.

➤ If you have Hashimoto's thyroiditis, you might have an adverse (jittery, headachy) reaction to L-tyrosine, L-phenylalanine, or DL-phenylalanine. If so, stop using those aminos.

➤ If you have active *hyper*thyroidism, you should *not* use L-tyrosine, L-phenylalanine, or DL-phenylalanine without medical advice.

➤ If you have PKU (phenylketonuria), do not use DL-phenylalanine, or L-phenylalanine.

➤ If you get migraine headaches, they may be triggered by L-tyrosine, DL-phenylalanine, or L-phenylalanine.

➤ If you have melanoma, do not use L-tyrosine or D- or L-phenylalanine.

➤ If you have low blood pressure, avoid GABA, taurine, or niacin, or use cautiously at low doses.

➤ If you have high blood pressure, ask your doctor about using low or moderate (500–1,000 milligrams) L-tyrosine, DL-phenylalanine, or L-phenylalanine. (These amino acids can raise blood pressure at higher doses in some people and lower it in others.) Also avoid licorice if your blood pressure is high.

BUYING YOUR SUPPLEMENTS

Most of your supplements can be found in ordinary health food stores and drugstores. Show a store assistant your master schedule. There are a few supplements that you'll need to order by phone or on the internet. See the "Resource Tool Kit" for a list of good sources for these supplements, including our own clinic's order line (800-733-9293).

Choosing Amino Acid Supplements

They can be produced in two forms. Most amino acids come in the L-form, identical to the amino acids found in food and, in fact, extracted from yeasts. There is also a D-form that is the mirror image of the L-form. It is not typically found in food but is produced in a lab and has very limited uses. Your supplement bottles will all specify which form of the aminos are being supplied. For example, tyrosine will be called L-tyrosine, and glutamine will be called L-glutamine. The only D-form recommended in this book is D-phenylalanine (which also constitutes half of the supplement DLPA). All of the manufacturers of these freeform, instantly absorbed aminos, made from fermented yeasts, provide equally high quality products. Carlson makes individual aminos as powders, without capsules, for vegans and those who need high potency or easy swallowing.

YOUR MASTER SUPPLEMENT SCHEDULE

Please make several copies of the master supplement schedule on pages 202–205 or write in pencil, so that you can revise your plan over time, as you change doses, start dropping supplements that you no longer need, or start trying new ones. In the master list, the supplements will appear in the order that they appear in the book, by chapter. Transfer onto the master list the special repair supplement and dose recommendations from the Action Steps at the end of the chapters that pertain to you: For "Lifting the Dark Cloud," see pages 50–52. For "Blasting the Blahs," see page 75. For "All Stressed Out," see pages 97–98. For "Too Sensitive to Life's Pain," see pages 116–117. For special sleep and addiction repair projects, see pages 248–249 and 283–285. (Also transfer recommendations from the adrenal, thyroid, and sex hormone tool kits that you and your practitioner feel apply to you.)

Supplements that are recommended for more than one mood problem will not appear a second time on the master list. Just insert your dosing recommendations into the place on the list where the appropriate supplement first occurs.

The Basic Supplements

Supplement	AM	B	MM	L	MA	D	BT*
☐ Multivitamin/mineral	—	2	—	—	—	2	—
☐ Calcium 250–500 mg	—	—	—	—	—	1–2	—
☐ Magnesium 200–400 mg	—	1	—	—	—	1	—
☐ Vitamin D 400 IU† (more if testing indicates a need)	—	1	—	—	—	—	—
☐ B complex 10–25 mg‡	—	1	—	—	—	1	—
☐ Vitamin C with bio-flavonoids (1,000 mg C and 300–500 mg bioflavonoids)	—	1	—	—	—	1	—
☐ Fish oil (300 mg combined DHA/EPA, 1,200–2,400/day)	—	2–3	—	2–3	—	—	—

*AM=on arising; B=with breakfast; MM=midmorning; L=with lunch; MA=midafternoon; D=with dinner; BT=at bedtime.

†Once you've tested your vitamin D levels, if you need doses up to 4,000 IU (quite common), get 1,000 IU vitamin D from *fish oil* source. See the "Resource Tool Kit," page 289, for testing and supplement sources.

‡Source Naturals or Country Life coenzymate brands are recommended.

The Special Repair Supplements

Supplement	AM	B	MM	L	MA	D	BT*

Lifting the Dark Cloud

❏ 5-HTP 50 mg (not 100 mg) — — — — — — —

❏ L-tryptophan 500 mg — — — — — — —

❏ Saint-John's wort 300 mg — — — — — — —

❏ SAM-e 400 mg — — — — — — —

Blasting the Blahs

❏ L-tyrosine 500 mg — — — — — — —

❏ L-phenylalanine 500 mg — — — — — — —

❏ A combination of — — — — — — —
L-tyrosine and
L-phenylalanine¥

❏ Extra† omega-3 fish oil — — — — — — —
(300 mg combined
DHA/EPA)

❏ Vitamin K 100 mcg — — — — — — —

❏ Grape seed extract 60 mg — — — — — — —

❏ Thyroid glandulars — — — — — — —

❏ Homeopathic thyroid,
as directed — — — — — — —

Easing the Stress

❏ Combination of GABA — — — — — — —
100–200 mg with taurine
and glycine‡

---

*AM=on arising; B=with breakfast; MM=midmorning; L=with lunch; MA=midafternoon; D=with dinner; BT=at bedtime.
¥True Focus by NOW Foods
†"Extra" means on top of the amounts of these nutrients that you get in your basic supplements.
‡GABAcalm by Source Naturals, True Calm by NOW.   *continued*

Supplement	AM	B	MM	L	MA	D	BT*
❑ GABA 500 mg	___	___	___	___	___	___	___
❑ *Calmes Forte*	___	___	___	___	___	___	___
❑ Inosital powder	___	___	___	___	___	___	___
❑ L-glutamine 500 mg	___	___	___	___	___	___	___
❑ Chromium 200 mcg	___	___	___	___	___	___	___

Too Sensitive to Life's Pain

Supplement	AM	B	MM	L	MA	D	BT*
❑ DLPA 500 mg (250 mg D-, 250 mg L-), or DPA 500 mg	___	___	___	___	___	___	___
❑ Freeform amino acid blend 700–800 mg	___	___	___	___	___	___	___
❑ Comfort Zone	___	___	___	___	___	___	___

Sleep Repair

Supplement	AM	B	MM	L	MA	D	BT*
❑ Melatonin	___	___	___	___	___	___	___
❑ Extra† calcium	___	___	___	___	___	___	___
❑ Extra† magnesium	___	___	___	___	___	___	___
❑ Extra† zinc, 50 mg	___	___	___	___	___	___	___
❑ Extra† vitamin C	___	___	___	___	___	___	___
❑ Extra† vitamin E 400 IU	___	___	___	___	___	___	___
❑ Extra† iron 15–20 mg (look for absorbable, non-toxic form—Ferrochel)‡	___	___	___	___	___	___	___
❑ Glycine 500–2000 mg	___	___	___	___	___	___	___
❑ Folic acid 1,000–5,000 mcg	___	___	___	___	___	___	___

---

*AM=on arising; B=with breakfast; MM=midmorning; L=with lunch; MA=midafternoon; D=with dinner; BT=at bedtime.
†"Extra" means on top of the amounts of these nutrients that you get in your basic supplements.
‡E.g., Iron Complex by NOW or Chelated Iron by Carlson.

continued

Supplement	AM	B	MM	L	MA	D	BT*

Addiction Repair

Supplement	AM	B	MM	L	MA	D	BT*
❏ *Alka-Seltzer Gold*	—	—	—	—	—	—	—
❏ Noni juice	—	—	—	—	—	—	—
❏ Milk thistle 300 mg	—	—	—	—	—	—	—
❏ Vitamin C powder	—	—	—	—	—	—	—

Adrenal Repair

Supplement	AM	B	MM	L	MA	D	BT*
❏ Licorice	—	—	—	—	—	—	—
❏ DHEA	—	—	—	—	—	—	—
❏ Pregnenolone	—	—	—	—	—	—	—
❏ Seriphos	—	—	—	—	—	—	—
❏ Glandular adrenal cortex	—	—	—	—	—	—	—
❏ Homeopathic adrenal cortex	—	—	—	—	—	—	—
❏ Rx cortisol	—	—	—	—	—	—	—

Sex Hormone Balancing

Supplement	AM	B	MM	L	MA	D	BT*
❏ Progesterone	—	—	—	—	—	—	—
❏ Black cohosh	—	—	—	—	—	—	—
❏ Rx estrogen	—	—	—	—	—	—	—
❏ Female Plus	—	—	—	—	—	—	—
❏ Rx testosterone	—	—	—	—	—	—	—
❏ Saw palmetto	—	—	—	—	—	—	—

Other Supplements

Supplement	AM	B	MM	L	MA	D	BT*
❏ _____	—	—	—	—	—	—	—
❏ _____	—	—	—	—	—	—	—
❏ _____	—	—	—	—	—	—	—
❏ _____	—	—	—	—	—	—	—

---

*AM=on arising; B=with breakfast; MM=midmorning; L=with lunch; MA=midafternoon; D=with dinner; BT=at bedtime.

Do You Have Trouble Swallowing Pills?

Those of you who hate swallowing pills can find sublinguals, chewables, powders, sprays, or liquids through knowledgeable health practitioners and employees of health stores. Your trouble swallowing is most likely due to an enlarged thyroid (the thyroid gland sits in your throat). That's been the case with a number of our clients whose trouble swallowing disappeared when their thyroid function improved. See the "Thyroid Tool Kit."

DIRECTIONS FOR TAKING YOUR SUPPLEMENTS

Once you are clear on which supplements to take and have used the suggestions here and in the "Resource Tool Kit" to purchase them, you'll be ready to start taking them. Here are some suggestions:

➤ Whether you have one or more than one mood type or other repair project to tackle, you can and should start taking all of your supplements at once, unless you are very sensitive and reactive to supplements, in which case add them in one at a time.

➤ When a range of doses is suggested in a chapter's Action Steps, please start with the lowest dose of all of your supplements. Do this to make sure you have no adverse reaction to too high an amount.

➤ If you've tried all your supplements at the lowest dose and tolerated them well but got little benefit from them, go up to the next highest dose and watch your reactions again. Do not increase over the maximum doses recommended here without expert consultation.

➤ Watch your reactions to the supplements carefully.

➤ At least for a few weeks, record your body's responses in a supplement/food/mood log to help you tune in and track progress or problems.

DEALING WITH ADVERSE EFFECTS
OF SUPPLEMENTS

Any supplement that has an adverse effect usually has it immediately. More rarely, an adverse reaction could develop after you'd been taking a supplement for a while. You could get a headache, nausea, loose bowels, or a worsening of a negative symptom that you already had, like sleeplessness or jitteriness. Do not ignore *any* adverse symptoms that start after you begin to use supplements. Stop taking the supplement(s) causing the trouble, right away.

Re the amino acids: If you take too much of any amino, you might get the very symptoms you're trying to alleviate. That's why I suggest you start

---

Supplement Troubleshooting Tips

Troubling Symptom	*Supplements That May Be Implicated*
Stomachache	hydrochloric acid (HCI), B complex
Headaches	L-tyrosine, DLPA, L-phenylalanine, DHEA, L-tryptophan or 5-HTP (rare)
Loose bowels	magnesium, vitamin C
Nausea	B complex, 5-HTP, L-tryptophan
Burping	fish oil (take the enzyme lipase to aid your fat digestion)
Light sensitivity	Saint-John's wort
Sunburn	Saint-John's wort
High blood pressure	licorice, tyrosine, L-phenylalanine
Jitteriness, insomnia	L-phenylalanine, L-tyrosine, licorice, fish oil, thyroid or adrenal supplements, B vitamins, chromium (rare)
Acne, oily skin	DHEA
Low blood pressure	GABA
Low energy, too sleepy	5-HTP, tryptophan, GABA, inositol

with the lowest dose available and build up as necessary. For example, a stressed nurse took 500 milligrams of GABA instead of starting with 100 milligrams. She got much more stressed for a few hours. On 100 milligrams she felt relaxed.

➤ If you have any adverse symptoms (such as a headache that starts only after you've taken certain supplements), check the "Supplement Troubleshooting Tips" above and stop taking or lower the dosage of the supplement that is the most likely culprit. If the symptoms don't stop quickly (in twenty-four hours), stop all supplements and, when the symptoms have disappeared, reintroduce your supplements one by one (once a day) until you find the culprit. (Our clients have to do this only rarely.) Try a 300-milligram capsule of milk thistle twice a day to assist with any trouble your liver may be having processing the supplements. This often helps overnight.

➤ If you mistakenly take your breakfast, lunch, or dinner supplements without food, the B vitamins in your multi may make you a bit queasy.

➤ To keep track of what you're taking, it can be very helpful to lay out your supplements either in small labeled plastic bags or in a plastic supplement container with dividers.

➤ It can be hard to remember to take the supplements between meals. Use an alarm watch, a pager, or a computer reminder, if you need help. If you forget your between-meal supplements, just take them with your next meal. Don't skip them. If you just can't do it, take all your supplements with meals and at bedtime. They'll still work, just not as strongly. You might need to increase your doses of amino acids, if you notice you aren't getting as much benefit when you take them with meals.

DIRECTIONS FOR ELIMINATING YOUR SUPPLEMENTS

At some point after you have corrected your imbalances and your symptoms are gone, you can begin to experiment very carefully with going off your special repair supplements, one at a time. If your original mood or other adverse symptoms come back (in a day or a week, or longer), you'll know that you still need to take that particular supplement for a while.

Eliminate it again in a month and see what happens. Continue to do this until you no longer need any of your special repair supplements, but be ready to take them again during stressful times, should you need to in the future. Continue with your basic supplements. After six months, experiment with varying your multi once or twice a year by trying a new one when your old multi runs out, to get a different ratio of nutrients.

READINGS

Atkins, Robert, M.D. *Dr. Atkins' Vita-Nutrient Solution* (New York: Simon & Schuster, 1998). A readable, fascinating tour of basic supplements.

Braverman, Eric, M.D. *The Healing Nutrients Within* (North Bergen, N.J.: Basic Health Publications, 2003). This is the most complete book on amino acid therapy I know.

Crayhon, Robert. *The Carnitine Miracle* (New York: M. Evans, 1998). This is a great book for vegetarians in particular.

Hausman, Patricia. *The Right Dose* (New York: Ballantine, 1989).

Sullivan, Krispin. *Naked at Noon: Understanding the Importance of Sunlight and Vitamin D* (North Bergen, N.J.: Basic Health Publications, 2003). See her Web site, www.krispin.com, for updated information on other supplements.

Lieberman, Shari, Ph.D. *The Real Vitamin and Mineral Book: Using Supplements for Optimum Health* (Garden City, N.Y.: Avery, 1997).

Murray, Michael T., N.D. *The Encyclopedia of Nutritional Supplements: The Essential Guide for Improving Your Health Naturally* (Rocklin, Calif.: Prima, 1996).

Holford, Patrick and Cass, Hyla, M.D. *Natural Highs: Supplements, Nutrition, and Mind-Body Techniques to Help You Feel Good All the Time* (New York: Avery, 2002).

Step 4

Getting Help with Special Mood Repair Projects

CHAPTER II

Moods and Meds

~

When Antidepressant Nutrients
Can Do a Better Job

If you're reading this chapter, you're probably either one of the people taking antidepressant drugs like Prozac, Zoloft, and Paxil or one of the many seriously considering it. These serotonin-boosting antidepressants are by far the most popular psychopharmaceuticals ever known. The use of these drugs, called "selective serotonin reuptake inhibitors" (SSRIs), to treat depression, anxiety, and associated mood problems has doubled in the past ten years and is expected to continue to rise. In fact, we pop up to 20 million tranquilizers each week in Britain, and a MORI survey recently found that 23 per cent of adults will take milder tranquilizers, such as benzodiazepines, for anxiety and sleep problems at some point in their lives.

If you're not using any of these antidepressants yet, you may be curious about whether you should try nutritional therapy first. If you're already on one of these drugs, you may be wondering if there are any natural remedies that would work better for you or that you could add to your drug therapy with benefit. We have worked with hundreds of clients either on or considering these specific drugs, and we've found that certain nutritional alternatives actually work better for most of them than the drugs do. But they don't work for everyone. The question is: Will they work for *you*?

In this chapter, I'll tell you about our clients' efforts to control their mood problems with SSRIs, about what has happened when they've tried the nutritional approaches, and about the scientific validation of the alternative strategies. I will also provide you with some specific suggestions on how to safely and comfortably wean yourself off prescription drugs with your doctor's help, should you choose to do so.

Before I begin, I want to caution you. If you are taking an antidepressant medication, do not discontinue it without consulting your physician. Some of these drugs can have very serious withdrawal effects that I'll mention in more detail later. More important, if your original depression was severe and your medication has helped, you need to be very careful not to risk a relapse. I know that many of you will say, "But my doctor doesn't know anything about natural remedies, so why should I bother talking with him or her?" While it's true that few medical schools offer courses in nutrition or natural therapies, more and more physicians are at least open to alternative treatment approaches. More to the point, they are often all too familiar with antidepressant side effects and are experienced in taking patients off unsuccessful drugs, but they also, understandably, want to be assured that alternative treatments are safe, effective, and well studied. I will be reviewing our clinic's approach and the science behind it so that both you and your physician can understand how nutritherapy can benefit you as it has so many of our clients. First, though, let's talk about why you might want to avoid or abandon antidepressant medications.

Where Do You Stand in the Controversy over Antidepressants?

The skyrocketing use of SSRIs has generated a great deal of controversy in the past two decades or so. Some think that these drugs are great, and have experienced real relief from serious mood problems because of them or know of people who have. Others are concerned about the side effects and potential long-term hazards of these drugs and feel that we're using them simply to medicate away our feelings when what we really need is some good counseling or a stiffer upper lip. As an addiction treatment specialist, I've always had an automatic bias against using drugs, which is one of the reasons that I've looked so hard and long for nondrug methods of dealing with mood problems. But over the years, I've had to rethink many of my attitudes about antidepressant drugs as I've come to understand why people want and need them so badly.

It's my clients, people perhaps like you, who have taught me this lesson, clients with intractable depression who started taking SSRIs very reluctantly, out of desperation, when nothing else had helped. Clients who were often ashamed of taking drugs but could find no other recourse and courageously reached for the lifeline that may very well have kept them from sinking.

I'm happy to tell you that you now have more than one option. The nutritional options, if they work for you, will be much safer and more effective than the drugs you've been using or considering. Since it will take only a few days to find out whether you're a good candidate for natural antidepressants, you won't have to wait long to make your decision.

Choosing Your Weapons Against Depression

There's no question that we're experiencing an unprecedented need for help with depression, anxiety, stress, and emotional pain in the West. It has touched almost every household in America. The question is, what should we do about it? How can we find the line between the emotional discomfort that requires biochemical remedies like nutrient supplements or medication and the emotional discomfort that indicates a need for counseling, a new job, or time to work problems through? Many people feel that SSRIs actually suppress important feelings that really should be processed in psychotherapy; and I have witnessed this with a few of our clients. Others feel that people who use SSRIs are exaggerating their upset feelings and should just "tough it out." That I have *not* seen (though I have heard of general practitioners who have inappropriately offered these drugs for minor and transient problems).

The vast majority of the people I've seen who have tried antidepressants *really needed* their biochemical assistance. They have not been using these drugs casually or for fun. I believe that the growing use of antidepressant drugs is a symptom of an epidemic of significant and crippling biochemical brain deficits caused largely by our increasingly stressful lifestyle combined with an inadequate diet. I'm also convinced that we need to rally every possible resource to fight this epidemic. Psychological, spiritual, pharmaceutical, and, of course, nutritional tools must all be considered.

If You're Not Currently on Medication, but Are Considering It

Since your dilemma might very well be at least partly psychological, what about starting with psychotherapy? You may already have done this. The drawback of psychotherapy (and/or spiritual counseling) alone is that it can take years before it becomes obvious that you also need help dealing with a biochemical problem. What about the all-meds approach? With this, there are the combined drawbacks of side effects, only partial relief, and the loss of the counseling you might need.

I propose the following strategy:

➤ Carefully study your own biochemical false mood symptoms on the Mood-Type Questionnaire in chapter 2.
➤ Try the nutritional remedies suggested in the chapters that address your particular false moods, as determined by your responses on the questionnaire.
➤ If you don't feel significantly better after two weeks on nutritherapy, see a counselor or psychotherapist. Be sure to consult someone who understands that there might be a biochemical component to your mood problem, is open to nutritional as well as pharmaceutical remedies, and can refer you to a doctor for medication if needed.
➤ If the nutritional tools do not benefit you and you have already tried psychotherapy, go directly to a psychiatrist or psychopharmacologist who can help you with a trial of medication.

Caution: Do not wait two weeks to see a counselor or psychiatrist if you are suicidal or desperately unhappy. Go now.

If You Are Currently Using an SSRI

If you're already on and benefiting from a drug like Prozac, you know that low serotonin is your brain's problem and identify with some or all of the symptoms on part 1 of the Mood-Type Questionnaire (or at least you did before you started using your drug): you may have already read chapter 3, which is all about the natural approach to serotonin boosting. (If you haven't, please do.) If so, you are probably wondering where you stand and why you're on an expensive and questionable drug when excellent natural alternatives are at hand.

This is my perspective: Although SSRIs can be helpful, I only rarely see them completely eliminate the depression and other mood problems caused by serotonin deficiency. They can have many disturbing or dangerous side effects, and they can be very difficult to withdraw from. Yet SSRIs do have a place in the armamentarium of treatment options for depression.

They have a place, but it should not be first place. They're best used as backups, when safer and more natural methods fail. However, if you're on a medication that is working well for you, with only minor or no side effects, especially if it has rescued you from very serious mood problems, I would be very reluctant to suggest that you go off it. However, if you are not getting the relief you need, then I believe that you should explore the nutritional options.

How Is Your SSRI Affecting You?

Are you disappointed? Perhaps, like some of our clients, you've found that medications helped you initially, then stopped working after a few months or years. This is the experience of about a third of those who try SSRIs. Or are you like most of the clients who come to us whose drugs still do help some, but not enough, and who want to be able to get rid of their mood problems *altogether?* (This is *not* too much to expect!)

Are You Living with Side Effects?

Our clients complain more about *lack* of effects than about side effects. But *all* of them have side effects to report. These are the most common:

Nausea	Feeling emotionally flat
No orgasm	Gaining weight
Jittery	Less interested in sex
Fatigued	Negative, even suicidal thoughts
Disturbed sleep	

Some of our clients who've tried SSRIs have had such adverse reactions to them that they've had to go off them within a month. Others have found that side effects came on more gradually. Many of them have wanted to get off SSRIs because weight gain, low energy, or sexual dysfunction were side effects they found unacceptable. Still others knew about the studies indicating that increased breast cancer and other tumor growth were associated with SSRI use.[1,2,3]

It's almost impossible to know for sure what the drawbacks of SSRIs really are. The FDA requires drug companies to provide only six weeks of testing to prove the safety and efficacy of their products. The drug companies have reported that dozens of side effects showed up during their short-term trials of SSRIs, but those reports obviously did not include the adverse reactions that showed up *after* six weeks. According to three physicians writing in the *New England Journal of Medicine,* "51% of approved drugs have serious side effects not detected prior to approval."[4,5] The FDA admits that it is not equipped to monitor drug effects in the long term, and little independent research on long-term effects of SSRIs is being done.

Some of the most frightening side effects of SSRIs, suicidal and homicidal thoughts and actions, are now firmly linked to Prozac, Paxil, and Zoloft.[6] Many cases have been settled out of court, and juries in the United States, Australia, and the United Kingdom have found against SSRI manufacturers, linking the use of SSRIs directly to both violent homicides and suicides[7] and confirming that violent tendencies were not present prior to SSRI use.

In 1992, we treated our first client on Prozac. After a recent suicide attempt, she had been rushed to a local hospital emergency room for treatment. The first question asked by the attending physician was, "Are you taking Prozac?" Evidently, the ER staff had become aware of the link between Prozac and suicide, but the patient had not.

All told, there have been hundreds of different adverse SSRI side effects reported to the FDA and its equivalents in other countries. The FDA received over 31,000 complaints against Prozac alone between 1987 and 1996 (including 121 drug-related deaths), and they acknowledge that this probably represents only a tenth of the actual incidence.[8] The list of these reactions is so long that I'm not going to be able to include it all here, but you can find it, provided by the FDA's freedom of information staff, posted at www.cris.com/~shddemon/prozac.reactions.[9] Many of these adverse effects are also listed in your SSRI prescription insert. Ask your pharmacist for one if you don't have it, or buy one of the many books that summarize drug side effects. (Be sure to also request a pharmacy search for any adverse reactions that might arise if you are taking any other drug with your SSRI.)

In reporting the grim facts of SSRI side effects, I'm not trying to deny the value that so many people have received from these drugs. I myself have witnessed these benefits and been grateful for them. I just want you to be alert to any mental or physical changes that might be attributable to your SSRI.

THE MOST DANGEROUS SIDE EFFECT: SEROTONIN SYNDROME

Some of our clients have found that their meds have caused the same kinds of problems that they had initially relieved. In fact, going off Prozac and Paxil totally cured a few of them of their depression and anxiety. Al-though their initial effects had been positive, apparently later the drugs had actually raised their serotonin level *too high.*[10]

The symptoms caused by having serotonin levels raised too high can often be very similar to those caused by having levels that are too low (sim-ilar to the symptoms on part 1 of the Four-Part Mood-Type Question-naire). This excess serotonin "syndrome" can be one of the most potentially dangerous effects of SSRIs, especially when they are combined with other serotonin-stimulating drugs (for instance, taking two SSRIs). We have rarely seen this syndrome result from SSRIs combined with nutrients, but we have rarely seen them used together over the long term. Usually our clients have only used them together briefly while tapering off SSRIs. In one study of five patients with OCD (not depression), combining SSRIs with the amino acid tryptophan caused adverse symptoms.[11] In another, larger study with depressed patients, these problem symptoms did not develop.[12]

The symptoms of serotonin syndrome can be mild, moderate, and/or severe,[13] with the severe forms responsible for most of the deaths associ-ated with SSRIs. Here is a list of the most severe symptoms of serotonin syndrome: "intense perspiration, fever, rapid heartbeat, very low blood pressure, and extreme fatigue . . ."[14] Also ". . . euphoria, drowsiness, sus-tained rapid eye movement, overreaction of the reflexes, rapid muscle contraction and relaxation in the ankle causing abnormal movements of the foot, clumsiness, restlessness, feeling drunk and dizzy, muscle contrac-tion and relaxation in the jaw . . . intoxication, muscle twitching, rigidity, high body temperature, mental status changes . . . [including confusion and hypomania], shivering, diarrhea, loss of consciousness."[15]

If you experience any of these symptoms while taking an SSRI, call your doctor or an emergency room immediately.

WITHDRAWAL PROBLEMS

Have you quit taking an SSRI and wondered whether the sudden appear-ance of disturbing symptoms was a temporary withdrawal reaction, a more sinister long-term reaction to withdrawing from the drug you'd been taking, or a return of your original false mood symptoms? Adverse symptoms that arise quickly are typically actual withdrawal symptoms—not signs of the return of your old depression or anxiety, which would typically take weeks or months to resurface.

What does it mean when a drug cannot be terminated without withdrawal symptoms? It means that the drug is addictive. Although SSRI manufacturers denied this possibility for years, in January 2002, both the FDA in the United States and its British equivalent identified Paxil as having significant addictive potential. Specifically, they insisted that the drug be accompanied by warnings of the serious withdrawal symptoms that could occur on termination. They also acknowledged that other SSRIs, including Prozac, had the same potential.[16]

Because of side effects or "no effects," many of our clients have attempted to quit their SSRIs before they come to see us. But they have sometimes had real trouble getting off these drugs. Most of the SSRIs (like most other mood-altering drugs) have biochemical hooks that can make them very difficult for certain people to give up. Although Prozac, which leaves the body slowly and gradually, is not as often a detox problem, the other SSRIs can set off quick withdrawal reactions in 50–86 percent of users. These reactions can include dizziness, confusion, flulike symptoms, GI problems, anxiety, depression, sleep problems, and even neurological symptoms such as tingling or electric shock sensations.[17]

Everyone is in agreement that withdrawal from all serotonin-stimulating drugs, other than Prozac, should be approached with caution. Fortunately, there is a way to make the transitions off SSRIs more comfortable.

NUTRITHERAPY: USING NATURAL ANTIDEPRESSANTS

Natural Help for Drug Withdrawal

Although I've heard clients describe their difficult *past* withdrawal experiences and seen the research documenting the withdrawal phenomena, I have rarely witnessed the problem firsthand. Why? Because at our clinic, we have been able to assist clients through a gradual, comfortable withdrawal process using the natural serotonin-building supplements 5-HTP or tryptophan. Typically, our clients have felt much *better*, not worse, as they've reduced the amount of the drug they'd been taking.

For example, our client Lisa, 33, had taken a total of twenty-six different medications over the previous fifteen years, often combining two to three at a time. She'd be very depressed for stretches, then she'd swing between depression and feeling great, sometimes several times a day. Her drug regimen always included at least one SSRI, which would typically help for six months and then stop working. Quite often, she had to go through very difficult withdrawals before she could switch from one set of drugs to another.

By the time she sought help at our clinic, Lisa had been on Wellbutrin (a mildly stimulating antidepressant), Klonopin (a tranquilizer), and Paxil (an SSRI) for eight months and was more productive than she'd been in a long time. Though her depressions continued to fluctuate in and out just as often, they were not as crippling. After reading about the amino acids in *The Diet Cure*, however, Lisa wanted to try nutritherapy instead of drug therapy. We encouraged her to go ahead with the experiment with her psychiatrist's willing participation. Lisa took 5-HTP and the stimulating amino acid tyrosine as she cut back on her Paxil and Wellbutrin, with virtually no detox symptoms. (Wellbutrin had been a very difficult drug for her to detox from in the past.) But the hard part was yet to come—Klonopin detox can be horrendous. To reduce the nasty side effects associated with cutting back on this tranquilizer, we recommended that Lisa take specific nutrients for extra support, including GABA, taurine, inositol, and glycine. Amazingly, Lisa was able to slowly taper off Klonopin relatively free of detox symptoms. I want to stress that Lisa was able to detox successfully partly because she was carefully monitored by her physician. I don't recommend that people go off even one medication on their own without medical monitoring.

How Well Do Natural Serotonin Boosters Perform Compared with the SSRIs?

Millions of 5-HTP, tryptophan, and Saint-John's wort takers can attest to the extraordinary mood-enhancing benefits of these natural remedies that I discuss at length in chapter 3. Their experience is supported by scientific research favorably comparing the benefits of these and other natural remedies, including exercise and light therapy, to the benefits of SSRIs. Here are a few of the scientific findings:

➤ *5-HTP* raised serotonin levels 540 percent, compared with Paxil's 450 percent and Prozac's 150–250 percent.[18] It also outperformed the SSRI Luvox as an antidepressant, 68 percent to 62 percent.[19]

➤ *Trytophan:* Between 50 and 60 percent of former SSRI takers relapse into depression, OCD, SAD, PMS, insomnia, bulimia, aggression, addiction, anxiety, and panic unless adequate tryptophan is made available.[20,21]

➤ *Saint-John's wort* has tested just as effective for depression relief as Prozac,[22] and *more* effective than Zoloft.[23]

➤ *Exercise* alone can raise serotonin levels nicely. A ninety-minute walk can increase levels by 100 percent. A daily forty-minute walk prevents relapse into depression (after a successful round of SSRI taking) twice as well as does taking Zoloft.[24]

➤ *Bright light* therapy can be a little more effective than Prozac in relieving winter depression (70 percent vs. 65 percent).[25]

Speed, Safety, and Effectiveness

In all the studies, the benefits of the natural approaches took effect more quickly than the benefits of the SSRIs and proved much safer. For example, 5-HTP is associated with 0 percent sexual dysfunction,[26,27] while the SSRIs are associated with 50–70 percent sexual dysfunction. In several studies, both Saint-John's wort and 5-HTP have had fewer side effects than the placebos!

This kind of research supports our clinic's experience of over fifteen years that natural methods can easily meet or exceed the benefits of SSRIs for many, perhaps most, people. Probably because our clients combine 5-HTP, tryptophan, or Saint-John's wort with so many other serotonin-supportive supplements and foods, plus light and excercise plus any needed counseling or medical care, they typically do much better off SSRIs than on them. And so should you. But, largely because patented pharmaceuticals are so much more lucrative as investments, there's been much less interest in promoting nonpatentable nutrients, despite their safety and effectiveness.

SSRIs and Nutrients:
The Saga of Serotonin Therapy

If natural antidepressant brain foods work so well, why aren't we just using them in the first place instead of the drugs? It's an interesting story.

Prior to 1989, although Prozac had been introduced with much fanfare, its pharmaceutical reps couldn't persuade the country's doctors to use it. Why? Because they were already sold on something else—the amino acid tryptophan, from which serotonin is made in the brain. Psychiatrists and other physicians resisted Prozac's lures, since over-the-counter tryptophan supplements were providing successful antidepressant and sleep aid with vir-tually no side effects. One of our medical consultants tells the story of how she finally agreed to try a tiny, 10-milligram dose of Prozac. The rep had in-sisted that a little Prozac could be useful "just to make the tryptophan work better." And it did.

Into this happy scene, one day in 1989, came a very badly contami-nated batch of tryptophan. The guilty Japanese amino acid manufacturer admitted later, in court, that it had knowingly sent the bad batch to the United States. It did enough damage (including killing over forty people) to terrify users and physicians all over the United States, prompt the FDA to call for a voluntary ban on sales, and create a huge new market for Prozac, which appeared on the cover of *Newsweek* magazine the next week. The Japanese company at fault, Showa Denko, never made another batch of tryptophan, but because of their "error," the other tryptophan-producing companies, with unblemished records, lost their U.S. markets. More important, millions of Americans and their doctors lost an irre-placeable resource for depression and insomnia relief.

In 1991, Prozac's U.S. manufacturer, Eli Lilly, published a study exon-erating tryptophan and acknowledging its benefits.[28] But few doctors saw it, and their fears persisted. Yet in other countries, like the United King-dom, Canada, and Finland, tryptophan sales and research never stopped, and no problems ever recurred. In fact, in these countries there has been much successful research on the use of tryptophan to treat "resistant" cases of depression, and scientific conferences on tryptophan research are held in Europe on a regular basis.

There is some very good news, though. In 1995, tryptophan became available again in the United States, by prescription from compounding pharmacies, and it was finally made available *without* prescription in 2000.

What About 5-HTP and Saint-John's Wort?

Although it has been widely used and highly regarded in Europe for decades, 5-HTP became available in U.S. health food stores and pharmacies only in 1997. Most of our clients can't tell the difference between tryptophan and 5-HTP. Moodwise, both can erase all symptoms of low serotonin, from de-pression and anxiety to insomnia and irritability. The third powerful natural serotonin booster, the herb Saint-John's wort, has also been extensively re-searched and used enthusiastically in Europe for at least twenty years. As I've mentioned before, it actually outsells Prozac in Germany, and it's been sell-ing strongly in the United States as well for many years.

What Makes the Nutrients Safer and More Effective?

In order to understand how 5-HTP and tryptophan can outperform the SSRIs, you need know how a serotonin-healthy brain should operate. First of all, it should be crammed with serotonin molecules, and these molecules should be alternately active, transmitting happy nerve impulses, and inactive, resting quietly in "reuptake" position. Eventually, the serotonin molecules will move on to be transformed either into melatonin, the chemical that puts us to sleep, or into an emotionally crucial chemical called 5-HIAA (5-hydroxyindole acetic acid), which I will soon describe in fascinating detail.

Now let's take a look at *your* serotonin-*depleted* brain: There you'll see only a few serotonin molecules—some active, some resting—with never enough to send adequate amounts of happy mood messages or, often, to convert to adequate amounts of melatonin or 5-HIAA. Enter the SSRIs, which can act to artificially prevent serotonin from going into resting (or reuptake) mode. Keeping what little serotonin you have active this way gives the illusion that you actually have more serotonin than you do, but it can also prevent serotonin from moving on to become melatonin or 5-HIAA.[29] Impaired sleep is a common side effect of SSRIs, and there is growing concern about the negative emotional impact of reduced levels of 5-HIAA.

What's wrong with damming up serotonin and blocking the production of the downstream brain chemical, 5-HIAA? Since this maneuver can make many people feel so much better, what's the problem? The chief concern is that 5-HIAA may be as important as serotonin for your emotional well-being. In fact, 5-HIAA can protect us from some of the most destructive of all negative moods, the ones that lead to violent crime, suicide, severe insomnia, and addiction.[30,31]

Most depressed and obsessive people are low in *both* serotonin and 5-HIAA. Further reducing their already low or marginal levels of 5-HIAA, as SSRIs tend to do, can trigger *new* and dangerous mood problems. As I mentioned earlier, several court cases have linked SSRI use to the recent rash of bizarre murder-suicides, and many experts believe that a lowered 5-HIAA level is the key contributing factor to these tragedies.

Here's where the nutrients have a potentially lifesaving advantage over the drugs: 5-HTP and tryptophan are both well-researched champions in *raising* 5-HIAA levels.[32,33] If you add 5-HTP or tryptophan to your SSRIs or replace your SSRIs with them, a more normal serotonin-related brain flow can resume and your 5-HIAA levels can rise. The B vitamin folic acid[34] and a lower-carbohydrate, higher-protein diet will also effectively help to raise your 5-HIAA levels.[35]

Now let's look at what happens when your serotonin-deficient brain is nourished by 5-HTP or tryptophan: Suddenly there are plenty of molecules transmitting away or resting quietly, as needed, and plenty are left over to convert into melatonin and 5-HIAA. Eventually, there is so much serotonin in your brain that you can stop taking your supplements. At that point, your restocked brain won't even miss them.

Combining SSRIs with the Aminos

The effectiveness and safety of 5-HTP and tryptophan have not escaped the notice of psychiatric and pharmaceutical researchers, who have begun to combine the nutrients *with* SSRIs. This combination has proven to both enhance the antidepressant drugs' effectiveness and reduce their side effects in most cases.

In a British study of severely depressed patients who had been unresponsive to at least four prior medications, tryptophan was given along with the SSRI Serzone. The depressive symptoms dropped more than 50 percent in what was ecstatically, if oddly, referred to as "an unusually high successful efficacy rate."[36]

A Canadian study found that 20 milligrams of Prozac combined with 2 to 4 grams of tryptophan speeded up antidepressant benefits and preserved the deep, or slow-wave, sleep that Prozac alone tends to disrupt[37]— and without any evidence of the excess serotonin syndrome![38] In the United Kingdom, standard psychiatric practice calls for the addition of tryptophan when SSRIs or other antidepressants don't work well.[39]

Our clients routinely take 5-HTP and tryptophan with their antidepressants (with their doctors' approval) in the process of tapering off their SSRIs, and they typically feel much better as soon as they begin adding the nutrients. If you're taking an SSRI that has not completely eliminated your adverse moods, you may want to talk to your doctor about adding one of these nutrients to your own drug regimen, even if you decide not to stop using the SSRI altogether. Be sure to watch for any sign of excess serotonin, though.

The Amino Acid Tyrosine Helps with the SSRI Side Effect of Low Energy

In addition to 5-HTP and tryptophan, there is another amino acid, tyrosine, that has benefited our clients who've used drugs like Zoloft and Paxil. Tyrosine can eliminate one of the most common side effects of these drugs: low energy.

Serotonin is the biochemical counterbalance to your brain's natural stimulants, the catecholamines. Raising serotonin levels via SSRIs can deplete the levels of these stimulating neurotransmitters as much as 60 percent.[40] This can cause low energy, apathy, twitches, tics, and sexual dysfunction. Tyrosine supplements provide the specific food that your brain can use to restore its balance by building up depleted catecholamines levels in minutes. This not only perks you up, it can help raise your 5-HIAA levels significantly as well.[41]

Check the low-catecholamine symptoms in part 2 of the Mood-Type Questionnaire if your energy is low, particularly if it has dropped while on SSRIs or if you get tired while taking 5-HTP or tryptophan (anything that raises serotonin can potentially lower catecholamines). This will help you determine whether you need to take tyrosine for a while. Tyrosine is usually taken in the early morning and midmorning. If you have any trouble getting to sleep or staying asleep, don't take stimulating tyrosine after three P.M. If you have no trouble sleeping, you can take 500 to 1,000 milligrams of tyrosine to counteract any midafternoon slumps you may be experiencing.

SWITCHING FROM SSRIs TO NATURAL ANTIDEPRESSANTS

If you would like to find out if amino acids would work for you instead of, or in addition to, the SSRI or similar drug that you may currently be taking, make a proposal to your doctor like the one we made to Joy's psychiatrist.

Joy had become angry, depressed, and negative at age 14. Though a straight A student, she started smoking pot for mood relief and got into trouble for it at school. At that point, her parents came to me for help. Since she would not cooperate with any nutritional suggestions, I referred her to a psychiatrist, who put her on Zoloft. Quick, but only partial, improvement ensued. She quit being hateful to her parents, but was still humorless, negative, and shut-down and continued to crave pot. I called the psychiatrist and proposed a trial of 5-HTP, starting with 1 capsule of 50 milligrams (the lowest dose) for two days. If there were no adverse effects at 50 milligrams, I suggested raising it to 200 milligrams a day—100 milligrams midafternoon and 100 milligrams at bedtime—for one week, along with her Zoloft. Suddenly Joy was her old self, happy to plan a vacation with her family and pleasant to be around.

The psychiatrist was surprised but pleased and encouraged her to continue on 5-HTP and a slightly lower dose of Zoloft. Things went well—so well that after a few months, her mom quit buying the 5-HTP. When I called to check in not long after that, Mom was full of the old complaints about Joy. When I reminded her about how well Joy had done earlier, Mom got her back on the 5-HTP, and her real daughter emerged again. I proposed that during the next summer vacation, Joy try her 5-HTP while gradually reducing the Zoloft. The goal was to see how well 5-HTP by itself could work for her. Her doctor agreed. Joy was fine during the gradual taper and did well completely off the Zoloft. However, in the winter (low-serotonin season), she needed to go up to 300 milligrams of 5-HTP. The next year, her mood was stable on 200 milligrams a day. After that, over a period of six months, she gradually needed less and less 5-HTP until she didn't need any at all.

Be Careful

Many people come to our clinic eager to get off their SSRIs. If you're in this boat, please don't just drop your SSRI overboard. Take the following factors into account:

1. Is now the right time in your life to try something new? Sometimes I advise clients currently going through upsetting times to wait till their lives have calmed down, if medication seems to have helped, before they launch into a drug taper. I often suggest, though, that they discuss with their doctor the option of taking some 5-HTP along with their SSRI until they are ready for the taper.

2. You must get professional advice about how to taper off. If the physician who prescribed your SSRI does not seem clear on how to taper you off it, consult with one who does, or find a pharmacist or psychopharmacologist who really knows the ropes to advise you and your doctor.

Pharmacists, now alerted to the extent of SSRI withdrawal problems, often have specific recommendations. Their Web site, www.pharmacyconnects.com, is for helping people withdraw from meds and identify adverse SSRI-related symptoms.

3. The best season for an antidepressant taper is not fall and it's not winter. These are low-serotonin times, when you'll have the strongest tendency to be depressed or anxious. The *best* time is spring or early summer, when your serotonin levels will naturally be at their height. You don't need to wait until spring, but you'd be most comfortable in the taper process then. While the sun still shines, you can try your wings with 5-HTP. Then, in the following fall, if your medless mood does drop, you can try more 5-HTP or get back onto your medication with or without 5-HTP, until the spring.

4. If you're taking medication *and* 5-HTP, work closely with a psychiatrist or psychotherapist who knows about the symptoms of serotonin syndrome to make sure you don't get mired in excess serotonin. Neither the scientific studies nor our clinic's experience indicate this possibility is of great concern, but no adverse symptoms should be ignored.

5. If you quit taking your SSRI *altogether*, monitor yourself to be sure that your low-serotonin symptoms don't return. Please post the list of low-serotonin symptoms from part 1 of the False-Mood Questionnaire on your fridge, and give copies to family members and friends. If these symptoms reappear, increase your 5-HTP or try the suggestions you'll read about next.

What If the 5-HTP Doesn't Work?

If your original mood problems return after a few weeks or months off your SSRI, you'll first want to increase your dose of 5-HTP. This supplement seldom fails, but it doesn't work for everyone. If, even at a higher dose, it fails for you, something is interfering with your brain's natural tendency to make plenty of serotonin out of 5-HTP. We've been watching closely for about eight years, trying to figure out why this happens, and we have identified several factors. If you don't get quick mood benefit from your 5-HTP, it is most likely to be for one of the following reasons:

You're one of those who does better on tryptophan than on 5-HTP. That's easy to find out: Stop your 5-HTP and take 500 milligrams of tryptophan for every 50 milligrams of 5-HTP you've been taking. You'll know in two days which is the right brain food for you. Tryptophan supplements can be ordered through our clinic's order line (800-733-9293), directly from Bios Biochemicals in the US (800-404-8185), or by a prescription from a compounding pharmacy.

If neither 5-HTP *nor* tryptophan works:

Your thyroid probably isn't producing enough of its hormones to allow you to digest or utilize 5-HTP or tryptophan. Up to 86 percent of depressed people have some kind of thyroid malfunction.[42] SSRIs, too, can be stymied by a low-thyroid condition, with over 50 percent of those who do not respond to antidepressants having low thyroid function.[43] Psychiatrists often combine thyroid meds with SSRIs to improve results. Clues: Are you often tired, easily chilled, and gaining unneeded weight? See the complete list of low-thyroid symptoms on pages 67–68 of chapter 4, and see the "Thyroid Tool Kit" for advice on how to get your thyroid function tested and corrected.

Some of our depressed low-thyroid clients have subnormal scores on their thyroid blood tests. Others have relatively normal blood test results but may have low levels of thyroid hormone (T_3) in their brains only.[44] If so, medication is required. Otherwise the brain can't use amino acids—or sometimes even SSRIs—to increase serotonin.[45] In these cases, the only way to know may be to get a trial prescription for some synthetic T_3 and see.

In our experience with clients given a trial of T_3 by their doctors or D.O.'s, the answer has come in a hurry. They either felt great, or they felt jittery and had heart palpitations. Dosing needs to go up gradually, and if you get benefit from your SSRI, you may need to keep taking it.

You may need Saint-John's wort. Especially when the thyroid is low, herbs and drugs often work better than nutrients do. (Herbs are like drugs in the mysterious ways they affect the brain and body.) But Saint-John's wort can effectively raise serotonin levels without depleting 5-HIAA levels.[46,47] As I mentioned earlier, Saint-John's wort is the antidepressant of choice in Germany, where it actually outsells Prozac.

Please read chapter 3 for detailed information on other factors that can interfere with natural serotonin building and how to use the natural antidepressants.

ACTION STEPS

1. Work with a psychotherapist who is open to the nutritional and, if needed, the psychopharmaceutical approach.

2. If you are *not* on an antidepressant, read chapter 3 to become very familiar with the natural solutions to the mood problems associated with low serotonin. Try them along with your basic supplements and good-mood foods and regular moderate exercise (unless exercise makes you tired).

3. Get bright light (150–200 watts or 2,500 lux within three feet of you) if you have winter depression. (See the "Resource Tool Kit," page 289, for light sources.)

4. *If you are on medication,* discuss with your doctor a one-week trial of 50–100 milligrams *5-HTP* twice a day—in midafternoon (by five P.M.) and at bedtime (by ten P.M.).

5. If your physician agrees and your trial week goes well, work with him or her to taper off your medication. In that case, you may need to increase your dose to as high as 150 milligrams 5-HTP in the afternoon by five P.M. and again by ten P.M. If your doctor is unsure about the appropriate antidepressant tapering procedure, suggest a review of the information on "discontinuation" on the Pharmacy Connects Web site, www.pharmacyconnects.com, or a consultation with a knowledgeable pharmacist or psychopharmachologist.

6. As you taper down on your medication, if adverse symptoms appear, increase your 5-HTP.

7. If all goes well off the drug, continue on your 5-HTP at the optimal dose you've discovered. After three to six months, experiment with gradually lowering your dose of 5-HTP. Start by tapering down 50 milligrams at a time (say, from 150 to 100 milligrams). Continue to try lowering your dose further, 50 milligrams at a time, every few months, but do not rush yourself.

8. Complete a gradual tapering off of your supplements. Or you can stop altogether at any time and see if any of your old symptoms come back. If they do, go back onto them and try tapering again in a month or two, until you no longer need 5-HTP, except perhaps in emotional emergencies or in midwinter.

9. Always go back if a lower dose exposes you to some of your old moods. Then try dropping your dose again in a few weeks or months.

10. If the 5-HTP does not altogether benefit you, switch to tryptophan, taking a 500-milligram capsule for every 50-milligram capsule of 5-HTP recommended.

11. Try Saint-John's wort, 300 milligrams three times a day, if neither 5-HTP nor tryptophan works for you.

12. If your energy is low and you identify with the symptoms in part 3 of the Mood-Type Questionnaire, try 500–1,500 milligrams tyrosine in early morning and midmorning.

13. If neither 5-HTP nor tryptophan works for you, check out the "Thyroid Tool Kit" for information on how to test and treat your *thyroid*. Use Saint-John's wort or an SSRI while you're testing and improving your thyroid function.

14. Review chapter 3 for other detailed suggestions on using serotonin-building nutrients.

RECOMMENDED READING

Barry, L., B.S.C. Pharm., and N. Kennic, Pharm., M.D. Pharmacy Connects, www.pharmacyconnects.com, April 2000. This Web site is the only detailed guide we could find on how to taper off various medications. Please share what the experts suggest with your doctor and pharmacist before you start your own withdrawal.

Glenmullen, Joseph, M.D. *Prozac Backlash* (New York: Simon & Schuster, 2000).

Hedaya, Robert, M.D. *The Antidepressant Survival Guide* (New York: Three Rivers Press, 2000).

Murray, Michael, N.D. *5-HTP* (New York: Bantam, 1998).

Tracy, Ann Blake. *Prozac: Panacea or Pandora?* (Salt Lake City: Cassia Publications, 1994, updated 2001).

CHAPTER 12

Sleep and Your Moods

〜

Getting the Kind of Rest You Really Need

You can't win any mood contests if you're losing sleep on a regular basis. Sleep is a vital recharging process for both your mind and your body, so a good night's sleep should leave you feeling not only rested but serene. If you don't get enough sleep—or don't sleep well—you'll suffer various physical consequences, but you'll also suffer emotionally. And you won't be alone: 80 percent of us are sleep deprived.[1]

More than half of our clients come to us with both mood problems *and* sleep problems. Some of the same biochemical imbalances that are causing their mood problems are often disrupting their sleep at the same time. Once these imbalances are corrected, normal sleep is restored along with normal mood. In this chapter, I'll go into detail on the biochemical mood/sleep connection and then get into the practical strategies that can counteract them successfully.

Of course, there are the outside factors, too, that may be keeping you up at night, such as wakeful children, marital discord, or an overly demanding job. But barring any real-life problems that may be sabotaging your sleep, the solutions outlined in this chapter should quickly start giving you the rest you need.

WHAT IS A GOOD NIGHT'S SLEEP?

Before we go any further, let's define the perfect snooze. Like many people, you may be so used to your own sleep patterns, however imperfect, that you don't know what you might be missing.

For most people, the best sleep takes eight hours, runs from dark to dawn—ideally from ten P.M. or earlier to six A.M. or so—and leaves you feeling great. You should actually start to feel sleepy within about three hours after the sun sets as your sleep-promoting brain chemicals are triggered by the reduced light. When you actually hit the pillow, it should take only a few minutes for you to get to sleep. Once you get to sleep, you should stay asleep through the night (without bathroom trips!). Ideally, you'll go through a series of vital sleep sequences that take at least eight hours to complete (children need twelve hours). At least six of those hours should be *uninterrupted*.

There are five stages of sleep that constitute a sleep cycle, and you need to go through four to five sleep cycles in one night. You'll usually pass through the first two superficial sleep stages in your first half hour of sleep. Then, hopefully, you'll drop into two progressively deeper sleep stages and stay there for most of the next few hours. This first half of the night, literally between ten P.M. and two A.M., potentially provides the most restorative sleep, because *only while you sleep deeply* can your immune system, your growth hormones, and other repair crews emerge to heal your body from the day's ravages. Finally, you dream in the REM (rapid eye movement) stage, which seems to be designed particularly for psychic repair. These five stages repeat throughout the night, though the second half of the night has more rapid ups, downs, and dreams than the first half.

If you sleep poorly, your mind and body are deprived of crucial cellular repairs that can be made only if you sleep long and deeply. You know what happens when you can't bring your car into the shop for its routine maintenance? You run it into the ground and shorten its "life span." Same thing here. So let's find out what's really keeping you up. But first let's get clear on what your particular sleep disturbance looks like.

WHAT IS YOUR SLEEPLESSNESS LIKE?

Do your sleep habits include any of the following basic flaws?

Are you a night owl? If so, like many people, you may not think that you have a sleep disturbance at all. You may actually consider your late nights a blessing. It can be fun—you get things done, you get some time alone when everyone else is asleep (unless you've spawned some baby night owls). But it's not fun in the morning if you need to get up so early that you can't get a full eight hours of sleep. Chances are, you are chronically undersleeping and feeling out of sync with your spouse—and the rest of the world. Being a night owl is a key symptom of either abnormally low serotonin or excessively high stress-coping hormones.

On the other hand, you may lie awake in frustration most nights for too long. Do you go over and over worries about the past day or the next day before you can finally get to sleep? Or do you just lie there? Do anxiety, pain, panic, or disturbing dreams wake you up in the night or too early in the morning? Or do you wake in the night or early morning "to go to the bathroom"? Do you take too long to get back to sleep or not get back to sleep at all? Are you a restless, thrashing sleeper or a light one? Do you wake up at the slightest sounds?

Are you proud to call yourself a "morning person" who wakes up very early no matter what time you get to sleep? Do you rarely get more than six hours of sleep a night? Do you wake up worried or anxious and have to get up and exercise or work on whatever is bothering you? Finally, are you one of the four million poorly adjusted shift workers who try to sleep during the day? Whatever part of your night's sleep you're missing, you're likely to find it in this chapter.

WHY AREN'T YOU GETTING ENOUGH SLEEP?

If you answered yes to any of the above questions, you are likely to have at least one deficiency in your body's sleep-producing chemistry. Let's start with the most common cause of sleep disturbance. It has to do with the brain chemical serotonin. But serotonin is an antidepressant, you might be thinking, what does it have to do with sleep? What you may not know is that this extraordinary biochemical mood marvel is also the only substance from which your brain can produce its most potent knockout drop: melatonin.

Your sleep is supposed to be induced by a biochemical concert that features gradually increasing levels of melatonin, starting in the afternoon and reaching crescendo at about ten P.M. Melatonin is produced out of serotonin by your pineal gland, a pea-size structure embedded deep within your brain. The pineal gland, which consists of pigment cells similar to those found in your eyes, is light sensitive. Very gradually throughout the afternoon and evening, as light gives way to darkness, the transformation of serotonin into melatonin is supposed to increase until it lullabies you to sleep. But here's the catch: Melatonin can be produced in adequate amounts only if you have enough serotonin on hand from which to make it.

YOUR FOUR NIGHTS IN SHINING ARMOR: 5-HTP, TRYPTOPHAN, MELATONIN, AND SAINT-JOHN'S WORT SUPPLEMENTS

5-HTP and Tryptophan

What can interfere with this crucial biorhythm? In my experience, the most common problem is lack of brain fuel. As you may know by now from reading chapter 3, your brain can't make serotonin without two key nutrients, tryptophan and 5-HTP. The amino acid tryptophan found in the protein-rich foods you eat converts into 5-HTP. 5-HTP converts into serotonin, and serotonin converts into melatonin. Unfortunately, it's not so easy to get enough of the tryptophan we need from food these days, so using supplements to produce melatonin can be critically important.

If you have the symptoms of low serotonin listed in part 1 of the Mood-Type Questionnaire, you probably don't have enough serotonin to get through the day, let alone the extra stores you'll need to get through the night. Fortunately, to make enough serotonin to convert to adequate melatonin, you can use supplements of 5-HTP. Over a thousand of our clients have discovered or rediscovered how good a good night's sleep can be by using 5-HTP. Whether their trouble has been getting to sleep, staying asleep, or both, this supplement tends to be the solution, side-effect free, and typically on the first night.

A client who'd been a thirty-year night owl and hated getting up exhausted in the morning to get ready for work sent us the following note a week after starting her supplements: "I feel sooooo good at night after only 50 milligrams of 5-HTP. I fall asleep easily in half an hour. I wake up refreshed, *with a sense of humor,* in plenty of time to get to work. After three days I quit drinking the morning cup of coffee I'd needed for thirty years."

Most of our sleep-deprived clients do very well with 50 to 150 milligrams of 5-HTP at bedtime. In the rare event that 5-HTP doesn't work for them, we recommend that they try 500 to 1,500 milligrams of a tryptophan supplement, which usually works better for them. Please keep in mind that the precise dose of both these nutrients may vary from person to person. Start with a single 50-milligram capsule at bedtime, and if that doesn't work in fifteen minutes, take a second or even a third capsule. Sometimes you'll need an additional capsule or more later, too, if you're prone to waking up in the night. And, especially if you have the mood symptoms of low serotonin, you'll want to add 1 to 3 capsules in the mid-afternoon both to get your serotonin levels up and to get a gradual melatonin buildup started.

You may be surprised by my recommending tryptophan as well as 5-HTP. Since it has been available for only a few years, after ten years off the shelves, tryptophan is not as easy to find as 5-HTP, which has been available in all health food stores and pharmacies for more than five years. Please read more about both 5-HTP and tryptophan in chapters 3 and 7, and find tryptophan ordering information in the Action Steps at the end of this chapter.

Many studies since the late 1970s have confirmed what our clinic has learned so happily about these two closely related sleep-promoting nutrients. For starters, they've been shown to raise the melatonin levels by 320 percent *in ten minutes.*[2] Here are a few representative quotes on tryptophan: "potent treatment for chronic insomnia,"[3] "76 percent experienced a markedly improved sleeping."[4] Regarding 5-HTP: "a significant increase in the duration of the night's sleep."[5]

Saint-John's Wort

This serotonin-, melatonin-boosting herb can be quite a good backup if, usually because of a thyroid malfunction, you don't respond well to 5-HTP or tryptophan. We very rarely need to recommend it but are glad to have it when we need it. In either capsule or more effective liquid tincture form, 300 to 600 milligrams (or a dropperful) at bedtime should do the trick. We often recommend 300 milligrams (or another dropperful) in the afternoon as well.

What About Melatonin?

You might be wondering why I don't recommend using melatonin supplements right off the bat. After all, they are also sold over the counter at health food stores and pharmacies. Some of you may indeed need to use melatonin if you don't find enough benefit from 5-HTP or tryptophan, if you are a shift worker with disrupted sleep cycles, or if you are suffering from jet lag. But if you have low-serotonin mood symptoms as described in chapter 3, I don't want you to skip the basic job of providing your brain with enough serotonin to do its crucial mood jobs—in addition to its job of converting to melatonin. By starting with 5-HTP or tryptophan, you are allowing your brain itself to decide how much of which mood and sleep chemicals it needs to make. By using these nutrient concentrates, you can most exactly duplicate the natural brain flow that culminates in the adequate production of both serotonin and melatonin.

Most of our clients have reported that this approach works just beautifully, but about 25 percent of the people who come to our clinic with sleep problems don't get enough help from either 5-HTP or tryptophan. Some of them don't have mood problems, just sleep problems. If you fall into either of these categories, it's time to start considering other options. The first one certainly would be to try adding melatonin to your regimen. *Note:* Don't drop your 5-HTP or tryptophan, though, if you have low-serotonin moods. Take melatonin in addition. It might help to take your 5-HTP or tryptophan along with your melatonin, but only on alternate weeks.

Testing and Restoring Your Melatonin Levels

In addition to being a super soporific, melatonin is a powerful immune system–promoting antioxidant, which partly explains why so much healing occurs during sleep (melatonin levels are low in breast cancer victims, for example). To determine whether low melatonin levels are interfering with your sleep, order a home saliva testing kit (see the "Resource Tool Kit" on page 289). Saliva testing is very accurate and convenient. One of the benefits of testing your melatonin levels is that you get to find out about your immune system as well as your sleep system.

Test your melatonin levels either at bedtime, if you can't get to sleep, or whenever you wake up sleepless in the night. Some people need to test their levels day *and* night, something we suggest for clients who seem to have melatonin reversal—that is, are sleepy in the daytime and too wakeful at night. (You might be particularly apt to suffer from melatonin reversal if you live in a dark climate, especially if you don't have bright light during the day in your home or work environment.)

Melatonin typically comes in .5-milligram (half-milligram) to 3-milligram doses. Because too much leads to morning grogginess, I like to suggest starting with as small a dose as possible. Try half of a 1-milligram capsule or sublingual tablet (placed under your tongue) at bedtime by nine-thirty P.M. and see if you get quickly to sleep.

When it comes to dosing melatonin, there are no hard-and-fast rules. Researchers have actually found that melatonin can be effective, given *any* time between noon and nine, and in doses from .3 to 10 milligrams. I have seen that many different doses and kinds of melatonin supplements can be helpful. If taking melatonin right before your targeted bedtime doesn't get you to sleep, try adding 1 milligram or more of *time-release* melatonin, taken at eight P.M.

Melatonin is typically a short-term repair tool. Stop after a week to be sure you still need it or to see whether you can use less. Since you are now supplying your brain with more serotonin (via the 5-HTP or tryptophan you're taking along with your melatonin), you should soon be producing enough melatonin on your own to get ideal sleep.

Caution: Some depressed people become more depressed on melatonin.

More Ways to Enhance Melatonin

In addition to taking amino acids and/or melatonin supplements, there are other ways to raise your melatonin levels.

Avoid Melatonin's Enemies. It's important to keep from suppressing your melatonin production by avoiding melatonin's most common enemies.[6]

Caffeine
Tobacco
Alcohol (may get you to sleep but wakes you up in the night)
Chocolate (especially dark)
Aspirin, Tylenol

Most antidepressants like Prozac, tranquilizers, and sleep medications (all promote shallow, not deep, sleep)

B complex near bedtime (especially B_{12})

Being close to (within three feet of) electrical appliances (like electric blankets!)

Using Darkness and Light to Raise Your Melatonin. As the natural light around you dims in the afternoon, your body will try to increase its production of melatonin. Avoid exposure to bright light close to bedtime, as it could retard this melatonin production. The darker the better as the evening wears on. Ideally, your rooms should be lit by no more than a reading light (directed on the page, not in your eyes!) or TV light (unless you're like me and can't get to sleep after watching TV). We need to mimic, as much as possible, the natural awake-in-the-light/asleep-in-the-dark sleep rhythm we were designed for. Remember, electricity is a modern invention, the human being is not.

Here's a surprise. Even though bright light at night can diminish your melatonin production, if you are around bright light early in the day, your melatonin levels will rise higher at night.[7] When you can't get out in bright natural daytime light (by far the best kind), you can use 150- to 200-watt incandescent bulbs—or full-spectrum fluorescent lamps that supply 2,500 or more lux (equivalent of 150–200 watts). You'll need to be within three feet of this light for the full effect. (This is also a great way to survive the winter blues.) More on this in the final section of the chapter, when I describe how to adjust to shift work or time zone changes. See the "Resource Tool Kit" for lamp shopping suggestions.

THE STRESS-SLEEP CONNECTION AND THE TRANQUILIZING AMINO ACID GABA

If test results and/or your response to melatonin supplements and light therapy indicate that melatonin is *not* the problem, what else could it be? It could be an imbalance in your stress hormones that could be making you superalert just when you need to be winding down and getting to sleep.

When you're under stress, your adrenal glands produce stress-coping hormones, notably adrenaline, which gets you ready to "fight or flee," and cortisol, which keeps you alert and increases your stamina. If your adrenals are pumping these hormones day and night, you may be too revved up when it's time to wind down. If you have enough melatonin, it can help rebalance your nighttime stress chemistry, but only up to a point.

If excess stress is your problem, inciting the release of too much adrenaline and other overstimulating chemicals, you'll want to try the amino acid GABA. GABA can have a relaxing effect on your entire body because it can instantly neutralize the surge of stress chemicals, allowing you to drift off to stages one through five. It can be used alone or in combination with 5-HTP, tryptophan, or melatonin, since it affects entirely different but complementary brain and body functions. (I talk a lot about GABA in chapter 5, page 89.)

GABA supplements come in various strengths: 100 to 500 milligrams of GABA can be found alone or combined two with other calming aminos, L-taurine and L-glycine. GABA is available in doses up to 750 milligrams, but I suggest that you start with 100 milligrams and go up only if you need to. Too much GABA can sometimes have a reverse effect and agitate you. *Caution:* GABA lowers blood pressure a bit, so if your blood pressure is already low, be careful.

The popular homeopathic formula Calmes Forte can also have a soothing effect, and it's worth a try if stress is clearly the problem but GABA is not the answer for you.

Checking and Correcting Your Cortisol Levels

One of the primary stress-coping hormones produced by your adrenal glands is cortisol. It is an even more potent hormone in some ways than adrenaline, but it is not agitating. It's strengthening, even superstrengthening. It's your wake-up-and-tackle-life's-challenges hormone. Cortisol's levels are supposed to be highest in the morning and lowest between about midnight and three A.M. Under intense stress, though, cortisol stays high day and night, subsiding only when the stress is gone or your adrenals can no longer keep up the surge. If its levels are high at night, instead of low, as they're supposed to be, you'll be kept up too late with a "second wind."[8] Or your cortisol levels could rise too early in the morning and wake you up prematurely. (Sometimes levels have been high for so long that the body just forgets to shut them off, even when the stress is over.)

A simple one-day home saliva test will reveal your bedtime and early morning cortisol levels. See the "Adrenal Tool Kit" for details on testing the levels of this vital indicator to determine if any of the following cortisol imbalances are interfering with your sleep:

➤ Most of our clients have been exhausted by too much stress. Their cortisol levels in the morning, at noon, and in the late afternoon are on the low side (and that's how they feel). But their bedtime levels may still be surprisingly high. Even if they're in the normal range at bedtime, if these levels seem to be higher than the levels earlier in the day, they may keep rising in the night and wake them up at some point. If this is your case, and testing finds that your cortisol is above normal levels in the evening when it should be dropping to its lowest levels to allow melatonin to rise, then a supplement containing a cortisol-regulating nutrient called "phosphorylated serine" (brand name Seriphos, *not* the same as the more readily available phosphatidyl serine), taken before dinner (approximately six hours before bedtime), should get you to sleep. Take it again six hours before you would typically wake up in the night or early morning, if middle-of-the-night wake-ups are also a problem. Seriphos encourages your pituitary gland to stop sending the order for more cortisol. After a month or so, this message should be permanently programmed, and you should not need any more Seriphos. *Caution:* Do not take Seriphos for more than three months total. Take a break for at least a week after each month's use. You don't want to turn your cortisol levels down too low.

➤ If your early morning cortisol levels are high (or at least quite high compared to the rest of your day's output), they can wake you up too early. But don't use Seriphos until you've investigated *why* your body is raising the levels of its top stress fighter. Your body may be putting up a fight at that time of day for a very good reason, and you could be getting an important wake-up call here. The typical reasons for early morning struggles are explained in the "Adrenal Tool Kit." In our clinic's experience, they are usually reactions to some kind of chronic yeast or parasite infestation or, sometimes, a bacterial infection, as odd as that may sound. Sometimes, though, you just need a bedtime snack to keep your blood sugar from dropping in the night, triggering an inopportune cortisol release.

➤ If your cortisol levels are too high most of the day *and* at night, you'll need to turn to chapter 5, "All Stressed Out," to figure out *why* your body is fighting so hard and what hidden and/or obvious stressors may be the causes. You'll need to get rid of the cause(s) before you can calm your system enough to get it to sleep.

Retest your early morning and/or bedtime cortisol again (whichever was abnormally elevated) in three months to see if your levels have dropped to normal.

THE SEX HORMONE FACTOR

Your adrenal glands not only make stress hormones, they also make sex hormones, including sleep-regulating estrogen and progesterone. Adrenals exhausted by stress coping often make insufficient sex hormones, which can lead to sleep disturbance. This is typically a factor for women with menopausal and premenopausal sleep problems. But men can be affected as well:

➤ Especially in premenopause (also called "perimenopause") and menopause, a common sex-hormone-related sleep problem is *low estrogen*. Estrogen is needed in your brain to stimulate the activity of serotonin. Low levels of estrogen can result in low serotonin, which you now know often means reduced melatonin. We have seen remarkable and quick sleep improvement in women who got no help from any nutrient supplements and so decided to take an estrogen-stimulating herb like black cohosh or natural micronized estrogen. Estrogen augmentation can also help to subdue the hot flashes that can so easily interfere with sleep. One of our most anguished insomniacs tried every one of our natural remedies, to no avail. Finally we asked her to measure her sex hormones with a saliva test. She was in menopause, and her estrogen levels turned out to be extremely low. She responded instantly to a prescription of 17 beta-estradiol. (Estrogen, unlike progesterone, is available only by prescription.)

➤ *Low progesterone* can prevent the GABA supplies in your brain from activating, thus not allowing you to relax enough to get to sleep. This could happen to you if you are male, but it's more likely to happen to you if you are a female under 35. For example, a sudden drop in progesterone during the week before your period (when progesterone should be at its highest peak) can contribute to PMS insomnia. After prolonged stress, especially around the start of menopause, progesterone levels sometimes drop too low all the time.

You may need more estrogen or progesterone, or both, but you don't have to guess. Turn to the "Sex Hormone Tool Kit," page 329, for advice on assessing and correcting any sex hormone imbalances.

Note: Raised melatonin can suppress ovulation and vice versa![9]

ADD GOOD FOOD AND ADDITIONAL NUTRIENTS TO YOUR SLEEP STRATEGY

Poor Eating Habits

If you are not eating well, regularly, or enough, your blood sugar may drop sometime between bedtime and the early morning. This can set off a bodily alarm and an attendant rise in stimulating cortisol and adrenaline as they attempt to raise your blood sugar. It could wake you up when you should be sleeping. So try eating more protein and fat through the day. Both keep your blood sugar levels stable and your brain supplied with sleep-promoting nutrients. Don't skip meals, and try a bedtime snack that combines protein, fat, and carbs (for instance, full-fat yogurt and fruit, or leftovers).

Protein

You can become deficient in the amino acids tryptophan and GABA by not eating enough protein, so eat at least 20 grams (3–4 ounces, or a palm-of-your-hand-size portion) three times a day.

Calcium and Magnesium Deficiencies

The soothing and relaxing minerals calcium and magnesium need to be taken regularly as part of your basic supplement support program. Both encourage serotonin production, but the basic amounts, listed in chapter 10, may not be high enough for you. Try adding more at dinner or at bedtime. Some people find magnesium more sleep promoting than calcium, others vice versa. *Note:* If your bowels get too relaxed, you've taken too much magnesium. If increasing these two minerals does not help within a few days, go back to your basic dose. If they have a reverse, stimulating effect (rare, but possible), stop taking them at bedtime right away.

Restless Legs? Not Enough Folic Acid, Vitamin E, or Other Nutrients?

Restless legs may be keeping you awake, along with many pregnant women, many women over 65, and more men. If so, your troubles are probably over; folic acid or iron deficiency anemia is typically the cause, and either type is easy to correct.[10,11] Most of us are deficient in folic acid, which, in addition to calming restless legs, may be the single most good-mood-promoting vitamin of them all. Folic acid comes only in tiny doses, so you may have to take many pills a day, if your basic B vitamin supplement doesn't provide you with enough. Meanwhile, check your iron levels. Ask your doctor for both an iron and a ferritin (more sensitive iron) test. If the amount of iron in your basic minerals doesn't do the job, you can add more.

Vitamin E can also be a big help at 400 IU taken with meals twice a day (maximum 1,200 IU a day).[12] For some people taking more of the mineral magnesium, 200–600 mg in any form but citrate (unless you're constipated) is the key. For others, it's the amino acid glycine. Both are natural muscle relaxers.

Food Allergies or Toxic Exposure

Is reflux, asthma, or indigestion interfering with your sleep? Please read chapter 7, "Out with the Bad-Mood Foods." These problems are almost always caused by allergic reactions to certain foods. The most common culprits by far are made from wheat flour (for instance, bread, pasta, and cookies) and cow dairy products, like milk and cheese. We have also had a few clients with insomnia caused by exposure to excessive levels of mercury or other heavy metals. An inexpensive hair analysis backed up by a blood test can rule this out. (See the "Resource Tool Kit.")

THE THYROID CONNECTION

There are three kinds of thyroid malfunction, and all three could affect your sleep.

1. *Hypo*thyroidism can make you sleep either too little or too much. A slow thyroid gland can interfere with sleep in some people because it does not put out enough of the T_3 that allows the brain to produce serotonin and melatonin. I talk a lot about this most common of thyroid problems in chapter 4.

2. *Hyper*thyroidism, with its excessively high levels of thyroid hormones, can keep you hyperawake. It can get your heart palpitating, too. In fact, your whole system can be racing when this energizing gland is turned up too high. (Do you have a history of workaholism or partying all night?) This is called Graves' disease. Please get a complete thyroid checkup if you have these kinds of symptoms. (See the "Thyroid Tool Kit," page 306).

3. *Thyroiditis,* a condition in which your immune system attacks your thyroid, can also cause disturbed sleep as the thyroid gland struggles to do its job under siege. You may not have heard of this problem, but it is not uncommon. Thorough blood testing that includes two measures of the immune system's antithyroid antibodies is vital. Please see the "Thyroid Tool Kit" for more details.

ADVICE FOR SLEEP APNEA SUFFERERS

Do you fall asleep easily during the day but have trouble getting a good night's sleep? Do you snore or stop breathing while you sleep? One of the causes of sleep apnea is serotonin deficiency. Studies using the amino acids tryptophan and 5-HTP have shown them to be helpful. Why? First, serotonin directly affects the function of our lungs.[13,14] Second, lots of oxygen is required for serotonin production, so if physical obstructions block oxygen flow, serotonin production can be diminished. Third, if a preexisting low-serotonin condition caused characteristic afternoon and evening carbohydrate craving, increased weight could easily result, contributing to obstructed breathing. Regarding other solutions to sleep apnea that have been found helpful:

➤ Food allergies are a common cause of a stuffy nose. See chapter 7, "Out with the Bad-Mood Foods."

➤ Low thyroid conditions, known to cause sleep apnea (and unneeded weight gain), can be identified and addressed successfully using the information in the "Thyroid Tool Kit."

➤ Among women, apnea most commonly occurs during menopause. Low progesterone is often involved, and saliva testing will identify if treatment with supplemental natural progesterone will help.

➤ High levels of the stress-related chemicals cortisol and norepinephrine are often present in apnea, as in other sleep problems.

➤ Excessive weight gain could be caused by overeating triggered by a number of factors other than low serotonin. Please explore the "Food Craving Tool Kit" for details.

SHIFT WORKERS AND TIME ZONE SHIFTERS

Because of your work or travel schedule, you may have to be up at night and asleep during the day, and are understandably suffering from sleep deficits as a result. Here are some tips that can help. For the few night-shift workers who've come to our clinic, we've relied on the expertise of the director of the lab that we use to test melatonin levels, William Timmons, N.D., of BioHealth Diagnostics. He has worked successfully with shift workers for years and I'd like to pass on his recommendations to you:

1. Use whatever melatonin-producing sleep aids you find most helpful during the hour before you head off to sleep: 5-HTP, tryptophan, Saint-John's wort, and/or melatonin. Melatonin itself is usually needed, especially when sleep schedules first start to change. Take 1 to 10 milligrams immediate release and/or time released, as needed. If you wake up groggy, you've taken too much. Reduce the dosage the next "night."
2. No matter what time you need to get to bed, to allow for eight hours of sleep, you'll need to make the light in your bedroom mimic darkening natural light. You'll need lightproof shades and only a dim reading (or TV) light for at least the last hour before you should be asleep. If you need to go into the brighter rooms in the house or hotel for a few minutes during the last hour, it's okay. (It can take some people up to fifty minutes for melatonin to be shut off again by bright light, but others are affected in five minutes.)
3. Shift workers: Set a dawn simulator lamp to start half an hour before whatever time you need to wake up. It will gradually mimic the morning light and wake you up without the stress of an alarm (though you can use one of them if you need to).
4. As soon as you wake up, turn on bright light in all the rooms you'll be using, and make it full-spectrum light (available in 100-watt bulbs or fluorescent tubes), if possible. (Travelers, just open the curtains.) Eat a good meal within an hour.

5. If your workspace is brightly lit, fine. If not, wear a head lamp or take breaks in brightly lit places or under your own therapeutic lamp or light box whenever you can (preferably at least every forty-five minutes) to prevent melatonin levels from rising again.

6. When you get off shift, exercise and eat a good meal three hours before you need to be asleep. A snack before bed is fine.

7. As long as you go to sleep after it's been dark in your bedroom for at least an hour, it doesn't matter when you go to sleep, so you should be able to switch from artificial dark to natural dark on your "weekends" (or, for travelers, back at home). Melatonin can help here, too.

DESPERATE MEASURES: SLEEP AND DRUGS

Alcohol and drugs can stimulate temporary serotonin releases, improving your mood and, by enhancing the melatonin conversion process, helping you get to sleep. One study showed that a whole joint of marijuana could raise a man's melatonin levels 4,000 percent![15] (No wonder marijuana can make people so lethargic.)

But artificial boosts can never get melatonin or GABA to *stay* at optimal levels, as the nutrients can. If your basic levels of serotonin and melatonin are just too low, over time the drugs will reduce them further, until they quit working or make you totally drug-dependent. Alcohol, for example, actually reduces melatonin after a few hours and wakes up most drinkers in the night. Drugs cannot provide the deep restorative sleep stages or even the dream (REM) stages that are so vital. Pot, for example, thoroughly blocks REM sleep. Despite all this, if the natural methods just don't work for you, particularly while you're exploring factors like stress, thyroid, or sex hormone imbalances that may take some time to correct, you may need to consider taking medication. To increase your serotonin and melatonin levels at bedtime, you can, hopefully only briefly, use prescription medications such as Trazodone. To compensate for low GABA, more traditional (and addictive) sedatives are usually prescribed.

If you have become dependent on any sleep-promoting drug, please turn to chapter 13 for advice on how to withdraw comfortably and safely.

A C T I O N   S T E P S

Your basic supplements are described in chapter 10 and listed on page 202 in a daily schedule. This is followed by a list of all the special supplements recommended in every chapter of the book. Check off the special supplements that you'll need from the Action Steps below. Then transfer them to the master supplement schedule, pages 203–205. Check the "Caution Box" on pages 199–200 for any contraindications before you add amino acids or Saint-John's wort to your master schedule.

1. Try 50–150 milligrams 5-HTP or 500–1,500 milligrams tryptophan at bedtime. If one doesn't work, try the other. (Tryptophan can be ordered on-line [www.dietcure.com] or by calling our clinic's order line at 800-733-9293.) You may also need 50–100 milligrams 5-HTP or 500–1,000 milligrams tryptophan in the late afternoon to start building up your melatonin levels. If neither works, try Saint-John's wort: 300 milligrams midafternoon and 300–600 milligrams at bedtime. (Tinctures like Nature's Answer work best at one dropperful each time.)

2. If needed, next try melatonin itself *along with* your tryptophan or 5-HTP. (It sometimes helps to take the aminos only every *other* week.) Start with .5 milligram and go up to 10 milligrams, as needed. Use time-release melatonin if your bedtime dose does not stop you from waking up in the night or early morning. Take it for a week, then stop to see if you still need it. Cut your dose of melatonin if you start getting groggy in the morning or are having any other adverse reactions.

3. Be sure to get bright light during the day. Go outside in spring and summer. Especially in winter, if you can't get outside, get bright indoor light (from 150- to 200-watt incandescent bulbs or fluorescent bulbs of 2,500 lux, preferably full spectrum) to within three feet of where you are sitting. For light therapy sources, see the "Resource Tool Kit," page 289.

4. Be sure that you're taking all your basic supplements, including relaxing calcium (500–1,000 milligrams per day) and magnesium (300–1,200 milligrams per day). To see if you need extra calcium or magnesium, try an extra 300–500 milligrams of each at bedtime separately, to see which is most helpful. (They typically come together in cal/mag supplements with twice as much calcium as magnesium. Try extra magnesium if you use such a formula.)

5. Try 100–500 milligrams GABA alone, or try it in a formula that combines 100 milligrams GABA with taurine and glycine, like Amino Relaxers by Country Life or True Calm by NOW. Always start with 100 milligrams and increase gradually if necessary.
6. Try the easily found homeopathic formula Calmes Forte to disperse stress at bedtime.
7. For restless leg syndrome, if the amounts in your basic vitamin/minerals aren't high enough to stop the problem, test for iron or folic acid deficiency. If found, try up to 30 milligrams iron, e.g., Iron Complex by NOW, or 5 milligrams folic acid. Or add extra vitamin E (up to 1,200 IU, total, per day). Be sure to try magnesium (200–600 milligrams), as well as glycine (500–2,000 milligrams).

Troubleshooting If the Above Nutritional Steps Don't Work

1. Test the levels of your stress hormones. See the "Adrenal Tool Kit."
2. Test your sex hormone output. See the "Sex Hormone Tool Kit."
3. Check for and treat any imbalances in your thyroid function as per the "Thyroid Tool Kit."

RECOMMENDED READING

Reiter, Russel, Ph.D. *Melatonin* (New York: Bantam, 1996).

Murray, Michael, N.D. *5-HTP* (New York: Bantam, 1998).

CHAPTER 13

Nutritional Rehab

The Missing Key to a Successful Recovery from Addiction

Alcohol and drugs are the refuge of the false mood beset. If you have identified strongly with some of the symptoms in the Mood-Type Questionnaire, you're automatically a potential candidate for some kind of addiction.

Like most people who come to rely on addictive substances, you probably are using them to relieve very real biochemical mood problems, whether you know it or not. Do you use cocaine or amphetamines because you can't get yourself going in the morning and rarely have the natural enthusiasm or focus you need? Is alcohol or tobacco the only thing that will turn off the stress? Is using Xanax the only way you can survive your anxiety or insomnia? Are marijuana or heroin the only pleasures that can make your life worth living? Whether you're reading this chapter because of a major or a minor problem with chemicals like these, I can help you identify the underlying mood or energy deficits that have drawn you to them in the first place. More important, I can give you alternatives that will turn off your addictive cravings as they naturally restore your sense of well-being.

My suggestions are based on three decades of practice in the field of addiction treatment. After founding and directing a number of San Francisco Bay Area recovery programs over the past twenty-five years, I have become truly expert in distinguishing the treatment techniques that get results from those that don't. Like most recovery professionals, I have found that psychological and spiritual approaches are valuable in many ways, but I have *not* found them to be effective for eradicating addiction—unless they are combined with the nutritional rehabilitation. The good news is that programs providing this vital treatment component are quickly proliferating. But before I get into the exciting story of nutritional rehab, I want to introduce you to the biochemical core of your addiction.

ENTERING THE ADDICTED ZONE

You may be one of the people who never knew how badly they'd been feeling until they had their first drink or toke and felt good for the first time in their lives. Most of our addicted clients tell me that they didn't even necessarily use alcohol or drugs to get high. They just wanted to "feel normal."

Why? Because most addicts are born with subnormal moods. For example, anyone born into a family where alcohol, drugs, food addictions, and/or significant mood problems exist can easily inherit deficiencies in the production of the natural mood boosters produced by the brain. Most of the alcohol- and drug-addicted clients I have worked with have come from families where addiction *and* depression or other mood problems have been notable. In many cases, stressful childhoods have further depleted their genetically deficient mood chemistry. Finally, as almost all adolescents do now, they experimented with alcohol, marijuana, or other drugs. But they were the ones who could never stop.

NO EXIT: HOW TREATMENT FAILS

Most people who find themselves trapped in addiction have tried to quit many times. The trouble is, they haven't found an escape route, only dead end after dead end.

Don't be discouraged or ashamed if, like them, you've already tried treatment and Twelve Step programs and "failed." In fact, you should be proud of yourself for trying. I want you to know that about 90 percent of those who try to quit—even with the most intensive and long-term treatment—are unable to do so. If you're among them, it's not likely to be your motivation that's lacking. Rather, like most recovering people, you have probably never been exposed to anything beyond the standard psychological and spiritual approaches to recovery. These approaches are excellent—I consider them important elements of any effective recovery program. But they don't address the *primary* cause of addiction, which is *physical*, not psychological or spiritual. Unless a program treats the biological core of addiction, it becomes a setup for relapse, shame, and despair.

Before we go any further, I'd like to tell you more about my experience working in the treatment field and why I began looking for new answers. In 1974, I became one of the first professionally trained psychotherapists in the country to be hired to work in a recovery home for alcoholics. Along with several other graduate psychology students, I started work at a treatment program in a beautiful four-story mansion in San Francisco. At the time, there was no treatment anywhere as we've come to know it. Alcoholics Anonymous was the only formal support available.

Our clients were workingmen of all ages and backgrounds who came "home" at night to eat together and attend Twelve Step meetings. They also met in informal support groups several times a week, but the director wanted to bring in professionals to develop more intensive therapeutic programs. We were free to experiment with *any* treatment techniques that might help. I'm proud to say that, among other things, we instituted the first family therapy programs, the first adolescent programs, and the first food addiction treatment programs in Northern California.

At the time, we thought that addictive cravings and mood swings were caused exclusively by emotional trauma or passed on from addicted fathers or mothers, who served as role models for this behavior. It followed logically that the new, humanistic psychotherapy techniques were the answer, and at first they really appeared to be working. There was no question that our counseling and education programs, combined with Twelve Step meetings, were helping to heal even the deepest childhood trauma and were making our clients more honest and open people. And there was no doubt that our programs helped them work things out with their spouses, children, and other family members.

For all its psychological victories, though, this approach was *not* helping many people overcome their cravings for drugs and alcohol. And it wasn't just our program that was failing; relapse rates were rising across America. As new addictive drugs like cocaine, crack, stronger marijuana, pills of all kinds, and heroin became widely available, relapse rates went up to 90 percent and higher. And they've stayed there ever since, despite all the creative effort and hard work of treatment professionals and the courage and commitment of their addicted clients.

This 90 percent figure is the inside story. It is the figure that all the treatment program directors I know of admit to. Some tell me their relapse rates are even higher.

The Biology of Relapse

If you have struggled with addiction and actually achieved periods of recovery, you know how good that can look from the outside. You work harder, you make it to more of your children's ball games, and you're more loving to your wife or husband. *But you don't feel good.* Your inner life stays unhappy no matter how happy your circumstances and the people you love become. Eventually that inner unhappiness drives you back to the relief of alcohol or drugs. If your outer circumstances—your work, home, family, and relationships—are also unhappy or stressful, relapse can happen faster, but 90 percent or more of all addicts relapse, regardless of

> their circumstances;
> which drugs they've used;
> how much they want to stay sober and clean.

Does relapse happen because of a fatally addictive, flawed personality? No! A forty-year Harvard University study disposed of that myth in 1983.[1] In studying six hundred men over the years, they found that there was no such thing as an addictive personality. *Any* personality type could become addicted. But there was an addic*ted* personality, one that could develop as people came "under the influence." The same study found that the addicted personality eventually disappeared in those who were able to stay sober.

So, if the reason people turn to drugs or alcohol is not because of an addictive personality, what can it be? Is it growing up in an addicted or otherwise disturbing or abusive family? No again. I remember how shocked I was when I first read the studies showing that children of nonalcoholic biological parents who were adopted into alcoholic families did not tend to become alcoholic themselves. But here's where it got even more interesting: Children born to alcoholic biological parents, adopted at birth into nonalcoholic families, *did* become alcoholic, at exactly the same rate as children of alcoholic parents who were raised by their biological parents. What this means is that it's not your upbringing that drives you to addiction as much as your genes—your inherited brain and body chemistries.

Scientists are now mapping the genes that predispose us to addiction just as they're mapping the genes that predispose us to heart disease and cancer. Not surprisingly, the key genes in addiction are the ones that program our brain's mood functions. If they are faulty, they can program deficiencies in particular brain sites that result in certain built-in bad-mood states. Depending on whether you've inherited deficiencies in serotonin, norepinephrine, endorphin, and/or GABA, you'll be attracted to drugs that affect that particular deficiency zone (or zones). If you don't correct these underlying biological malfunctions, you can't fully recover from your addiction.

SEARCHING FOR NUTRITIONAL RECOVERY

Of course, back in the 1970s, when gene mapping was still mere science fiction, the biological causes of addiction remained very much a mystery. Yet I had a nagging feeling that some factor was being overlooked. I thought I had found it in 1979 when I read Dr. James Milam's famous book *Under the Influence*, in which he reported that more than 95 percent of alcoholics had very low blood sugar levels (were hypoglycemic) and that sweet and starchy foods affected them just like alcohol. Milam reported that these carbs gave them a pleasant rush, followed by a mood crash and cravings for more. Milam ran an inpatient program and found that his recovering clients greatly benefited from being fed a diet that eliminated sweets and most white-flour starches. Our outpatient clinic started giving the same dietary recommendations in 1980 and saw some equally exciting results. Some of our clients were finally able to beat their addictions once they began cleaning up their diets. Much to our frustration, however, we were not successful with everyone. Inexplicably, the majority of our clients were simply unable to give up sweets, starches, and caffeine, no matter how hard they tried. Their depressions and mood swings continued—along with their new food addictions—all clearly contributing to their eventual relapses into alcohol and drug use.

THE AMINO CAVALRY ARRIVES

In 1986, I came across the work of addiction and genetics researcher Kenneth Blum, Ph.D., who had developed strategies to correct addictive brain patterns using certain proteins, or amino acids, in the form of supplements and had impressive clinical studies to back them up.

At the same time, I learned about the work of Joan Mathews-Larson, author of the marvelous book *7 Weeks to Sobriety*, who was successfully using Blum's methods and other nutritional strategies in her outpatient alcoholism recovery clinic in Minneapolis. At my direction, my nutritionist, a Ph.D. with both clinical and research skills, designed a trial program of amino acid therapy for our clients.

I will never forget the first time we ever used the amino acids. My client, James, a postal worker, was about to lose his job and family because of addiction to crack cocaine. He'd already been in an inpatient treatment program, but, like *more than 90 percent* of crack addicts, he relapsed immediately after leaving it.

James, along with his wife and parents, participated in our outpatient program of individual, group, and family counseling. He also went to Cocaine Anonymous and Narcotics Anonymous meetings and had a sponsor. But he could not stay clean.

He ate well most of the time and liked to work out, though, like most recovering addicts, he overate sweets when he was off drugs. We asked him if he'd like to try something new to help with his drug (and sweets) cravings and the low energy and depression he experienced when he wasn't on crack. He was desperate to quit and happy to agree. In fact, he was intrigued, because he had been an athlete and had used amino acids for muscle building. In addition to a multi-vitamin/mineral supplement, we gave James three amino acids to be taken between meals, three times a day. A week later, James came back to report in—totally clean for the first time in months.

Frankly, we hadn't expected much, so the story that he told us was astounding. He'd gone to work a few days after starting his amino regimen and was given the worst possible assignment—driving a truck to San Jose, an hour away, with his drug-using buddy. As soon as they were out of the yard, his buddy showed him a joint of "caviar" (a crack-and-marijuana combination that James usually found irresistible). James broke out in a cold sweat, fearing he'd smoke it, get caught, and be fired. Ten minutes later, he suddenly realized that he'd forgotten that his friend had drugs in the cab at all! He really wasn't tempted, so he didn't use, either that day or for another month. That was a miracle for him.

When he did use drugs a month later, it was because he'd gotten depressed, suddenly, after drinking what he thought was a harmless 7UP at a party. That taught him what a potent drug sugar could be for him. It picked up his mood and energy briefly, then dropped him into a danger-ous depression very fast, one that he needed cocaine to "fix."

James became the first of many addicts to beat the statistics by taking a few amino acids and other nutrients and eating healthy food—added to a program of good counseling and Twelve Step support. (A nice bonus of nutritional recovery is that since it eliminates interest in sweets and starches as well as alcohol and drugs, our recovering clients no longer gain up to thirty pounds in their first month of sobriety.)

Holistic Recovery: Finding Emotional, Spiritual, *and* Physical Support

I recommend that you get all the support you possibly can: group, family, and individual counseling, education, Twelve Step meetings, and, of course, nutritional rehabilitation. You and the people close to you deserve all the help you can get to heal the damage caused by the ordeals associ-ated with addiction—physical, emotional, financial, and otherwise. Your life may need to be completely overhauled, and that can't be done with-out help. Most treatment programs still provide only the standard emo-tional and spiritual recovery tools, but there are a growing number of nutritionally sophisticated programs opening up all over the country. I list them in the Action Steps at the end of this chapter.

You may need inpatient care. Some standard residential programs will cooperate with you, if you bring in your own supplements and re-quest high-quality food. Unfortunately, others will actively discourage you from pursuing nutritional recovery. If possible, find a program that is at least neutral about the inclusion of a nutritional component in your treatment plan, but try to get permission *in writing* from the program director to bring in *unopened* bottles of supplements before you commit yourself. If you just can't find a treatment program that will allow you to take supplements, you can still try to eat well, and you can take advantage of the psychological and spiritual help available. Just start your nutritional recovery work the minute you get out.

If you can find an outpatient program that can provide enough support, staff members typically don't care what your nutritional habits are, but don't be surprised if they don't share your enthusiasm.

NUTRITIONAL REHAB: GETTING STARTED

To start your own nutritional recovery program, I'd like you to ask yourself the same two basic questions that we ask at our clinic. This will help you figure out which of your four mood-enhancing brain chemicals are deficient and which nutrients will do the best job of restoring them.

1. What are the substances you turn to regularly to alter your moods? List them all. No matter how minor they may seem, each can tell part of the story: coffee? diet soda? chocolate? bread? chips? cigarettes? wine? marijuana? cocaine? Xanax? Vicodin? . . .
2. What do you get from these substances? In what way do you feel better after you've used them? Exactly what mood states are you using them to relieve or change?

The point is not to focus on your negative behaviors or the negative feelings you may feel or express when you're under the influence. What you're looking for now is the *positive* influence these drugs have at least on your inner experience of yourself. The fact is that you use them to feel *better*, not to wreck your life or anyone else's. Don't let shame keep you from exploring why you use them. Get input from the people you're close to, if you're able to be open at this point about your problem with addiction.

It doesn't matter, at first, which specific mood-coping substance is your problem. What matters is *how that substance changes your mood chemistry.* Does it give you a lift, an energy surge? Does it give you confidence or a sense of humor? Does it relax you, take the edge off, or allow you to go to sleep?

Following is a modified version of the Mood-Type Questionnaire from chapter 2. Look closely at the list of false mood symptoms again and then check off the substances that you use to relieve those symptoms in the next column. Then note the amino acids and other nutrients in the third column that can eliminate the false moods and the need for mood-altering substances.

PART 1. UNDER A DARK CLOUD?

Which of the following negative symptoms do you use addictive substances to relieve?	Which substances make those symptoms go away?	Nutrients that can help:
❏ negativity, depression with dark thoughts	❏ sweets	5-HTP
❏ worried, anxious, shy	❏ starches	L-tryptophan
❏ low self-esteem	❏ fatty foods (chips, milk, eggs)	Saint-John's wort
❏ obsessive thoughts	❏ chocolate	melatonin
❏ obsessive behaviors	❏ alcohol	
❏ SAD (fall/winter depression)	❏ marijuana	
❏ PMS moodiness	❏ tobacco	
❏ irritable, impatient, angry	❏ Ecstasy	
❏ panic/anxiety attacks; PTSD	❏ other _____	
❏ phobias		
❏ hate hot weather		
❏ night owl		
❏ insomnia		
❏ find relief from the above symptoms in exercise		
❏ fibromyalgia, TMJ		
❏ have or have had suicidal thoughts and/or plans		

continued

PART 2. DRAGGING YOURSELF THROUGH LIFE?

Which of the following negative symptoms do you use addictive substances to relieve?	Which substances make those symptoms go away?	Nutrients that can help:
❏ depression: the flat, bored, "blah" kind	❏ sugar	L-tyrosine
❏ lack of physical or mental energy	❏ chocolate	L-phenylalanine
	❏ caffeine	SAM-e
❏ lack of drive, enthusiasm	❏ aspartame (NutraSweet)	omega-3 fats
❏ difficulty focusing, concentrating	❏ alcohol	
	❏ cocaine	
❏ need a lot of sleep, slow to wake up	❏ other uppers	
	❏ marijuana	
❏ easily chilled, cold hands or feet	❏ tobacco	
	❏ other _____	
❏ tend to put on weight too easily		

continued

PART 3. ADDICTED TO PAINKILLERS?

Which of the following negative symptoms do you use addictive substances to relieve?	Which substances make those symptoms go away?	Nutrients that can help:
❑ very sensitive to emotional and sometimes physical pain	❑ sweets	DL-phenylalanine (DLPA)
❑ tear up or cry easily (e.g., in movies or during commercials)	❑ starches	D-phenylalanine (DPA)
	❑ chocolate	
	❑ alcohol or tobacco	B vitamins
	❑ heroin	vitamin C
❑ avoid dealing with painful issues	❑ marijuana	magnesium
	❑ other _____	5-HTP
❑ find it hard to get over losses or get through grieving		
❑ crave pleasure, comfort, reward, enjoyment, or numbing		

continued

PART 4. ADDICTED TO "DOWNERS"?

Which of the following negative symptoms do you use addictive substances to relieve?	*Which substances make those symptoms go away?*	*Nutrients that can help:*
❏ driven, overworked, pressured, too many deadlines	❏ sweets	GABA
	❏ starches	
	❏ alcohol	taurine
❏ have trouble relaxing or loosening up	❏ tobacco	glycine
	❏ marijuana	
❏ tend to be stiff, uptight, tense	❏ Valium or other tranquilizers	glutamine
		chromium
❏ easily upset or frustrated, snappy	❏ painkillers	
	❏ other _____	adrenal support
❏ easily overwhelmed, just can't get it all done		
❏ weak, shaky at times		
❏ sensitive to bright light, noise, odors		
❏ use smoking, drinking, eating, or drugs to relax, calm down		
❏ worse if you skip meals or go too long without eating		

Some substances, like Xanax or crack, have very limited and predictable effects. But consider marijuana: it has a reputation for pleasure enhancing and for slowing us down, mellowing us out, and putting us to sleep (or knocking us out with its now mammoth THC content). But when I asked the 300 participants at an international Marijuana Anonymous conference how many of them used marijuana for its "mellowing" effect, only half of the hands came up. The other 150 marijuana addicts had depended on marijuana for its *stimulating* effects. They'd done their laundry on it. It had helped them focus on projects or even exercise! So among the suggestions that follow, look into the downer, the upper, or the painkiller sections, depending on which effect(s) marijuana has on you.

Alcohol is another drug that can do anything: put you dancing up on tables or put you in the recliner in front of the TV, or both. Like marijuana, alcohol can also be an effective painkiller. *Tobacco* can do it all, too. Even stimulants like Ritalin or amphetamine can calm some people while they stimulate others.

It always goes back to the same crucial question: "How do your favorite substances make *you* feel?" They're your favorites for a real reason, a powerful reason. Don't dismiss your need for them as just self-indulgence or weak willpower. Really think about that "buzz" or "high," and put more words to it. The symptom questionnaire will help, so work with it carefully to find out what is *really* involved in your addiction. If you're addicted to more than one drug, or use substances that can have more than one brain effect, you'll probably need more than one set of supplements. It's very common, for example, to use one set of supplements for stimulation in the morning *and* another set of supplements later in the day for relaxation. One set takes care of the biochemical deficiencies that drew you to drugs like coffee or speed in the morning, while the other set corrects the deficiencies that drew you to alcohol at night.

NUTRITIONAL REHAB OVERVIEW: A RECOVERY DIET PLUS SUPPLEMENTS

Before you start on any aminos, be clear on what your entire nutritional recovery program will look like. Don't minimize the importance of the right foods and the basic supplements.

Junk Food vs. Recovery Food

Please *memorize* both the bad-mood foods and the good-mood foods in chapters 7 and 8. Replacing bad-mood junk foods with good-mood healthy foods is vital if you are to stay in and enjoy recovery. Sweets, refined starches, and unhealthy fats can all have druglike effects on your brain that can contribute hugely to unstable moods and relapse. Because they're really more like drugs than foods, they can addict you accordingly. If this is a major problem for you, see the "Food Craving Tool Kit" for specific advice about food addiction. Otherwise, just turn to chapter 8 for suggestions. *Hint:* Have at least three meals a day that include eggs, chicken, fish, meat, fresh vegetables, butter, and olive oil—then add some fresh fruit, beans, or whole grains, as needed.

No Food vs. Recovery Food

I have seen more relapses caused by skipped meals than by any other single thing. If you don't plan your day's food in advance—all three meals, plus healthy snacks—you can count on the kinds of bad moods that can lead to relapse, often that very day. If you drink coffee in the morning, you'll likely kill your appetite and skip breakfast, so please quit coffee or switch to decaf and taper off, but whatever you do, don't use caffeine *before* you eat breakfast (or any other meals).

Using Nutrient Supplements for Recovery

➤ Addiction depletes you badly. You'll need all of the basic nutrients to build yourself back up again. The basics are spelled out in chapter 10, on page 202.

➤ In addition, go over the specific suggestions in every section of this chapter that relates to you and your particular addiction, whether they apply to uppers, downers, painkillers, or some combination of the three. Then identify your individual nutrient protocol in the Action Steps at the end of this chapter by checking off the specific supplements you'll need to use.

➤ Over the next six to twelve months, you'll use the amino acids and the other special nutrients indicated to gradually restore whichever brain and body functions your alcohol or drug use has been targeting.

➤ You may need some additional nutrients over the short term, during your first two weeks of detox, particularly with alcohol, opiates, or tranquilizers, where a more severe detox reaction can be expected. You'll need medical backup, too, if you'll be detoxing from tranquilizers or heavy alcohol use, to be safe from potential seizures. You'll always need liver support from marvelous milk thistle supplements.

ESCAPING YOUR DOWNER ADDICTION

Which drugs do you use to calm down, to relax, to sleep, to stop a panic attack? Alcohol, marijuana, tobacco, Valium, Xanax, Ativan? Alcohol and prescription tranquilizers can be dangerous to detox from. Please see a "detox doc" for medical supervision and a medical taper. See the "Detox Box" in this chapter and be sure to read about dealing with stress chemistry in chapter 5, and consult the pertinent recommended books listed on page 286 before you actually detox from these drugs or alcohol. Also, see the special notes on alcohol, marijuana, and tobacco on page 271.

Note: Withdrawal from prolonged tranquilizer use can be long, complex and treacherous, with many unpredictable physical and emotional

---

Your Downer Recovery Protocol

➤ Try GABA, 100–500 mg between meals, four times a day. Try a formula combining GABA with the other soothing, anti-seizure aminos—taurine and glycine—such as True Calm by NOW or Amino Relaxers by Country Life. These are low potency, though, so you'll probably need to start with 4 or 5 capsules or tablets at a time. GABA is available alone in 500 mg tablets. See what combination works best for you.

➤ You may also need 5-HTP or tryptophan. Read chapter 3 to learn about how low serotonin can cause anxiety of all kinds (including panic) and sleeplessness.

➤ Use 3–6 mg of melatonin if sleep is a problem and the above aminos do not get you to sleep.

➤ Experiment with extra magnesium to help relax your system (with albion-chelated magnesium from Carlson or Solgar, you won't get loose bowels even at doses over 800 mg).

symptoms, including panic and suicidal impulses. If oral amino acids do not substantially relieve your symptoms, try to work with one of the detox treatment providers listed later in the chapter who uses intravenous (I.V.) amino acids and high dose vitamin C. Also, be sure to read Ashton's and Trickett's recommended books on how to most successfully taper off of these drugs.

Eileen's Story

We used to be justifiably scared by the reputation of Valium and Xanax for long, dangerous withdrawals. But a 75-year-old beauty taught us that, surprisingly often, we had nothing to fear. Eileen had been addicted to Xanax for four years. Her doctor would not take her off it for fear of withdrawal seizures, though she complained of the awful effects it was having on her: she was always dropping things, she couldn't drive, and the quality of her sleep (the original reason she had been put on Xanax) had grown worse than ever. Although Xanax initially boosts the levels of the brain's natural tranquilizer, GABA, it often ends up depleting it. This was obviously what had happened to Eileen. She was miserable. After straightening out her diet and building her up for a few months with the basic nutrients, we had her detoxed and sleeping comfortably on her own in less than a week on a supplement that combined the relaxing (or inhibitory) amino acids GABA, taurine, and L-glycine. GABA and taurine specifically can protect against brain seizure, the greatest danger in withdrawal from these kinds of drugs.

We had a knowledgeable doctor standing by with a prescription for a different tranquilizer in case we got into trouble as she tapered off of Xanax. But we never needed the help. Over a period of seven days, he lowered her dose of Xanax while she took increasing doses of the three-amino blend four times a day. The first night, Eileen didn't sleep at all, as expected. The second night, she got a little restless sleep. But the third night, she slept for four hours and said it was the best sleep she'd had in years. From there on, it was clear sailing as her Xanax dose dropped lower and lower and her sleep got better and better. She quit dropping things. Best of all, she started driving again, something she'd had to stop because of Xanax's side effects. Eileen stayed on her amino acid blend for a few months, in a gradually diminishing dose, until she didn't need them at all. That was ten years ago, and she's still sleeping and driving perfectly.

Troubleshooting: Check Your Adrenal and Thyroid Functions and Rule Out Pyroluria

If GABA and the other recommended supplements don't eliminate your problem quickly, read chapter 5, test your levels of adrenal stress hormones and build yourself up as needed, using the protocol in the "Adrenal Tool Kit" on page 317. You might also need to check your thyroid. The "Thyroid Tool Kit" will tell you how. An impaired thyroid can prevent the aminos from working and sometimes even trigger anxiety and panic attacks. If stress, anxiety, and inner tension have long been part of your false mood picture, you may also have a genetic condition called pyroluria that blocks the absorption of key nutrients to the brain. I discuss it on pages 303–305, where you'll find a symptom questionnaire and the nutritional suggestions for correcting this problem that affects over 40 percent of alcoholics.

ESCAPING STIMULANT ADDICTION

What drugs do you use for a lift, to raise your spirits and energy, to help you focus? Do you favor caffeine, cocaine, speed, diet pills, Wellbutrin, Phentermine, marijuana, alcohol, tobacco? There's a whole chapter (chapter 4) on why you may have been drawn to those stimulants in the first place. You should read it before you prepare for detox.

The most well-known stimulants have no dangerous withdrawal symptoms, yet cocaine, crack, and/or speed are called hard drugs because they can be so hard to quit, anyway. Many addicts can't even make it through thirty days in an inpatient treatment program without them. In a local residential program for crack-addicted women with children, only 1 out of 250 were able to stay clean.

This exceptionally high failure rate can be attributed to the fact that cocaine and amphetamines have such an overwhelming impact on our energy chemistry. The crash that tends to drive so many recovering stimulant addicts into relapse comes from a sudden, critical depletion of their naturally stimulating brain chemicals. In the course of the addiction, the levels of these *natural* stimulants, the catecholamines, have been exhausted after a period of overactivity forced by cocaine or speed. (And chances are their levels weren't that swift to begin with.) Detoxing from these drugs leaves the brain and body on empty. *No* gas. That's why recovering people are so tired and need to sleep a lot at first. Their bodies badly crave some form of artificial stimulation to keep going, so they turn to

Your Stimulant Recovery Protocol

The key: 1,000–2,000 mg L-tyrosine, three times per day, between meals, starting the minute you wake up.

Some people do better with a combination of 500–1,000 mg L-tyrosine and 500–1,000 mg L-phenylalanine. (Try True Energy by NOW for a combination formula.) See what works best for you. You'll also want to increase your energizing omega-3 fish oil supplement dose by at least 1 capsule with each meal beyond the basic dose. Last, add SAM-e, a brain chemical that is often depleted in stimulant addicts.

	AM	B	MM	L	MA	D
L-tyrosine 500 mg or	2–4		2–4		2–4	
L-phenylalanine 400–500 mg or combine the above	2–4		2–4		2–4	
Omega-3 fish oil 300 mg DHA/EPA (1–2 in addition to your basic dose)		3–4		3–4		3–4
SAM-e 200 mg	4		4			
Milk thistle 300 mg		1				1

coffee, tobacco, and sugar, all of which will deplete them even further after giving brief bursts of relief. Depression and exhaustion continue, with the added burdens of increased weight.

Fortunately, the exhausted brain can quickly absorb the amino supplements tyrosine (and L-phenylalanine) to create, once again, its own natural supply of stimulation. With amino acids and the basic vitamins, minerals, and fatty acids, the crash usually dissolves along with the cravings, typically on the first day.

Raymond Brown, Ph.D., a San Francisco psychologist and addiction specialist, conducted a study in 1989 comparing groups of cocaine addicts who had been given an amino acid formula high in tyrosine and L-phenylalanine with those who got no amino acid supplementation. The results were dramatic: The success rate after ten weeks for those on the amino acid formula was 80 percent; for those not on aminos, it was 13 percent! Says Brown, "I would never again try to work with addicts without amino acids."[2]

Troubleshooting: Check Your Thyroid and Adrenal Functions and Consider the Possible Role of Food Allergy

If tyrosine and the other supplements listed above don't work for you, what's the problem and what can you do? You need to figure out why your energy was sagging in the first place. Why were you drawn to uppers rather than to downers? Please see chapter 4 for a complete rundown. Here I'd just like to summarize the most common underlying causes of energy problems.

1. The need for stimulants often signals a thyroid and/or adrenal deficiency problem. Stimulant drugs can do some of the same things that thyroid and/or adrenal hormones are supposed to do: they speed up metabolism in the body and the brain. Detailed directions for testing and treating low thyroid and/or adrenal function can be found in the "Thyroid Tool Kit" and the "Adrenal Tool Kit."
2. Intolerance to certain grains is another common cause of low energy and depression, often dating back to childhood, that can underlie stimulant drug addiction. As part of your detox, go off foods made from the grains wheat, rye, oats, and barley for two weeks, then eat lots of them again on day fifteen. If your energy improves when you're not eating the bread and pasta but drops dramatically when you're back on them again on day fifteen, I recommend that you stay off these grains permanently. (See chapter 7 for more on testing for this exhausting food reaction.)

ESCAPING PAINKILLER ADDICTION

Whether it's chocolate, alcohol,[3] marijuana,[4] tobacco,[5] codeine, Vicodin, heroin, or methadone you're using, your preexisting biochemical inability to tolerate pain and discomfort is where your need for these drugs most likely started. Chapter 6, "Too Sensitive to Life's Pain?," is all about the endorphins, your natural painkillers—the ones that your painkilling drugs work by overstimulating. I want you to get very familiar with that chapter.

At our clinic, we have worked with many clients who, needing release from physical and/or emotional pain, became addicted to alcohol or drugs. Obviously, some painkillers are easier to part with than others.

Heroin and, particularly, methadone are the most difficult drugs to detox from of any I've ever encountered. Nutritional supplements and a healthy diet (as soon as you can eat) can improve the nasty withdrawal from these

---

Escaping Painkillers

I advise the following supplements and guidelines for recovering from all types of painkiller addiction:

1,000 mg vitamin C powder or capsules, taken to bowel tolerance* and 400 mg magnesium four times a day† (for the worst days in week one only)

	AM	MM	MA	BT
GABA 500 mg (week one only)	2	2	2	2

	AM	MM	MA	BT
DLPA 500 mg	4	4	4	

	AM	MM	MA	BT
If DLPA makes you at all tense or jittery, substitute D-phenylalanine 500 mg	2	2	2	1

	AM	MM	MA	BT
5-HTP 50 mg	1–2	1–2	2	2–3

	AM	MM	MA	BT
Freeform amino acid blend 700–800 mg	3	3		

Test adrenal function (see the "Adrenal Tool Kit"). If it is low, begin ear acupuncture before detox, to prevent more severe and prolonged withdrawal reactions.

---

*Bowel tolerance means start with 5 grams every hour until you get diarrhea.
† Relaxing magnesium can loosen bowels at high doses, use albion-chelated magnesium by Solgar or Carlson to avoid this.

two drugs, and drugs like them, but it won't eliminate it. The drug buprenorphine can be used successfully as a taper (through a detox doc). Although there are some legal restrictions to its use, I have seen it work very well, and a group of U.S. detox docs has lobbied successfully to ease the legislative roadblocks. But by far the best detox results from the use of IV aminos. Be sure to see the "Detox Box" in this chapter for more on this and other suggestions for withdrawal.

The first few days and nights are inevitably tough. *GABA* is probably the most helpful amino during these early days. It relieves some of the anxiety and muscle cramping. *DLPA* (or the less stimulating *DPA*) builds up your brain's endorphin (natural opiate) levels, while *5-HTP* can help with both endorphin boosting and sleep. Another aid is high-dose *vitamin C*. At high enough doses, vitamin C (like DPA) can inactivate the enzyme that breaks down endorphin. In a study comparing it with conventional detox methods, 50 percent of heroin addicts on vitamin C had only mild detox symptoms, and only 15 percent had severe symptoms. Of the C-less group, 57 percent had severe symptoms, and only 7 percent experienced mild symptoms.[6] *Acupuncture* is also famous for increasing endorphins and helping with opiate recovery especially after detox is over (though 20 percent may be resistant to its effects).[7]

➤ Because it takes fifteen to nineteen amino acids to create the endorphins and enkephalins, another very helpful supplement is a blend of amino acids that quickly supplies the brain and body with many easily assimilated building blocks. Look for a formula that contains at least nine of the essential freeform amino acids, from which the total twenty-two can be produced. Take them for the first month or so of recovery, longer if you need to.

Troubleshooting: Physical Pain, Psychological Pain, Adrenal Exhaustion, and Other Concerns

➤ If you are suffering from chronic physical pain, more than nutritional help is needed, though building up your natural painkiller levels will help enormously. One of our clients had been an athlete all his life. By age 65, he was suffering constant pain in his knees and hips from overdoing it. His use of prescription painkillers had been creeping up for three years. However, when he started taking the amino acid DLPA, he was able to cut his Vicodin in half the first week. He was able gradually to reduce it further over the next few months, until he had successful knee surgery. Every night after surgery, the DLPA kept him from going back to a high dose of Vicodin, and later, with the cause of the pain reduced by the surgery, he was able to go off the Vicodin altogether.

➤ To get through severe psychological pain, you'll need regular, ongoing counseling. The best place to start is in a good twenty-eight-day intensive treatment program. Most severe Vicodin, heroin, and methadone addicts will want inpatient support through the withdrawal process and to get immediate help with any psychological pain that may arise when the drugs are removed. See suggestions in Action Steps at the end of the chapter.

➤ If you're suffering from adrenal exhaustion and the intolerable accompanying feeling of being overwhelmed, you must test and repair your adrenals' ability to handle stress, or you won't be able to tolerate life without drugs. Please study the "Adrenal Tool Kit" for help in what may be a crucial recovery project.

➤ If you are a driving type A but have low pain tolerance and possibly suicidal depressions, please rule out the possibility that you have overly high histamine levels by getting a blood histamine level test. Our clinic rarely sees this type, but you'll find good information on it in Joan Mathews-Larson's book *7 Weeks to Sobriety*.

➤ Narcotics Anonymous meetings, particularly in big cities, are filling up with a new kind of heroin addict, lured by the drug's capacity to provide painless weight loss. If you are using opiates for weight loss, please get *The Diet Cure* and read it right away. Without the motivation to stop dieting, and some healthy but effective alternative ways to stop overeating, if that is your problem, you won't be ready to detox.

SPECIAL CONSIDERATIONS FOR RECOVERY FROM ALCOHOL, MARIJUANA, AND TOBACCO

Alcohol

Whatever your use of alcohol, the key to recovery involves figuring out exactly how alcohol is "working" for you. Is it an upper (a stimulant or antidepressant)? Is it a downer (a stress reliever, relaxant, sedative, or sleep promoter)? Is it a physical or emotional painkiller? Or is it all three? Alcohol's ability to affect many parts of the brain and body is extraordinary. That's why it's been so popular for so many thousands of years. If you're using alcohol to boost more than one of your brain's mood-enhancing chemicals, you'll want to identify all the nutrients you'll need and take them all together right from the start. Many people take all four of the amino acids that feed the four major neurotransmitters. How many of the sections on the Mood-Type Questionnaire did you check off? Review the suggestions in all relevant sections of this chapter (recapped in the Action Steps) and put all the supplement recommendations together on your blank master supplement schedule on pages 202–205 in chapter 10. For example, if you use alcohol both to relax and to kill pain, you'll want to put both GABA and DLPA (or DPA, if you tend to be hyper) on your list. You might also need to include 5-HTP, if sleep is a problem. If alcohol gives you some needed energy, you might need tyrosine in the morning, too. You'll also need to consider some other key nutrients in addition to your basics.

For excellent information on nutritional recovery for alcoholics, read *7 Weeks to Sobriety* by Joan Mathews-Larson. For example, Dr. Larson alerted our clinic to the fact that 44 percent of alcoholics have a condition called pyroluria, which can block the benefits of certain nutrients; see page 303.

The Blood Sugar Stabilizing Program

Another of the primary reasons people get addicted to alcohol is that their blood sugar levels tend to drop too low, too often. Over 95 percent of alcoholics are hypoglycemic.[8] When they experience a drop in blood sugar, the code red "get a drink" signal turns on as the brain begins to fail from lack of fuel. No amount of willpower alone can turn it off. Reversing hypoglycemia is a vital job if you're going successfully to escape alcoholism.

Alcohol acts just like sugar biochemically, only more so. It contains more calories per gram, and it gets into your bloodstream faster. For people whose blood sugar levels tend to be low, this can be irresistible. Fortunately, your brain can also burn the amino acid glutamine for instant relief, but instead of causing toxic addiction, glutamine is actually good for you. We recommend that alcoholics take glutamine between meals to keep their blood sugar stable (and their cravings at bay) throughout the day and evening. It tastes slightly sweet, so in a pinch, if an alcohol craving appears unexpectedly or you've skipped a meal or forgotten to take your supplements, you can just open up a capsule of glutamine and let it dissolve under your tongue. The large blood vessels there will pick it up and deliver it ASAP to quiet things down in your brain. Glutamine also benefits your liver and your digestive tract, both common targets of alcohol toxicity.

The mineral *chromium* is another blood sugar stabilizer. Both chromium and the aminos are deficient in most alcoholics, as is *zinc,* a mineral crucial for your brain function. *Zinc* is also required for a normal appetite, something many alcoholics lose along the way. You'll need a good appetite to enjoy the healthy foods you're going to be eating. (Without three good meals a day plus snacks, you won't be able to keep your blood sugar stable and your cravings subdued.) These two supplements will help stop your cravings, not only for alcohol, but for sweets and starches too. (Sorry, no white-flour pasta, bread, bagels, and so on. You might as well pick up a beer!)

The Omega-3 Fats, DHA, and EPA

Alcoholics start out depleted in omega-3 fats. Without them, they often become depressed, use alcohol for temporary relief, become addicted, get more depleted and depressed, and crave more alcohol! Heredity can be a major factor here: Do you come from people who inhabited the shorelines of cold northern waters? Do you have Scandinavian, Irish, Scottish, Welsh, or Native American ancestry? Japanese or other northern Asian coastal ancestry? If so, you are likely to have a hereditary need for the vital omega-3 fats that can be found only in fish. You may lack the enzyme that can convert other omega-3-rich foods, like flaxseeds, into the EPA and DHA constituents found directly in fish oil. If so, you are doubly in need of fish oil supplements. Be sure to take the basic fish oil recommendations in chapter 10. For a few months, you might need to take extra fish oil. (If this higher dose overstimulates you, cut back to the basic dose.)

Food Allergy or Yeast Overgrowth

Grain-based beers and liquors can become irresistible for people with allergies to the grains wheat, rye, oats, and barley. If you also crave bread, pasta, and the like, allergy addiction is even more likely a possibility. Avoiding certain grain-based foods as well as alcohol may be an essential part of a successful recovery effort. In chapter 7, I discuss the grain allergy issue and how to do a home test to see if it's a problem for you.

If you've had a history of antibiotic use, you may have developed an overgrowth of yeast as a result. Following is a list of the most common symptoms of yeast overgrowth. Since yeast feeds on alcohol, as well as on sugar and high-starch foods, you may need to kill it off to stop the cravings. Medications like Diflucan can do it, and there are natural yeast-killing regimens available as well. Protocols should always include the daily use of good bacteria like acidophilus and bifidus. See the Action Steps at the end of this chapter for specific yeast-killing suggestions.

➤ Crave alcohol, sweets, and/or high-starch foods.
➤ Often feel bloated, with abdominal distension (especially after eating above substances).
➤ Are foggy headed.
➤ Feel depressed.
➤ Suffer from yeast infections.
➤ Used antibiotics extensively (at any time in life).
➤ Used cortisone or birth control pills for more than one year.
➤ Have chronic fungus on nails or skin, or have athlete's foot.
➤ Experienced recurring sinus or ear infections as an adult or child.
➤ Have itching around the groin, vagina, or anus.

SAM-e
SAM-e levels are low in many alcoholics. If you still feel depressed and crave alcohol after two weeks on nutritional rehab, try 800 milligrams, twice a day, for one bottle. If it helps, cut the dose in half and use more as long as you need to—until going off it does not bring on cravings.

Troubleshooting: Adrenals, Thyroid, or Pyroluria
➤ Your stress-coping adrenal glands may be shot. Alcohol forces a temporary release of stress-coping adrenal hormones, which may be one key reason that you need it. Be sure to read chapter 5 to explore this potentially important issue.
➤ If alcohol gives you a lift, don't forget to check chapter 4 to explore whether your thyroid, which should be giving you a natural lift, needs some help that will relieve you of your need for alcohol.
➤ More than 40 percent of alcoholics may have a condition called pyroluria, whose unusual symptoms are listed on pages 303–305 along with treatment suggestions.

Marijuana

If you find yourself getting defensive about your marijuana use and dismissing its darker addictive side, just remember that marijuana growing is no longer a cottage industry. It is one of the biggest and most profitable businesses on earth. It drives one hundred pot-heads a month to the detox center at the Haight Clinic in San Francisco, begging for help in escaping from their "natural" drug. Marijuana is not a natural plant now. It's been hybridized to a potency thousands of times greater than it had in the early 1960s, when it really was just a "weed."

Just as many people can drink alcohol without getting addicted, many people are also able to smoke some marijuana without getting addicted. But, particularly if you come from an addictive family, you may have the gene that makes any strictly social use of marijuana—as well as alcohol or any other drug—impossible. Marijuana addiction is common. Chapters of Marijuana Anonymous have sprung up all in the past fifteen years. You may be able to find meetings near you, and you'll find good information by going on-line, www.marijuana-anonymous.org.

Marijuana's most potent, mood-altering ingredient, THC (tetrahydrocannabinol), is fat-soluble; it lodges in the fatty cell walls of your brain cells and lingers in your body longer than other drugs or alcohol. This means that marijuana can significantly alter your brain and your mood even between highs. This is why people can have consistent personality changes after they start smoking marijuana but have no awareness of it. The tendency for marijuana to store and build up in your brain means that if you've been a heavy marijuana smoker, it can take a year or more to get marijuana completely out of your system and get you back to your real self. The fog will clear only gradually. Be patient. My client Zack, who had smoked marijuana daily from the time he was 12, took nine months to function at his peak. During his first month off, he didn't crave marijuana anymore, but he still couldn't stick with a job, although he stayed marijuana-free, attended Twelve Step meetings and counseling, and did nutritional repair work. At three months, he started junior college, and though his grades were mediocre, for the first time in years he completed a quarter! He finished the next quarter, too, and actually got decent grades. In his third quarter, he got all As. His brain was back.

Some marijuana addicts go into withdrawal mode right away. Others take longer, as the drug gradually leaves its sites in the brain and body.

Zack had a detox experience with night sweats and insomnia, but not until ten days after he quit smoking marijuana.

Since marijuana concentrates in the cell walls all over the brain, it can affect any and all neurotransmitters. To choose the best supplements for you, take those that relate directly to the reason you smoke. Do you use marijuana for energy, to relax, to kill pain, or for all three reasons? Use any of the nutritional protocols that apply to you in this chapter, whether for upper, downer, painkiller addiction, or all three.

At the clinic, we saw a couple who had smoked lots of marijuana together for years. She was overweight and lethargic and used marijuana for energy, while her husband was hyper and driven and used it to calm down. She lost her marijuana cravings on naturally energizing L-tyrosine, and he lost his on the relaxing GABA/taurine/glycine supplement called True Calm. In addition to taking supplements and making dietary improvements, try to exercise and use a sauna to stimulate more sweat, because sweating will speed up the detox process through your skin (an organ that rids the body of toxins, very much like the liver).

Tobacco

I have found the drug tobacco to be one of the fiercest and most complex addictors of all. Again, as is true for marijuana, huge corporate financial resources have gone into making tobacco ever more addictive, increasing both the nicotine and the sugar content of this formerly "natural" drug. Sweeteners account for the majority of a cigarette's additives. Other additives include arsenic and other poisonous chemicals.

In deadliness, tobacco far exceeds heroin and cocaine. It kills ninety thousand smokers per year in the U.K. Because we at the clinic regard tobacco as such a formidable drug, we often wait one to three months before withdrawing addicts from it completely. During this detox preparation period, we build up our clients physically so that they can develop the physiological strength to successfully withstand withdrawal. Age and length of use are key factors. At our outpatient clinic, we regularly detox smokers under age 30 in one month or less. A smoker in his or her 60s, with severe health problems and a history of drug addiction and poor nutrition, can take six months to detox. If you go into an inpatient facility, though, consider giving up tobacco while you are freeing yourself of your other addictions. Research tells us that quitting tobacco while you are going off other drugs improves your chances of recovery. See if you can find programs that are smoke-free.

To conquer your own tobacco addiction once and for all, you'll need to address the most common co-addictors, sugar and caffeine. At the clinic, we treat them in combination as one drug. All three destabilize blood sugar levels, forcing adrenaline and endorphin releases. Serotonin, norepinephrine, and other crucial brain chemicals are also typically depleted by this trio. Please be sure to know your mood type(s)—are you using tobacco as an upper, a downer, a painkiller, or all three? Consult any of the sections in this chapter that apply to you, to gather appropriate supplement resources for your particular detox. Choosing the right amino supplements for detox is a matter of determining what you get from using tobacco and its co-drugs. Is tobacco a *stimulant* for you? If so, as you withdraw from it, does depression set in? Or does tobacco function mainly as a *tranquilizer* for you, making you feel calmer when you smoke and anxious and stressed when you try to quit? Or does tobacco both speed you up *and* slow you down? If so, your detox supplement plan will be more extensive as you follow both the upper and downer protocols.

If you use tobacco to deal with stress, I advise you to check out your adrenal function right away. The adrenals are often exhausted in tobacco addicts, and restoring their proper functioning is crucial to a successful detox. If you can't handle stress without tobacco, you won't be able to stay off it. If supplements like GABA don't do the trick, be sure to read chapter 5 on stress recovery and test your adrenal function as per the "Adrenal Tool Kit," page 317.

Before you actually stop using tobacco, begin the detox process by eliminating your intake of caffeine, sugar, and any other drugs or alcohol as you start taking your nutritional supplements, eating a recovery diet, and exercising regularly. Sugar cravings lead to most of the weight gain that people commonly experience when they stop smoking, but with this detox program, those cravings usually disappear by day two. If your weight does rise, it should drop again within six months. If it doesn't, check your thyroid function as per the "Thyroid Tool Kit." Caffeine cravings and headaches might take a few more days to eliminate. By the time you go on to eliminate your tobacco use, your cravings for tobacco will also have been reduced. At our clinic, the tobacco detox clients who follow this program are surprised to find that within a few weeks, they are reaching for fewer cigarettes without any conscious effort. The single most successful amino acid protocol we've used combines 1,000 milligrams of enlivening tyrosine,

1,000 milligrams of soothing taurine, and 1,000 milligrams of blood sugar–stabilizing glutamine taken before breakfast, midmorning, and late afternoon.

Hypnotherapy can be an effective tool in withdrawal from tobacco use. We have found that three sessions, on days one, three, and seven of the actual tobacco withdrawal week, have been very useful to most of our clients. These sessions target the behavior patterns associated with smoking and create new ones. Combining hypnotherapy with nutritional therapy can make all the difference for those who are struggling with stubborn tobacco habits. *Acupuncture* detox using ear points and large needles can also be helpful.

DETOX TECHNIQUES FOR DIFFICULT DRUG WITHDRAWALS

➤ *Medication.* If you've had seizures when you've tried to stop drinking alcohol in the past or have been drinking very heavily for some time without a break, see a doctor for help with a taper on tranquilizers to prevent this most dangerous detox symptom. Ditto for tranquilizers, the only dangerous detox other than alcohol detox.

➤ *IV Amino Acid Drips.* When we see someone who cannot be withdrawn safely or relatively comfortably from a drug by using oral amino acids and other supplements, we suggest they look into the only safe and comfortable detox we know of, an intravenous drip of amino acids and other nutrients developed by Nobel Prize–winning physician William Hitt, M.D. A 35-year-old man addicted to the potent tranquilizer Klonopin could not be detoxed at all, even in a hospital, until he was given aminos intravenously at the Hitt Clinic in Tijuana, Mexico, the world's first intravenous amino acid detox facility. Three years later, the man was still Klonopin-free. He'd suffered almost no discomfort while receiving amino acids six hours a day through an intravenous drip for ten days. His mother, who had taken him down to the clinic, confirmed the story. Since then, I've heard many similar stories from people who have been to the Hitt Clinic. Its success with notoriously difficult-to-detox-from drugs like methadone and Klonopin is extraordinary. The procedure provides many times more aminos than can be absorbed orally and

The Detox Box

Here is a list of natural strategies you can use at home to help you through the discomforts of early withdrawal from opiates and benzo-diazepines (and alcohol, if needed). Do not go through a potentially dangerous detox without medical backup and reliable people in the house with you.

➤ Two baths per day for three to four days, then once a day, until detox discomfort is over.
  1. Epsom salts (4 cups per bath).
  2. Digestive enzymes (open 4 capsules of digestive enzymes, or 2 enzyme teabags into hot bathwater).
  3. 3 droppers of kava extract if you feel agitated.
  4. 2 bags of Detox Tea by Traditional Medicinals.
  Baths are not only soothing, they help your skin detox along with your liver and reduce the overacidity of your body, which causes much of the distress in detox. Scrub well under a shower afterward.
➤ Take Alka-Seltzer Gold to further alkalinize (deacidify) your system.
➤ If you have, or can find, a holistic doctor who is set up to administer IV drips, ask for daily infusions of vitamins and minerals for your first week of detox with lots of extra vitamin C. The "Meyers cocktail" is a good basic recipe that such doctors are familiar with. Otherwise take vitamin C ascorbate, 1,000 mg per hour, powder or capsules, to bowel tolerance (until your bowels become loose).
➤ GABA 500 mg capsules (1–2 at a time) as needed, up to four times a day, specifically to help with early detox symptoms (anxiety, cramping, and insomnia). *Watch for blood pressure drops if you get too much GABA.*
➤ Noni juice (medicinal juice from a tropical fruit)—2 tablespoons (it's nasty tasting), then 1 tablespoon every four hours until detox is over.
➤ Daily massage.
➤ Ear acupuncture: raises endorphin levels and reduces some of the early, and lots of the later, detox discomfort.

also includes many vitamins and minerals that also make detox easier. This procedure has been available only at Dr. Hitt's clinic in Mexico, across the border from San Diego—until recently. But now it's also available in clinics in Beverly Hills (310-724-6300), New Orleans (985-645-0045), Phoenix (602-808-0030), and Fort Lauderdale (954-714-9155). Call 800-287-0906 for information on other U.S. IV detox sites.

➤ See the Resource Tool Kit for UK detox support on page 289.

Treatment Resources

Harmony Devon

Coombe House, Coleford, Crediton, Devon, EX17 5BY,
tel: +44 (0) 1363 85023, e-mail:
harmonydevon@harmonyrehab.com,
www.harmonyrehab.com

Provides a holistic recovery process up to 90 days in length including healthful gourmet meals and nutrient supplement programs individually designed by their nutritionist.

Medical and psychiatric consultation and extensive counselling and educational programs also provided in a beautiful setting.

Twelve Step Programs

Alcoholics Anonymous
PO Box 1, Stonebow House, Stonebow, York Yo1 7NJ, tel: 01904 644026,
www.alcoholics-anonymous.org.uk

Narcotics Anonymous
202 City Road, London, EC1V 2PH, tel: 020 7251 4007,
e-mail: ukso@ukna.org, www.ukna.org, Helpline: 020 7730 0009
or e-mail: helpline@ukna.org

Marijuana Anonymous
Tel: 020 7565 5663 or www.marijuana-anonymous.org

ACTION STEPS

Your basic supplements are described in chapter 10 and listed on page 202, in a daily schedule. This is followed by a list of all the special supplements recommended in every chapter of the book. Check off the special supplements that you'll need from the Action Steps below to create a master supplement schedule for your whole personal mood cure program. For any contraindications, see the "Caution Box" on pages 199–200 before you add any amino acids, Saint-John's wort, or SAM-e to your master schedule.

Detox Support Suggestions

➤ See "Detox Box," page 279, for home detox suggestions.
➤ Get medical monitoring from a detox doc for withdrawal from tranquilizers or alcohol or for a buprenorphine taper from opiates, if needed. To find a detox doc, look in the Yellow Pages under "Physicians" for addictionologists or physicians with a specialty in addiction and recovery.
➤ Also look on the web for details of detox treatment centers in the U.K. The European Association for the Treatment of Addiction (EATA) has an on-line directory of treatment services, counsellors and links to other useful U.K. organizations and helplines—European Association for the Treatment of Addiction (UK), Waterbridge House, 32–36 Loman St, London SE1 0EE, tel: 020 7922 8753, e-mail: secretariat@eata.org.uk, www.eata.org.uk

Nutritional Supplement Protocols

In addition to the basic supplements already listed on page 202 on your blank supplement schedule, add the following supplements appropriate for you:

The Downer (Tranquilizer) Protocol

❑ *Consult a physician regarding the safety of detox and a planned taper, if needed.*

	AM	B	MM	L	MA	D	BT*
❑ True Calm by NOW, or Amino Relaxers by Country Life (100 mg GABA combined with L-taurine and L-glycine)	1–4		1–4		1–4		1–4
❑ Add GABA 500 mg, as needed (e.g., at bedtime for sleep)			1		1		1
❑ Extra magnesium (200 mg)	1–2		1–2		1–2		1–2
❑ If sleep is still a problem, try 50 mg 5-HTP and/or melatonin 3 mg, at bedtime					1–2		1–2
❑ Milk thistle 300 mg		1				1	

*AM=on arising; B=with breakfast; MM=midmorning; L=with lunch; MA=midafternoon; D=with dinner; BT=at bedtime.

The Upper (Stimulant) Protocol

	AM	B	MM	L	MA	D	BT*
❏ L-tyrosine 500 mg	2–4		2–4		2–4		
L-phenylalanine 400–500 mg	1–2		1–2		1–2		
Or a combination of L-tyrosine and L-phenylalanine	2–4		2–4		2–4		
❏ Milk thistle 300 mg		1				1	
❏ Omega-3 fish oil 500 mg DHA/EPA (1 per meal in addition to your basic dose)		3		3		3	
❏ SAM-e, if above doesn't relieve depression		800		800			

*AM=on arising; B=with breakfast; MM=midmorning; L=with lunch; MA=midafternoon; D=with dinner; BT=at bedtime.

The Painkiller Protocol

Detox: See the "Detox Box," page 279.

❏ Extra vitamin C week one only. Take more than your basic dose of vitamin C as per the "Detox Box"

❏ Extra magnesium, 200–400 mg as needed

❏ GABA, 500 mg in week one, take as per the "Detox Box," then as needed

	AM	B	MM	L	MA	D	BT*
❏ DLPA (DL-phenylalanine) 500 mg		4		4		4	
❏ If DLPA makes you tense or jittery, use DPA (D-phenylalanine) 500 mg	1–2		1–2		1–2		1–2
(Order hard-to-find DPA at 800-733-9293)							*continued*

---

*AM=on arising; B=with breakfast; MM=midmorning; L=with lunch; MA=midafternoon; D=with dinner; BT=at bedtime.

	AM	B	MM	L	MA	D	BT*
❏ 5-HTP 50 mg	1–2†		1–2†		2†		2–3†
❏ B complex 50 mg			1†		1†		
❏ Milk thistle 300 mg		1				1	
❏ Freeform amino acid blend 700–800 mg	3		3				
❏ Ear acupuncture for as long as needed							

---

*AM=on arising; B=with breakfast; MM=midmorning; L=with lunch; MA=midafternoon; D=with dinner; BT=at bedtime.
†For the first week only.

The Alcohol Protocol

Consult a detox specialist (M.D. or otherwise) regarding detox safety before you stop drinking, especially if you have ever had seizures when stopping in the past.

	AM	B	MM	L	MA	D	BT*
❑ Glutamine 500 mg	2–3		2–3		2–3		2–3
❑ Chromium† 200 mcg	1		1		1		1
❑ Omega-3 fish oil 500 mg DHA/EPA (cut back if sleep is affected)		2–3		2–3		2–3	
❑ Milk thistle 300 mg		1				1	
❑ Zinc 50 mg		1				1	
❑ SAM-e, if above doesn't relieve depression		800		800			

*AM=on arising; B=with breakfast; MM=midmorning; L=with lunch; MA=midafternoon; D=with dinner; BT=at bedtime.
†Not needed if your basic multi is NOW True Balance.

The Yeast Protocol

➤ Call our order line (800-733-9293) for information on how to kill yeast naturally and which supplements you'll need.

➤ A health practitioner can order a stool or blood test to measure your levels of yeast and yeast antibodies. A medication such as nystatin or Diflucan can also kill yeast effectively. (Diflucan is hard on the liver.)

The Tobacco Protocol

Add hypnotherapy or ear acupuncture to whichever other supplements your detox nutritional protocol calls for.

Troubleshooting for All Recovery Efforts

➤ If you do not get the serenity, stamina, and energy you need to free yourself of alcohol or drug cravings by following the above suggestions, check your adrenal and thyroid functions (see chapter 5 and the thyroid section in chapter 4). Test and treat as needed, using the "Adrenal Tool Kit" and "Thyroid Tool Kit" at the back of the book. Opiate addicts in particular should test their adrenal function and, if it is low, should begin adrenal restoration ASAP (before detox, if possible) to prevent more severe and prolonged withdrawal reactions.

RECOMMENDED READING

Mathews-Larson, Joan, Ph.D. *7 Weeks to Sobriety* (New York: Fawcett Columbine, rev. ed., 1997).

Grant, Charles, M.D. *End Your Addiction NOW* (New York: Warner Books, 2002).

Ketcham, Katherine, William F. Asbury, Mel Schulstad, and Arthur P. Ciaramicoli. *Beyond the Influence: Understanding and Defeating Alcoholism* (New York: Bantam Doubleday Dell, 2000).

Blum, Kenneth, Ph.D., and Payne, James. *Alcohol and the Addictive Brain* (New York: The Free Press, 1991).

Miller, David, M. A. *Overload: Attention Deficit Disorder and the Addictive Brain* (Duarte, Calif.: Hope Press, 2000, www.hopepress.com).

Trickett, Shirley, *Free Yourself from Tranquilizers and Sleeping Pills* (Berkeley, Calif.: Ulysses Press, 1997).

Ashton, C. Heather, *Benzodiazepines: How They Work and How to Withdraw* (Boston: Benzodiazepine Awareness Network, 2002, www.benzo.org.uk).

The
Mood Cure
Tool Kits

Resource Tool Kit

Finding Practitioners, Testing, Supplements, Special Foods, Products, and Services

Medical Help

Look for holistically oriented doctors, D.O.'s (osteopathic physicians who have an M.D. equivalent plus special skills adjusting the body), nurse practitioners, and physician's assistants (both have M.D. privileges). *Note:* Holistically oriented physicians have a wide variety of approaches to medicine. They may or may not wish to cooperate with the Mood Cure suggestions. Interview carefully to make sure that the practitioner you are considering is familiar with the thyroid testing or other medical help you're looking for. In addition to the following referral organizations, the Yellow Pages (paper or on-line) under "Physician," "Nutrition," or "Holistic" will often yield clues. Another good source of leads is your local health store personnel.

➤ **British Holistic Medical Association (BHMA):** 59 Lansdowne Place, Hove, E. Sussex BN3 1FL, tel: 01273 72 5951.

Acupuncturists

These doctors of Chinese or Japanese medicine cannot prescribe medicine, but they may use saliva testing, and they certainly use needles and often herbs and supplements to balance adrenal and sex hormones and help many other problems. Check the Yellow Pages and look for an experienced practitioner (more than ten years) with some training in China, if possible.

➤ **British Acupuncture Council, The:** 63 Jeddo Road, London W12 9HQ, tel: 020 8735 0400.

Holistic Nutritionists*

Avoid nutritionists who rely on fasting or vegetarian diets. Look for someone who is familiar with the use of amino acids.

➤ **The Nutrition Clinic:** 1 Harley Street, London W1G 9QD, tel: 020 7589 4394, fax: 020 7589 9186, e-mail: antony@thenutritionclinic.com, www.thenutritionclinic.com. Clinic specialising in the use of nutritional treatment of mood disorders in line with the approach used in this book. Experienced in the use of diet therapy, amino acid therapy, vitamins, minerals and essential fatty acids and other remedies to combat stress-induced conditions. All supplements detailed in *The Mood Cure* that are available in the UK are available via The Nutrition Clinic.

➤ **British Association of Nutritional Therapists (BANT):** 27 Old Gloucester Street, London WC1 3XX, tel/fax: 0870 742 150, www.bant.org.uk.

➤ **The Food and Mood Project:** PO Box 2737, Lemes BN7. Set up by Mind, the mental health charity, to help people explore the relationship between what they eat and how they feel. To arrange a consultation at one of the clinics in Brighton or Lewis contact: Amanda Geary, tel: 01273 478108, e-mail: amanda.geary@foodandmood.org. For details of their newsletter, lectures, workshops, and on-line support groups visit: www.foodandmood.org

➤ **British Society for Allergy & Environmental & Nutritional Medicine (BSAENM):** for publications—PO Box 28, Totton, Southampton, Hants SO24 2ZA, tel: 02380 812124; for information—PO Box 7, Knighton LD7 1WT, tel: 0906 302 0010.

---

*As distinct from registered dietitians, who are not well versed in the holistic approaches.

Practitioners of All Kinds Who Use Nutrients for Mood Problems

➣ **Society for Complimentary Medicine:** 3 Spanish Place, London W1U 3HX, tel: 020 7487 4334.
➣ **Centre for Traditional Chinese Medicine, The:** 78 Haverstock Hill, London NW3 2BE, tel: 020 7284 2898.
➣ **British Homeopathic Association, The:** 15 Clerkenwell Close, London EC1R 0AA, tel: 020 7566 7800, www.trusthomeopathy.org.
➣ **The College of Homeopathy:** 32 Welbeck Street, London W1G 8EU, tel: 020 7487 4322.

Nutrition Education

➣ **The Institute for Optimum Nutrition (ION):** 13 Blades Court, Deodar Road, Putney, London SW15 2NU, tel: 020 8877 9993. (Founder Patrick Holford has written extensively on mood and nutrition.)
➣ **Centre for Nutrition Education:** Suite 1, Dudley House, High Street, Bracknell RG12 1LL, tel/fax: 01344 360 033, www.ns3.co.uk, e-mail: enquiries@ns3.co.uk.
➣ **Plasket Nutritional Medicine College:** 14 Southgate Chambers, Launceston, Cornwall PL15 9DY, tel: 01566 77 37 31, www.pnmcollege.com.
➣ **Raworth Centre, The:** 20-26 South Street, Dorking, Surrey RH4 2HQ, tel: 01306 742 150, www.raworth.com.
➣ **Food Mood Project:** (see page 290).

Holistic Clinics That Treat Mood Problems

➣ **The Nutrition Clinic:** 1 Harley Street, London W1G 9QD, tel: 020 7589 4394, fax: 020 7589 9186, e-mail: antony@thenutritionclinic.com, www.thenutritionclinic.com. (see page 290).
➣ **The Breakspear Hospital:** Hertfordshire House, Wood Lane, Paradise, Hemel Hempstead HP2 4FD, tel: 01442 261 333. International environmental treatment unit for laboratory diganosis of chemical poisoning and environmental illness, and medically supervised nutritional detox programmes.

➤ **Harmony Devon:** Coombe House, Coleford, Crediton, Devon, EX17 5BY, UK, tel: 01363 85023, e-mail: harmonydevon@harmonyrehab.com, www.harmonyrehab.com. Provides a holistic addiction recovery process up to 90 days in length including healthful gourmet meals and nutrient supplement programs individually designed by their nutritionist. Medical and psychiatric consultation and extensive counselling and educational programs also provided in a beautiful setting.

TESTING LABS

The following labs are great sources of testing of all kinds, referrals to practitioners in your area who use their testing and consultation services, and treatment information for practitioners. Most of these labs will work with a wide variety of practitioners, including nutritionists, acupuncturists, chiropractors, and naturopathic doctors.

➤ **Individual Wellbeing Diagnostic Laboratory:** 1 Cadogan Gardens, London SW3 2RJ, tel: 020 7730 7010, www.iwdl.net. Offer a range of tests including salivary adrenal testing, blood thyroid profile, and food intolerance tests.

➤ **Great Smokies Diagnostic Laboratory:** Health Interlink Ltd, Interlink House, Unit B Asfordby Business Park, Welby, Melton Mowbray, Leicestershire LE14 3JL, tel: 01664 810 011, fax: 01664 810 012, www.health-interlink.co.uk. All tests need to be authorised and requested by a practitioner. Call to find the nearest practitioner to you who is experienced in the use of their testing.

➤ **Biolab:** The Stone House, Weymouth Street, London W1N 3FF, tel: 020 7636 5959. All tests need to be authorised by a medical doctor. One of the foremost labs in the world for nutrient level testing.

➤ **The Doctors Laboratory:** 58 Wimpole Street, London W1M 8LQ, tel: 020 7460 4800, www.tdlplc.co.uk. Offer a wide range of tests. All tests need to be authorised and requested by a practitioner.

➤ **ALCAT (UK) Ltd:** Centenary Business Centre, Hammond Close, Nuneaton, Warwickshire CV11 6RY, tel: 024 76 320 333, fax: 024 76 320 444. Offer comprehensive and accurate food intolerance testing, which requires blood sample.

➤ **York Nutritional Laboratory:** Murton Way, Osbaldwick, York
YO19 5US, tel: 07904 690640, www.allergy-testing.com. Provides
allergy-testing service by post.

Testing for Vitamin D Levels

Blood Test. Available through physician's order. Ask for the 25 (OH)D test,
also called 25 hydroxy OHD (*not* the 125 OHD test).
Saliva Test. Contact Diagnos-Tech's (www.diagnostechs.com) to order a
home testing kit.

Allergy Testing

There are a few testing methods that we use when allergy symptoms persist even after the most common allergens have been tested by elimination
and challenge. None are perfect.

➤ **ALCAT.** This blood test seems to give somewhat more accurate
results than other allergy blood tests.
➤ **Great Smokies Diagnostic Laboratory:** Comprehensive antibody
assessment (blood test) shows fairly good accuracy. (See contact info
above.)
➤ **Applied kinesiology.** A muscle test developed by chiropractors, this
test can determine if your muscle strength declines when you are
exposed to certain foods. Many kinds of holistic practitioners can test
you this way.

SUPPLEMENTS

Sources for Most Supplements Mentioned in
The Mood Cure

➤ Your local health store and many drugstores.
➤ Recovery Systems (my clinic) order line: 800-733-9293 or
www.moodcure.com.
➤ **The Nutri Centre:** 7 Park Crescent, London W1N 3HE,
tel: 020 7436 5122. Shop stocks or can order the supplements
mentioned in this book. Also available by mail order.

➤ **Nutri-Link Ltd:** 24 Torquay Road, Newton Abbot, Devon TQ12 1AJ, tel: 01626 205 417, fax: 01626 205 418. Stocks a vast majority of supplements mentioned in the book.

➤ **The Nutrition Clinic:** 1 Harley Street, London W1G 9QD, tel: 020 7589 4394, fax: 020 7589 9186, e-mail: antony@thenutritionclinic.com, www.thenutritionclinic.com. Supplies all supplements detailed in *The Mood Cure* that are available in the UK.

Yeast or Parasite Elimination Supplements

➤ Call our order line for the tests and supplements used at my clinic: 800-733-9293 or consult an experienced alternative health practitioner.

➤ Always retest after your elimination program is complete.

Zinc Status by Ethical Nutrients

➤ Available through most health food stores or order lines. (Zinc Tally by Metagenics, the same supplement by a different name, may be ordered from our order line or from any private practitioners who carry supplements.)

Vitamin D from Fish Oil Source

➤ Solgar or Carlson Labs, 1,000 IU (the one you want has a *small* amount of vitamin A listed on back of the label but is not an A and D supplement).

Omega-3 Fish Oil

Some sources:

➤ Carlson's Super DHA has 700mg DHA/EPA per cap.

➤ NOW's Super EPA has 600 DHA/EPA per cap.

➤ Best buy is Kirkland Fish Oil (300 mg DHA/EPA per cap).

Herbs for Menopausal Symptoms

➤ Change-O-Life by Nature's Way or other herbal formulas that emphasize black cohosh, for relief of hot flashes and the like.

L-Tryptophan

➣ Recovery Systems order line: 800-733-9293 or www.moodcure.com.
➣ Bios Biochemicals: 800-404-8185; www.biochemicals.com.

THERAPEUTIC LAMPS

You can buy full-spectrum lamps in a variety of desk or floor models, or you can buy bulbs to replace those in your current fixtures from one of the following outlets or your local hardware or health store. ParaLite, Verilux Happy Eyes, and Ott-Lite are just a few of the brand names in full-spectrum lighting. You can also make your own therapeutic light using two or three full-spectrum regular incandescent bulbs (at least 100-watt equivalent each). *Note:* If you have significant mood swings, especially if you know that you are bi-polar, do not use the 10,000 lux light boxes and use even the lower light sources very carefully. Bright light can set off manic (hyper, irritable) moods.

➣ The Combo Box by American Environmental is the brightest and safest light we could find. It contains both 3000 lux full spectrum tubes and 10,000 lux narrow spectrum tubes. Order it through NEEDS (www.needs.com).
➣ The Healthy House, Cold Harbour, Ruscombe, Stroud, Glos, GL6 6DA, tel: 01453 752216, fax: 01453 753533, www.healthy-house.co.uk.

FOODS AND SOURCES

Protein Powder

Be sure that each tablespoon contains 12 or more grams of protein. Egg, whey, or rice powder are best.

➣ Nutribiotics Organic contains 12 grams rice protein per tablespoon (available from your local health food store; for a number of on-line sources, check www.nutribiotic.com/wherebuy.htm).
➣ Jarrow Organic contains 12 grams rice protein per rounded tablespoon (available from your local health food store; for a number of on-line sources, check www.jarrow.com/sales.htm).

DHA Eggs

➤ Widely available in health stores and some supermarkets, these eggs are high in the omega-3 fats and vitamin E.

Celtic Salt

Call our clinic's order line or search on-line.

Goat's Milk Products

Many stores and supermarkets sell goat's milk and cheese. Health stores sell wonderful varieties of goat cheese (feta, cheddar, ricotta, etc.) and yogurt.

Organic Cow's Milk Products

Allergic to milk? Try raw milk products to see if your allergy is just to processed milk. Your allergy might be to pasteurized, homogenized milk or to hormones, chlorine, iodine, antibiotics, and other additives that get into conventional milk.

Coconut Milk and Oil

Canned and preferably whole fat (first press) and without preservatives.

➤ Thai Kitchen coconut milk is one of the best available in stores.
➤ Nonhydrogenated coconut cooking oil can be found in health food stores or on our or other order lines.

Quick Wheat-Free and Gluten-Free Specialties

➤ Wild Rice, Fall River: www.frwr.com. Fully cooked, ready to serve—just heat and serve.
➤ Polenta in precooked rolls (Food Merchants Brand organic: www.quinoa.net)—just heat and serve.
➤ Pasta: We like Tinkyada, Ancient Harvest (corn and quinoa), or Pastariso (rice) spaghetti, fettuccini, macaroni, penne, or angel hair made from rice. Bean-based pastas can also be tasty.

➤ Garbanzo flour: Higher in protein than grain flours and can be used with rice or other flour to increase protein in baking.
➤ Garbanzo miso: The others have gluten.
➤ All-Purpose Flour Blend, Gifts of Nature—tastes and acts like wheat flour. Use for all baking and thickening sauces. Bean flour increases protein.

General Food Sources

➤ **Farmers Markets:** ask in local health food stores or www.lfm.org.uk for farmers markets in London.
➤ **Fresh Water Filter Co.:** tel: 020 8597 3223. Produces a superior under-the-sink filter. Cartridge needs to be replaced every three months or so, depending on use. The company provides an automatic invoicing service to remind you to replace cartridge.

The customer services department of food stores hold lists of products which are free from certain ingredients suitable for those on special diets.

Asda: 0500 1000055   Safeway: 01622 712899
Boots: 0115 9506111   Somerfield: 0117 935 9359
Co-op: 0800 0686727   Tesco: 0800 505555
Marks & Spencer: 020 7268 1234   Waitrose: 01344 824975
Sainsbury: 0800 636262

➤ **Against the Grain Ltd:** Claridge House, 29 Barnes High Street, London SW13 9LW, tel: 020 8876 6247.
➤ **AllergyCare:** 1 Church Square, Taunton, Somerset TA1 1SA, tel: 01823 325023.
➤ **Allergyfree Direct Ltd:** 5 CentreMead, Osney Mead OX2 0ES, tel: 01865 722003, fax: 01865 244134, www.allergyfreedirect.co.uk.
➤ **Barbara's Kitchen:** PO Box 54, Pontyclun, South Wales CF72 8WD, tel: 01443 229304, e-mail: enquiries@barbaraskitchen.co.uk, www.barbaraskitchen.co.uk.
➤ **Blissful Buffalo (milk & meat):** Belland Farm, Tetcott, Holsworthy, Devon EX22 6RG, tel: 01409 271406, www.blissfulbuffalo.fsnet.co.uk.
➤ **Buxton Foods Ltd.:** 12 Harley Street, London W1N 1AA, tel: 020 7637 5505, fax 020 7436 0979, e-mail: sales@stamp-collection.co.uk, www.stamp-collection.co.uk.

➤ **Delamere Direct (goats milk):** Yew Tree Farm, Bexton Lane, Knutsford, Cheshire WA169BH, tel: 01565 632422, e-mail sales@delameredairy.co.uk, www.delameredairy.co.uk.

➤ **Dietary Specialities Direct:** Freepost NWW 2474A, Warrington WA5 5ZW, tel: 07041 544044, fax: 07041 544055, e-mail: info@nutritionpoint.ltd.uk, www.glutenfree-dsdirect.co.uk.

➤ **Eskley Sheep Milk:** Lianbaddon Farm, Michaelchurt, Eskley, Hereford HR2 0PR, tel: 01981 510294, info@sheepmilk.co.uk, www.sheepmilk.co.uk.

➤ **Everfresh Natural Foods:** Gatehouse Close, Aylesbury, Buckinghamshire HP19 3DE, tel: 01296 425333.

➤ **General Dietary Ltd.:** PO Box 38 Kingston upon Thames, Surrey KT2 7YP, tel: 020 8942 8274, fax: 020 8942 8274.

➤ **Sustain – the alliance for better food and farming:** 94 White Lion Street, London N1 9PF, tel: 020 7837 1228, fax: 020 7837 1141, www.sustainweb.org.

RECOMMENDED READING

The following suggestions focus mostly on mood and nutrition, some on more severe problems than *The Mood Cure* covers.

Ross, Julia, M.A. *The Diet Cure* (New York: Viking, 2000).

Mathews-Larson, Joan, Ph.D. *Depression Free Naturally* (New York: Ballantine, 2001). Also see Dr. Larson's Web site, www.healthrecovery.com, especially for good information on pyroluria and high-histamine problems.

Slagle, Patricia, M.D. *The Way Up from Down* (New York: St. Martin's, 1992). The first book on amino acids and mood.

Braverman, Eric, M.D. *The Healing Nutrients Within* (North Bergen, N.J.: Basic Health Books, 2002). This new edition focuses on amino acid therapy for a wide variety of problems, including mood. Order from www.pathmed.com.

The Journal of Orthomolecular Medicine. To order, call 416-733-2117 (or search archives at www.orthomed.org/jom/jom.htm).

Abrams, Hoffer, M.D. See all his books, such as *Healing the Mind the Natural Way* (New York: Putnam, 1995).

Pfeiffer, Carl, M.D. *Mental and Elemental Nutrients* (New Canaan, Conn.: Keats, 1975). One of many outstanding books on his pioneering work.

Werbach, Melvyn, M.D. *Nutritional Influences on Mental Illness* (Tarzana, Calif.: Third Line Press, 1991). A compendium of helpful research studies.

Edelman, Eva. *Healing for Schizophrenia: A Compendium of Nutritional Methods* (Eugene, Ore.: Borage Books, 1996).

Kalita, Dwight, M.D. *Brain Allergies* (New Canaan, Conn.: Keats, 1987).

Amen, Daniel, M.D. *Change Your Brain, Change Your Life* (New York: Three Rivers Press/Crown, 2000) and *Healing ADD* (New York: Berkley, 2002) about moods related to ADD, brain injury, and other brain adversities. See his dazzling Web site, www.brainplace.com.

Other Information Sources

➤ **Bristol Cancer Help Centre:** Grove House, Cornwallis Grove, Clifton, Bristol BS8 4PG, tel: Admin & Reception: 0117 980 9500, Helpline: 0117 980 9505, www.bristolcancerhelp.org.

➤ **North West Mind:** 21 Ribblesdale Place, Preston PR1 3NA, tel: 01772 821734.

➤ **Northern Mind:** Pinetree Centre, Durham Road, Birtley, Chester-le-Street, County Durham DH3 2TD, tel. 0191 490 0109.

➤ **South East Mind:** 1st Floor, Kemp House, 152-160 City Road, London EC1V 2NP,tel: 0171 608 0881.

➤ **South West Mind:** Pembroke House, 7 Brunswick Square, Bristol BS2 8PE, tel: 0117 925 0960.

➤ **Trent & Yorkshire Mind:** 44 Howard Street, Sheffield S1 2LX, tel: 0114 272 1742.

➤ **West Midlands Mind:** 20-21 Cleveland Street, Wolverhampton WV1 3HT, tel: 01902 424404.

➤ **Mind Cymru:** 3rd Floor, Quebec House, Castlebridge, Cowbridge Road East, Cardiff CF11 9AB, tel: 01222 395123.

➤ **Schizophrenia Association of Great Britain:** International Schizophrenia Association, Bryn Hyfrd, The Crescent, Bangor, Gwynnedd LL57 2SAG, tel: 01248 354048, e-mail: sagb@btinternet.com, www.binternet.com/~sagb.

PYROLURIA PROTOCOL

Testing and Treatment for Pyroluria

This is a relatively unusual condition in the general population (11 percent), but is more common in some groups that tend to have the most stubborn mood problems. For example, approximately 40 percent of alcoholics have pyroluria. If you answer yes to fifteen or more of the following questions, test the level of pyrroles in your urine with a kit ordered from Bio Center Lab, 800-494-7785. Excess pyrroles reduce levels of zinc and vitamin B_6, as well as pantothenic acid, niacin and manganese. Measure your zinc level using Zinc Tally or Zinc Status (see under "Supplements," page 293). If this diluted zinc-containing liquid is held in your mouth for ten seconds and has no particular taste, your zinc levels are probably quite low. Our clinic always uses the "tally" with incoming clients, and this is how we discovered pyroluria. Some clients, even after they had been taking zinc supplements for several months (50 mg), could not taste the tally. The questionnaire and urine testing confirmed pyroluria. One pyroluric had her first vivid dreams in twenty years the first night she raised her B_6 and zinc doses. Also consider a hair analysis that will show manganese levels, and a blood test for zinc. I am just getting familiar with this condition, but I can see that it is a very important one for certain people, affecting stress levels and mood generally and preventing full response to nutrient therapy until it is addressed. For a more thorough explanation of causes and remedies, I refer you to the information and the nutrient protocol designed by the clinician who alerted me to pyroluria, Joan Mathews-Larson, Ph.D. It is contained in chapter 5 of her excellent book *Depression Free Naturally* (New York: Ballantine, 2001), as is the following questionnaire.

IDENTIFYING SYMPTOMS
OF PYROLURIA

yes   no

❑   ❑   When you were young, did you sunburn easily? Do you have fair or pale skin?

❑   ❑   Do you have a reduced amount of head hair, eyebrows, or eyelashes, or do you have prematurely gray hair?

❑   ❑   Do you have poor dream recall or nightmares?

❑   ❑   Are you becoming more of a loner as you age? Do you avoid outside stress because it upsets your emotional balance?

❑   ❑   Have you been anxious, fearful, or felt a lot of inner tension since childhood, but mostly hide these feelings from others?

❑   ❑   Is it hard to clearly recall past events and people in your life?

❑   ❑   Do you have bouts of depression and/or nervous exhaustion?

❑   ❑   Do you have cluster headaches?

❑   ❑   Are your eyes sensitive to sunlight?

❑   ❑   Do you belong to an all-girl family or have look-alike sisters?

❑   ❑   Do you get frequent colds or infections or unexplained chills or fevers?

❑   ❑   Do you dislike eating protein? Have you ever been a vegetarian?

❑   ❑   Did you reach puberty later than normal?

❑   ❑   Are there white spots/flecks on your fingernails, or do you have opaquely white or paper-thin nails?

❑   ❑   Are you prone to acne, eczema, or psoriasis?

❑   ❑   Do you prefer the company of one or two close friends rather than a gathering of friends?

❑   ❑   Do you have stretch marks on your skin?

❑   ❑   Have you noticed a sweet smell (fruity odor) to your breath or sweat when ill or stressed?

❑   ❑   Do you have—or did you have, before braces—crowded upper front teeth?

❑   ❑   Do you prefer not to eat breakfast or even experience light nausea in the morning?

yes no

❏ ❏ Does your face sometimes look swollen while under a lot of stress?

❏ ❏ Do you have a poor appetite or a poor sense of smell or taste?

❏ ❏ Do you have any upper abdominal, splenic pain? As a child, did you get a "stitch" in your side when you ran?

❏ ❏ Do you tend to focus internally (on yourself) rather than on the external world?

❏ ❏ Do you frequently experience fatigue?

❏ ❏ Do you feel uncomfortable with strangers?

❏ ❏ Do your knees crack or ache?

❏ ❏ Do you overreact to tranquilizers, barbiturates, alcohol, or other drugs—that is, does a little produce a powerful response?

❏ ❏ Does it bother you to be seated in a restaurant in the middle of the room?

❏ ❏ Are you anemic?

❏ ❏ Do you have cold hands and/or feet?

❏ ❏ Are you easily upset (internally) by criticism?

❏ ❏ Do you have a tendency toward morning constipation?

❏ ❏ Do you have tingling sensations or muscle spasms in your legs or arms?

❏ ❏ Do changes in your routine (traveling, new situations) provoke stress?

❏ ❏ Do you tend to become dependent on one person whom you build your life around?

❏ ❏ Are there severe mood problems, mental illness, or alcoholism in your family?

This questionnaire was originally developed by author, researcher, and clinician Carl Pfeiffer, Ph.D., an inspired pioneer in the field of biochemistry, mood, and nutrition.

Thyroid Tool Kit

Testing and Rebalancing

I f the natural thyroid-promoting methods that I described in chapter 4 fail you, as they do many people in our experience, you'll need the help of a physician. Yet despite the fact that thyroid medication has been a top-selling drug in the United States for years, many physicians still refuse to take low-thyroid symptoms seriously, frequently even refusing to do thorough testing. If you suspect that you have a thyroid problem, you're probably going to have to be assertive, no matter how emotionally flattened you feel, in order to get the medical help you need. If your current doctor refuses to help, see the "Resource Tool Kit" for suggestions on how to seek out a more holistic doctor, N.D., or D.O., who will pay more attention to your symptoms, order complete thyroid testing, interpret the results sensitively, and treat you effectively. Before you go to see a doctor, though, (1) prepare a good thyroid-relevant family history, (2) check off and copy the list of your low-thyroid symptoms on page 67, and (3) bring in the results of at least three days of the following home test.

TESTING

The Home Temperature Test

Your underarm (or basal) temperature, taken first thing in the morning, can be a good indicator of your thyroid function. If your basal temperature is below 97.8 degrees in the cool of the morning before you start moving around and raising it, your thyroid may be in trouble. If your *oral* temperature tends always to be low, the likelihood of a thyroid problem is even greater.

This method has been used for many years, since before a study confirming its accuracy was conducted by Broda O. Barnes, M.D., champion of the holistic approach to thyroid treatment (results of the study were published in the *Journal of the American Medical Association* in 1942).[1]

1. Buy a nondigital thermometer (a basal, or fertility, thermometer is easier to read than a regular oral one). Do not use a digital thermometer, which is not as accurate under the arm.
2. As soon as you wake up, turn bright lights on, stay in bed, and keep your eyes open for thirty minutes (going to the bathroom, if you have to, and reading are fine).
3. After thirty minutes place the thermometer under your armpit. Leave it there for ten minutes, staying quietly in bed with your eyes open.
4. Do this for three mornings or more (they don't have to be consecutive mornings) to get an average temperature.

If you are a menstruating woman, basal temperature testing is most accurate during days 1–4 of your period. Avoid taking your temperature around your ovulation (midcycle), because ovulation causes your temperature to rise for a few days.

If you're in menopause or are male, any morning is fine. Even if you are having hot flushes, your basal temperature should not be affected.

If this axial (underarm) temperature is subnormal (under 97.8 degrees), your thyroid function is probably too low. (Low temps may mean that your early morning cortisol and/or testosterone levels are low as well.)

Be sure to take at least three morning temps to get a consistent average. It's a good idea to continue to take them at least monthly during thyroid treatment, too, to make sure they go up to normal. Often, rising basal temps are the first sign of a reviving thyroid function.

Office Tests

A thyroid-knowledgeable doctor will carefully examine your thyroid gland itself. If your physician does not touch this gland located at the base of your neck, find another who will. You should also expect to have your ankle (Achilles' tendon) reflex tested (that is, tapped with a mallet). This is another concrete indicator of thyroid function. If your foot doesn't bounce, your thyroid can't, either.[2] If this reflex is slow or nonexistent, keep testing it throughout your thyroid therapy until it starts to respond.

The right physician will be impressed by your symptom list, family history, and basal temperatures and will be eager to do an exam and order blood and other tests.

Lab Testing

We've found thorough lab testing to be invaluable in establishing a baseline, convincing medical professionals, and confirming our clients' intuitive feelings that "something, maybe my thyroid, is wrong." Before you test, though, please remember that your *symptoms* are the most reliable indicators of your thyroid function. That said, here are my best suggestions after watching a few thousand clients go through thyroid testing and treatment. Please be sure to get no less than the most basic *five thyroid blood tests* and a *salivary adrenal function test.*

➤ *TSH (thyroid stimulating hormone).* This test, the only test that all physicians are happy to order, measures the signal that your pituitary gland, your brain's master endocrine gland and your thyroid's boss, is sending to your thyroid, telling it to make more or less of its hormones. If your thyroid is making plenty of its hormones, your pituitary will send very little TSH, your score will be lower, or "normal," and your thyroid function will appear to be normal, too. According to our medical consultants and many other experts, including Great Britain's much-published A. P. Weetman, M.D., the ideal TSH score is 1–2.[3] In January 2001, the American Association of Endocrinologists announced that any TSH score above 3 be considered an indication of probable hypothyroidism. Most laboratories, unfortunately, still use the old figures with "normal" ranges going from 0.4 to as high as 6.

➤ T_4 (free). This blood test measures the amount of the less active thyroid hormone that you have ready to convert to the more active T_3 form in your cells. Most M.D.'s and D.O.'s will fairly readily order this test for you along with the TSH. (The "free" forms are the bio-available forms.)

➤ T_3 (free). This blood test measures the levels of the most active thyroid hormone. Though many M.D.'s balk at ordering it, be sure to get it. Psychiatrists routinely use T_3 testing to monitor their use of medication for depression. We've had many clients with low T_3 and normal T_4 levels who were not converting T_4 to T_3. Since T_3 is the most active hormone, its levels are critical. (Total T3 testing is also a useful indicator.)

➤ *Antithyroglobulin and antithyroperoxidase.* These two blood tests measure the number of antibodies (immune system attacker cells) you may be making to attack your own thyroid gland and thereby suppress your thyroid hormone production. If you turn out to have elevated antibodies, you probably have autoimmune thyroiditis or hyperthyroidism. I discuss both conditions on pages 314–315.

➤ *TRH.* If all your test results are normal, but your symptoms are not, the TRH (thyrotropin-releasing hormone) test can identify whether your pituitary is giving your thyroid the right signals.[4]

Urine or Saliva Tests for T_3 and T_4

Both T_3 and T_4 levels can be tested most accurately through a *urine testing* process. Most of our clients with low-thyroid symptoms whose blood tests show "low normal" results for T_3 and/or T_4 have had *below* normal results on this urine test.

Saliva Testing for Adrenal Function Is Essential!

The thyroid typically alters its function during stress, slowing down and converting its more active hormone, T_3, to inactive, or reverse, T_3 (reverse T_3 can also be measured through *blood testing,* though we have only *very* rarely found it useful). That's one of the key reasons the adrenal test is among the most valuable tests we've ever found for helping explain the drained and overwhelmed feelings that our depressed clients often suffer. If stress has been a significant problem in your life, treating your thyroid alone, without checking your adrenal function, can backfire. This has happened to some of our clients with low-thyroid symptoms who became more stressed and jittery instead of more energized when they started a trial of thyroid medication. When we discovered the adrenal connection, that stopped happening. See the "Adrenal Tool Kit" for information about adrenal testing, interpretation, and treatment. If your adrenals test low, start revving them up even *before* you start your thyroid medication, if possible. Sometimes correcting adrenal function takes care of the thyroid problem as well. (Hydrocortisone has been used successfully as a complete cure for thyroiditis, for example, according to the Broda Barnes Foundation.)

INTERPRETING AND TREATING TEST RESULTS

Re TSH Test Results

If your TSH is over 3, your physician should give you a trial of medicine. Don't forget that the endocrinologists' definition of the normal range went down from below 6, to below 3 in 2001.

If your score is between 2 and 3, you may have an argument with your physician about whether you "really need" a trial of thyroid meds. Let your symptoms, basal temps, and other test results be your guides. The physicians we consult consider the ideal TSH range to be between 1 and 2. One of them, Richard Shames, M.D., author of *Thyroid Power,* has worked successfully with our clients since 1989. And be sure to mention British expert A. P. Weetman, M.D., who advocates treating for symptoms and any TSH over 2. (You can print out his articles on MedLine to show to your M.D.)

If your TSH is below 1, your physician may want to cut your medication (if you're already on it) or test you for *hyper*thyroidism (*over*active thyroid). The latter is a fine idea. The former may not be, if you feel worse at a lower dose of meds. The controversy is very strong on how low the TSH can go before your thyroid is turned off for good by medication (something we've never seen happen).

Regarding T_3 and T_4 Test Results

Most holistic (complementary or alternative) physicians feel that even low normal (bottom third or so of the reference range) blood test results clearly justify a trial of medication, if symptoms exist. For example, if your T_3/T_4 score is 1.9 and the "reference range" is 1.5–3, you are in the low normal range. When either T_3 or T_4 or both are in this lower normal range, the evidence is pointing strongly in the direction of a problem, assuming that your symptoms point that way, too. Ask for a ninety-day trial of thyroid medication. (You might also mention the fact that psychiatrists often prescribe thyroid medication trials to treat depression, with no prior testing at all.) This is neither a dangerous nor an unreasonable request. You'll feel better, worse, or nothing within a month. If you feel better, you'll stay on the medicine and your doctor will monitor you via retesting until you're both satisfied with your dose. If worse, you try a different dose, or a new medicine, or stop altogether and look for another cause for your symptoms. (Don't forget to check your adrenals!)

If your T_3 or T_4 scores are too high, you may well have hyperthyroidism, particularly if your TSH is low. See page 315.

TREATING YOUR THYROID

The Medication Story

You'll want to have a good idea of specific strategies to pursue, if you and your physician are convinced by symptoms, history, physical exams, and lab test results that you need help in the thyroid department. Even if your test results show no abnormalities, keep in mind that test results are not as reliable as real-life symptoms. Just ask your physician for a three-month monitored trial on one of the medications I'm about to list. If your symptoms warrant it, most holistic physicians will be happy to help you with such a trial.

A 1997 article in the *British Medical Journal* by Dr. Weetman encouraged M.D.'s to provide a ninety-day trial of thyroid medicine even if *no* test scores were abnormal, *if low thyroid symptoms were present*.[5] This is what was always done before blood tests for thyroid function were developed in the 1960s. One of the physicians who treated thyroid problems entirely by symptoms in those days was the physician Broda O. Barnes. He became an author, educator, and champion of the symptom-based approach to thyroid treatment after blood testing became popular and M.D.'s were discouraged from using any other gauge for assessing thyroid problems. The Broda O. Barnes Foundation was established to educate physicians and the general public about Barnes's sensible methods. It continues to give regular conferences and consultations and distribute books and tapes on the subject. We recommend their foundation's national list of Barnes-educated physicians to people who call us from outside of our area in California, and it has usually been helpful to them. A small fee is charged for these lists. (Their number is 203-261-2101, and their Web site is www.brodabarnes.org.)

Dr. Barnes strongly preferred the natural thyroid medicine made from pigs' thyroids. We have noticed, after fifteen years of observation, that perhaps half our clients do well on this regimen. The other half do better on the synthetic thyroid hormones T_4 and/or T_3. Some do best with a combination of animal *and* synthetic medicines. The important thing is to stick with it. Find another doctor if necessary, but keep with it until you find the right medication at the right dose to eliminate your symptoms without *any* adverse effects. Here is a list of the medications that our clients have used successfully over the years.

Glandular Thyroid by Prescription

This extract from pigs' glands contains not only the hormones T_3 and T_4 but also T_1 and T_2, whose somewhat obscure roles may include protection from dry skin and breast and uterine cysts. Armour Thyroid, or the hypoallergenic Naturthroid or Biothroid, can be just perfect at the right dose. However, finding the right dose is a process of trial and error. If you feel no difference after a few weeks at the dose you begin with, ask for more. If more causes you to be sleepless, feel jittery, or have heart palpitations, your doctor will cut your dose or try another medication. If too little happens, he or she will raise your dose again. For some people, porcine thyroid is too stimulating, because pigs' thyroids produce quite a bit more of the active hormone (T_3) than human thyroids do, in relation to T_4. Yet inexplicably, for some of our clients these glandular medicines have no effect at all, and synthetics do a better job.

Synthetic T_4

Levoxyl and Synthroid are two of the many synthetic brands of generic and nongeneric levothyroxine (T_4). Most physicians prefer to start with T_4, which can convert to the more active T_3 as needed. If you have allergies, be aware that some T_4 products also contain acacia and/or lactose. The generic versions of T_4 may be at least as effective as Synthroid, or more so. In fact, a recent outcry about Synthroid's lack of uniform quality has led to an investigation by the FDA, which has demanded that Synthroid reapply and go through formal trials to prove its viability (something it never did to begin with, having been grandfathered in originally). Sometimes one form of synthetic T_4 is more effective than another. Try them all if you have to.

As T_4 is the less active thyroid hormone, if you don't get results at any dosage (many of our clients don't), you'll need to add some synthetic T_3.

Synthetic T_3

Much research confirms the usefulness of T_3 medication for depression. Short-acting Cytomel (brand name) taken one to three times a day, or better yet *time-release T_3*, can be very effective. Your physician will be careful to start you at a low dose and will go higher only if you seem to need more. (Remember, too much T_3 can make your heart race.) Cytomel's one disadvantage, for some people, is that it (like your own natural T_3) dissipates quickly, along with its benefits, before the next dose is due. If you are not entirely pleased with its effects, try the time-release form, which your physician can order through a compounding pharmacy. (Compounders make up, or compound, special orders to physician specification.) If your Yellow Pages don't list one under "Pharmacies," see the "Resource Tool Kit" for advice on finding compounders outside your area (they ship). Broda Barnes–trained physician Gary Ross, M.D., recommends the time-release product from Women's International Pharmacy for our clients, and it works beautifully.

Once your physician has started your trial of medication, keep working with him or her until you get the right medication at the right dose to relieve your depression and any other low-thyroid symptoms you may have. You may have been "down" so long that you have no idea how much better you might be able to feel. Keep taking your basal temperature, reviewing your original emotional and physical low-thyroid symptoms and retesting. When everything is normalized, you're at the right dose of the right medicine.

Special Treatment Considerations for Thyroiditis— When Your Thyroid Antibodies Test Too High

Hashimoto's thyroiditis is a major problem in the United States. Many experts say that it is the primary cause of all of the most common kinds of thyroid dysfunction. Thyroiditis can produce not only the usual symptoms of hypothyroidism, but additional, more agitated symptoms (including seizure), because the thyroid is at war in this disease. If you have

---

Too Much Iodized Salt?

Excess iodine is a well-established cause of both low thyroid and thyroiditis. Researchers in the United States, Japan, and Greece have found that increased iodine from iodized salt has led to sharp increases in the incidence of thyroiditis. In Greece, for example, where iodine was only recently added to salt, goiters (neck swelling associated with low thyroid) have become much less common, but thyroiditis has become much more so. Because of this, I don't advocate the use of lots of ordinary table salt, or even most sea salt, which is usually just a coarser version of table salt. All contain added iodine (and low levels of minerals other than sodium). I do suggest real, natural "celtic" sea salt.

Hashimoto's, your thyroid gland is under attack by immune cells (antithyroid antibodies) that are being sent out by mistake to subdue it. Your thyroid may be capable of making plenty of its hormones, but the antibody attack interferes with consistent production and delivery. So if you're feeling like an emotional battleground, you are one. Hashimoto's thyroiditis can inflame, create lumpy scar tissue in, and ultimately destroy your thyroid gland. It can turn into *hypo*thyroidism, when your gland can't put out adequate amounts of its hormones anymore, and you're just feeling low much of the time. Yet it can also be associated with *hyper*thyrodism.

I suspect thyroiditis when one of our clients has symptoms such as nervous, tense depression; trouble swallowing pills; feels "wired," especially after ingesting caffeine or the amino acid L-tyrosine; and has other mood and sleep issues that don't resolve quickly on our nutrient supplements and good mood foods. Thyroiditis almost always requires medical intervention, at least for a while and *always* requires adrenal testing. In fact, treating adrenal exhaustion with replacement cortisol has entirely corrected thyroid function in many cases. (See the "Adrenal Tool Kit.")

Viral reactions and allergic reactions may be triggers. Common allergy-provoking foods made from wheat, rye, oats, and barley have been firmly linked to Hashimoto's thyroiditis. In fact, a recent Italian study found that eliminating these grains stopped the autoimmune attack on the thyroid altogether.[6] Studies also show that soy contributes to higher rates of thyroiditus. You'll get directions in chapters 7 and 8 on how to find out if grains, soy, or any other foods are problematic for you and your thyroid.

The most successful medication for our clients with Hashimoto's has started with T_4 (some form of levothyroxine), then added time-released T_3 (or Cytomel), as needed. Animal thyroid has less often been a successful medication for thyroiditis in our experience. Being so similar to human thyroid, it may continue to stimulate the immune system attack, whereas the synthetic hormone doesn't seem to. Adjust your dose as needed and retest all your thyroid hormone levels *including your antibodies* every three to twelve months (your TSH more often, at first). You should also get tested for anemia, which is quite common with Hashimoto's. Extra B_{12}, folic acid, and iron may be needed in addition to your basic supplements. If you find you have B_{12} anemia, B_{12} shots can be very helpful. Be sure to also take a multi-mineral supplement that contains selenium and zinc.

Treating Hyperthyroidism (When Your Tests Indicate Too Much Thyroid Activity)

Our clinic has had so few hyperthyroid clients that I am not familiar with all the treatment options. Some medications can turn down the thyroid without destroying it. When it's been turned down for a while, you'll develop hypothyroidism (low thyroid) and need to go on one or more of the meds I describe above. Hyperthyroidism can often be an autoimmune problem and respond to the approaches mentioned in the previous section on thyroiditis, like eliminating allergy foods. One of our hyperthyroid clients had very serious long-standing food allergies *and* a major parasitic infection with exhausted adrenals underlying her problem.

Can You Recover and Stop Medication?

After a year, you can try a few months off your medication (you'll be tired at first until your own thyroid kicks back in). Results vary. If your benefits last, stay off medication. If not, go back on it. Thyroid expert Nathan Becker, M.D., a University of California at San Francisco endocrinologist, tells us that about one-third of his patients can go off medication successfully after a year.

RECOMMENDED READING

Educational materials (and training conferences) from Broda O. Barnes Foundation: 203-261-2101; www.brodabarnes.org.

Shames, Richard, M.D., and Karilee Halo Shames, R.N., Ph.D. *Thyroid Power: Ten Steps to Total Health.* (New York: HarperResource, 2001).

Shomon, Mary J. *Living Well with Hypothyroidism* (New York: Avon/ Wholecare, 2000).

Adrenal Tool Kit

_~_

Testing and Rebalancing

Find a Health Practitioner First. Please use the suggestions in the "Resource Tool Kit," page 289, to find a holistic M.D., N.D., or D.O., acupuncturist, chiropractor, and/or nutritionist who is already familiar with the saliva testing and treatment described here or is willing to work closely with lab-testing consultants to learn the ropes. The labs themselves are good sources for referrals to competent adrenal-balancing professionals. Most of them won't sell adrenal function test kits except through professionals anyway. You'll want help in this process, I assure you.

Consider Acupuncture. Acupuncturists have been treating the adrenal glands for thousands of years. Get acupuncture treatments from an experienced practitioner, preferably one with at least some training in China. Try to find an acupuncturist who uses saliva testing and knows Chinese herbs. These professionals can also measure your adrenal function through your pulses and treat you with needles and herbs along with the other methods suggested in this kit. Not only are the adrenal glands directly supported through acupuncture, but acupuncture is famous for its ability to raise endorphin levels, and we know that these pleasure-producing endorphins are depleted by stress and are needed to help regulate cortisol.

Acupuncturists call the pulse that registers the vitality of your adrenal glands your "adrenal/kidney meridian." (The Chinese regard the kidneys and their neighboring adrenals as a single gland.) If your burnout is severe, your pulse will be very weak or unsteady, in which case you should consider being treated with needles and herbs. If you dislike needles, the same work can be done by hand, with acupressure. You can even work your own adrenal points and meridians using your acupuncturist's suggestions or using self-acupressure guidebooks.

TESTING

Office Tests

Even before you order saliva testing, ask your practitioner to do an eye examination to see if your pupils contract easily and completely in bright light. Many low-adrenal people are very sensitive to light, even wearing dark glasses indoors, because their pupils can't contract. Also, check for whether your blood pressure follows the normal pattern both lying down and then standing up. (This is called "orthostatic blood pressure testing.")

Lab Tests

All of the following tests can be ordered through the labs listed in the "Resource Tool Kit."

Saliva testing is a lifesaver! It's been available since the early 1980s, and its results correspond amazingly well to our clients' actual experience. It turns out that saliva contains easily measured amounts of most hormones, including cortisol and DHEA, another hormone produced by the adrenal glands that helps us better cope with stress. That's why most research on these hormones is done using saliva testing now. Because only the free, or active, forms of these hormones get into the saliva, this test is equivalent to the most sophisticated and expensive blood tests of "free" hormone levels.[1] Many studies have confirmed the reliability of saliva testing for hormones. In fact, most scientific research on hormones is now done using saliva in preference to blood. It's certainly more convenient!

Your body always keeps a certain level of cortisol in your bloodstream, highest in the morning, to allow you to face the day, and lowest at night, to allow you to sleep. Saliva testing will tell you and your health consultant exactly what kind of depletion or excess your adrenal stress hormones may be evidencing and when. It will also show you which stage of stress burnout you're in.

Are you in early, stage one, stress burnout, when your cortisol levels are too high all the time? In stage two, when they're starting to drop too low? Or in stage three, when they're too low most or all of the time? Labs have determined what the normal cortisol output in a twenty-four-hour period is, so they can compare it to *your* output on what is a typical day for *you*. Most tests measure the levels of cortisol and DHEA in at least four samples of saliva, which you'll collect while at home or at work: early morning through bedtime. Keep a log of food, mood, energy, stress, and activities on the test day. That will help you and your practitioner interpret the results. You'll need to retake this test as you recover (at least twice in the following year). *Note:* If you're sick or experience any sudden, unusual stress, wait to test until after you've felt "normal" for a week, or the immediate stress has passed, to measure a *typical day*.

Men: Ask for a single test that measures the two stress hormones *plus* estrogen and testosterone. That way you'll have a baseline should you take a remedy like DHEA, which could affect the levels of either of these sex hormones. Be sure to monitor levels by *retesting* in a few months. (If sleep is a problem, ask for a melatonin and progesterone measurement, too.)

Women: I recommend testing for cortisol and DHEA, *plus* estrogen, progesterone, and testosterone. If you no longer have periods, or have normal periods and are under age 35, a one-day test might do. If you are still menstruating and are having significant problems like irregular periods, severe PMS, or infertility, consider measuring these hormone levels during your whole cycle. (See the "Sex Hormone Tool Kit" for details.) Getting baseline levels of your sex hormones will help keep you from creating imbalances by using supplements of DHEA, for example. Be sure to retest in a few months. (Ask for a melatonin test, too, if sleep is a problem.)

Urine testing. Pharmasan can test your adrenaline levels.

Additional Lab Tests: Blood Testing

Thyroid—Because the thyroid is easily affected by cortisol levels and vice versa, if you are exhausted and have cold hands and feet and unneeded weight gain, *be sure* to get tests for your T_3, T_4, TSH, and two thyroid antibodies. (See the "Thyroid Tool Kit" for more on this.)

Vitamin D—Vitamin D is an important regulating hormone for adrenal
function (and bone building). An accurate *blood test* produced by Di-
asorin Labs is available: it's called 25-OHD or 25 hydroxy OHD (*not*
125 OHD). Lab One has the best price on it.

Pregnenolone—It can be useful to test for this primary adrenal hormone
from which cortisol, DHEA, and all of the other adrenal hormones are
made.

Other Testing to Identify Internal Stressors

Testing for Food Allergies

Irritating foods may be the most common stressors there are. Wheat and
dairy are the likeliest culprits. Elimination and challenge is the most accurate way to test for common food allergies, and I explain how to do this
simple home test on page 140 in chapter 7.

Stool Tests for Yeast, Parasite, or Bacterial Overgrowth

Most standard labs are typically not very good at finding these tiny invaders. If you have the following symptoms, get blood candida antibody
test—or don't bother with this test, just go ahead and do a yeast kill. If
your symptoms persist, get a stool test. If you turn out to have parasites,
you'll typically have to kill them first before you can get to the yeasts.

➤ Often feel bloated, abdominal distension.
➤ Are foggy headed.
➤ Feel depressed.
➤ Suffer from recurring yeast or bladder infections.
➤ Used antibiotics extensively (at any time in life).
➤ Used cortisone or birth control pills for more than one year.
➤ Have chronic fungus on nails or skin, or have athlete's foot.
➤ Had recurring sinus or ear infections as an adult or child.
➤ Have itching, rashes.

It's important to know which parasites—or, more rarely, toxic bacteria—you
have in order to decide what to use to get rid of them. We use the following labs pretty successfully, but no lab can guarantee results, especially
with parasites. Be sure to retest one month after you have completed a
yeast, parasite, or bacterial kill-off program with a competent professional.

Testing for Heavy Metals

A hair analysis of levels of potentially toxic metals (like mercury) is inexpensive and easy to order. Urine, blood, and stool tests are also available and should be used for confirmation. Heavy metals can be removed using nutrients with the help of an experienced practitioner or one who can get suggestions from lab consultants.

INTERPRETING TEST RESULTS AND APPLYING THE ULTIMATE ADRENAL REPAIR STRATEGIES

Are You in Stage One of Overstress— Did Some or All Four of Your Cortisol Samples Show Extremely High Levels?

➤ *If your excessive stress is just starting,* you're still likely to be making plenty of stress-coping cortisol. And this is a good, potentially lifesaving thing. But if your stress has gone on *too long* and your cortisol levels have stayed too high for too long, the catabolic, or body-destroying, effects of cortisol may have begun to take a toll. Having excessive elevations of your own cortisol is like getting too many cortisone shots. Your immune system, bones, brain, heart, and muscles can all suffer. And even if the stress that triggered the cortisol flood has ended, your glands may have adapted (in as little as three weeks) and may continue to put out what is now excessive amounts of unneeded cortisol. Some signs of stage one: sleep disturbance, a wired feeling, loss of appetite, weight loss, memory loss. (You may remember this feeling from stressful times earlier in your life, if you don't have it now.)

➤ *If you have no obvious current stressors,* it's time to find out what hidden problem is raising your cortisol and what to do about it. (Remember, your diet is your most likely hidden stressor.) You may need a bedtime snack if your blood sugar is dropping at night and triggering a bedtime cortisol surge that keeps you awake. Or you may need to use phosphorylated serine (brand name Seriphos), the only nutrient we know of that's been tested (at Diagnos-Techs) and shown to safely lower cortisol. (Tranquilizers do, but they also prevent you from going into the deep, restful sleep cycle you need so badly to recover from stress exhaustion.) Take Seriphos about six hours before your bedtime to help get to sleep. It may also be taken *at* bedtime if cortisol levels are too high in the early morning and wake you up too early. Seriphos is a combination of the minerals phosphorus and calcium with the amino acid serine. It reduces the ACTH (pituitary) messages that order your adrenals to release emergency amounts of cortisol. Read the label carefully—pregnant and lactating women can't use it, for example. *Caution:* Do not take Seriphos for more than a month at a time. You don't want to turn your adrenals down too low.

➤ *If your cortisol is too high in the morning, or high-normal, even though the rest of your day's scores are low,* you must test for parasites, which tend to become more active at night, stimulating the adrenals to kick up your cortisol levels just when they should be dropping at the end of the day. I know that it sounds bizarre, but so far, our clients who have high morning cortisol levels have all had parasites or, in one case, a nasty bacteria, just as Dr. Timmons, the head of BioHealth Diagnostics, told us they would. In this case, don't use Seriphos— you'll need plenty of cortisol till you get rid of your parasites (or, occasionally, a bacterial or yeast overgrowth).

Eliminating Yeasts, Parasites, and Bad Bacteria

Whether your cortisol is too high or too low, yeasts, parasites, or bacterial overgrowth could be the reason. It takes three to four months using a non-medical protocol to kill these bugs. Prescription antiparasitic antibiotics or antifungal (yeast) drugs work quickly, or you can use a combination of herbs and medications to kill off these creatures. For a written description of antiyeast and antiparasite protocols, or for the yeast or parasite elimination supplements that we actually use at our clinic, call 800-733-9293 and/or consult the experienced alternative health consultants of Diagnos-Techs.

Yeasts and parasites can be hard to kill. Many people try unsuccessfully for years with special diets and supplements that never seem to work. The reason that I recommend only our clinic's protocols is that I just don't know of any other really effective natural alternatives. I do know that medications, though they can be hard on your liver, are often required to get rid of parasites and bacteria. Yeast overgrowth, which is much more common, can usually be killed off with nonprescription supplement protocols, like those we use at our clinic, but you may need to or choose to use meds like Diflucan or Sporanox, especially if you have a very bad case. Add milk thistle to protect your liver if you decide to use any drugs. If you have no health professional to help with this kill-off, ask Diagnos-Techs for referrals and see the "Resource Tool Kit" for other suggestions.

Are You in Stage Two?
Adrenal Exhaustion Really Begins Here

Depending on how long you've been besieged, and how sturdy your adrenals are, you may move at some point from stage one into stage two. Your cortisol levels during the day will look uneven, some still high, others quite low, and that's probably how you'll be feeling. If your cortisol levels are dropping *below* normal, you'll also need to consider the supplements I'll describe next for stage three.

Are You in Stage Three,
the Deepest Stage of Adrenal Exhaustion?

This is where most of our clients, hundreds of them, have landed by the time they come in to see us. Overall cortisol and DHEA levels are low or *sub*normal, all or most of the day. And they definitely *feel* subnormal. Afternoon levels are usually the lowest of the day.

Raising Cortisol Naturally

Adrenal cortex glandulars. Cortisol is made in the outer "cortex" of the adrenal gland. Over-the-counter products made from animal adrenal glands can be very helpful, and you can find them easily yourself, or a professional can order high-quality adrenal cortex products by companies like Bezwecken. Allergy Research has a product called Organic Adrenal Cortex, available at health stores. Use such products during the times of day that your test results show you to be low in cortisol.

Whole adrenal glandulars. Please be cautious about taking easy-to-find *whole* adrenal glandular supplements. The adrenaline they contain (made in the medulla, or inner part of the gland) can make your problem worse by overstimulating you, adding to your stress level and exhausting your adrenals further. If you tend to be at all tense, you won't like them, but if you're feeling burned out and exhausted, you may actually *need* more adrenaline and benefit from them.

Homeopathic remedies. These treatments for glandular problems are called sarcodes. Their lowest doses are indicated by higher numbers. For example, Dolisos International Labs (800-365-4767) makes a 6C-strength homeopathic adrenal cortex, which is mildly elevating and sustaining (for stage two), and a 4C, which is strongly elevating (for stage three).

Licorice. If you have *normal* to *low* blood pressure, not *high* blood pressure, you can sometimes raise your cortisol levels in a hurry by using this surprisingly potent herb in the form of whole licorice root capsules or liquid extracts. "Glycyrrhiza" is the name of the chemical in licorice that has this pro-adrenal effect. (Do not get the kind of licorice used for ulcers, without glycyrrihiza.) It slows down the conversion of cortisol into other hormones, allowing levels to build up. Licorice should be taken one to two times a day right before the time of the drop shown on your test results. *Caution:* If you take licorice after three P.M., your sleep may be affected. Use licorice only short-term, for one to three months. Reduce or stop your dose as you no longer need it, particularly if your appetite decreases or if you feel too speeded up. If you get heart palpitations or high blood pressure, stop at once (we have rarely seen this reaction). *Caution:* Do not use licorice if you have high blood pressure or high estrogen levels. Licorice can raise both.

Pregnenolone is available over the counter. The usual doses recommended are quite low—10 to 50 milligrams per day, but one of our most exhausted clients ever responded to nothing, including thyroid medication, until she tested low in pregnenolone and tried an unusually high dose (130 milligrams). Then she was transformed. This hormone is used by the adrenals to convert to over thirty hormones, notably cortisol, progesterone, and DHEA, so supplementing with it can take a big burden off your adrenals. Some people, though, seem to experience no benefit from it at all. It's available in capsules or the more potent drops, over the counter. Pregnenolone seems to work best for men and menopausal women. *Caution:* Don't use pregnenolone if your progesterone or estrogen is too high or if you are hyperthyroid. If you are taking progesterone in any form, be sure to test your progesterone and estrogen levels before using pregnenolone.

For Stage One, Two, or Three of Adrenal Exhaustion, if DHEA Levels Are Too Low

We have seen some chronically stressed and fatigued clients respond strongly to DHEA supplements within a week. It is available as capsules or drops over the counter. We use low levels (5 to 25 milligrams, one or two times a day, along with meals), but follow your practitioner's advice on dosage and your own responses. *Caution:* Do *not* take DHEA without first testing your levels. If you have hormonally linked illness, such as breast or uterine cancer, endometriosis, or prostate cancer, test your testosterone and estrogen levels first. Then retest every three to six months if you decide to take DHEA because it can convert to both these hormones and you don't want to create new imbalances. It tends to convert more to testosterone in women than in men in our experience and that of the lab directors at BioHealth Diagnostics and Pharmasan.

Prescription Cortisol

Here, our medical consultants rely on the work of William Jeffries, whose *Safe Uses of Cortisol* is such an invaluable guide. He suggests making up the deficit between what your cortisol output should ideally be for a whole day (approximately 23 to 42 milligrams per milliliter), and what your test shows you to actually be producing. For example, a stage three client who tested at "8" was given 20 milligrams of prescription Cortef. She had a very quiet, stress-free life, so this modest increase of cortisol was enough for her. But when she broke her foot and got a bad case of the flu in the same week, she needed extra cortisol, and her doctor raised her dose to 40 milligrams a day to match what her own body would normally have produced had her adrenals not been so fatigued. Remember, your cortisol levels should ideally rise to meet stressors, then subside as the stress abates.

Your adrenals' cortisol levels naturally rise highest in the morning and drop gradually through the day and night. Supplementation should restore this normal rhythm as well.

Cortef is a brand name for hydrocortisone. (Hydrocortisone, another name for cortisol, without additives is available at compounding pharmacies.) The other kind of prescription cortisol is cortisone acetate. Dr. Jeffries typically suggests low doses of 2.5 to 5 milligrams of Cortef or the equivalent, two to four times per day.[2] Prescription cortisone can cause the "moon face" (swelling of the face) and other side effects, but only with consistent use of 50 to 150 milligrams or more per day—far in excess of natural amounts typically produced by the adrenals themselves or recommended by Dr. Jeffries.

One of the few clinicians in the country, other than Dr. Jefferies, expert in the use of medications that correct cortisol levels is Professor Virgil Stenberg, Ph.D., of the University of North Dakota; his research has confirmed the value of appropriate doses of this medication combined with a careful diet, for conditions such as rheumatoid arthritis and fibromyalgia. He uses a technique called "microdose therapy" in which high doses are used very briefly in "pulses" and extraordinary, often permanent, relief follows. His clinics can be reached at 800-743-8381 or www.microdose.com.

Thyroid note: If you still feel tired even after building up your adrenals, be sure to test and treat your thyroid as per the "Thyroid Tool Kit." These glands work as a team.

RETESTING AND MONITORING

Make sure that all your stress repair work is really paying off and not backfiring. For easy and inexpensive follow-up tests, you can order a single cortisol test at the time of day you're most concerned about—the time when you had your most abnormally high or low levels. We had one client whose midafternoon levels kept seesawing. At first her levels were quite subnormal at four P.M. After she'd done some cortisol boosting with licorice, she felt great for a while, but then she started having trouble sleeping. It turned out that her own adrenals had kicked in and she no longer needed the licorice. But she had not retested in three months as planned, so in month four we told her to do so. Sure enough, her cortisol levels had gone from too low to too high. I suggest you retest two to three times in the first year and at least once a year thereafter, or sooner if you start feeling overly stressed again. Decrease your supplements or prescription cortisol as you build yourself back up. Your hormone retests will guide you in this as well as knowing when to eliminate any DHEA or pregnenolone you might be taking.

Special testing considerations for men and women. Your adrenals make at least half of your sex hormones (more if you are over 40). Stress can throw your sex and stress hormone levels way off. In rebuilding your stress-coping hormones, you may consider using pregnenolone or DHEA supplements that can also alter your sex hormone levels, so it's crucial that you get baseline sex hormone testing now and a retest later to make sure you don't create imbalances. For example, DHEA can convert to both estrogen and testosterone. Too much of either hormone can cause real problems.

How Long Will It Take to Rebuild Your Stress-Coping Capacity?

Depending on how deeply depleted you adrenals are (saliva testing will be a big help in determining that), you could be feeling much better that week or recuperating gradually over a six-month period. Miranda was feeling much less overwhelmed after two weeks on her improved diet and basic supplements. But after the terrorist attack in New York in 2001, she crashed badly. At that point none of the over-the-counter supplements did anything for her, and she needed prescription cortisol to pull her out of her slump. That helped right away, but it took two weeks on it before she started going for morning walks again. And she had to insulate herself from stress as much as possible for two months while she built herself up. She was on 15 to 22 milligrams of hydrocortisone three times a day for six months. Then she gradually lowered her dose and went off it. But she kept it around and used it if she started to feel too upset or got sick, just for short periods. She retested her adrenals every three to four months, until they were consistently in the normal range.

To Find Adrenal-Balancing Supplements

Licorice, DHEA, and pregnenolone can all be found in most health stores or ordered through our clinic's order line or others listed in the "Resource Tool Kit."

RESOURCE INFORMATION

Jeffries, William. *Safe Uses of Cortisol* (Springfield, Ill.: Charles C. Thomas Publishing, 1996).

Wilson, James L. *Adrenal Fatigue. The 21st Century Stress Syndrome* (Petaluma, Calif.: Smart Publications, 2001).

Microdose therapy information: Dr. Virgil Stenberg; clinic information and workbooks are available through his central Arizona office, Microdose International, 800-743-8381.

Practitioner's Manual and tapes (BioHealth Diagnostics Lab, 2001). Only for health practitioners ordering tests from the lab. 800-570-2000.

Thie, John F., and Keith Marks. *Touch for Health: A Practical Guide to Natural Health Using Acupressure Touch and Massage* (Marina del Rey, Calif.: De Vorss, 2002).

Sex Hormone Tool Kit

Testing and Rebalancing

Sex hormone imbalances are legendary causes of mood swings. Think of PMS, postpartum depression, or the variety of unpleasant moods that can be part of "the pause" for both men and women. Imbalances and deficiencies that cause emotional and physical problems can be alleviated safely. It takes careful work, though, with a knowledgeable practitioner who can help you assess whether your hormonal output is too low or too high, overall, or at times, and if your hormones are interacting in the ideal ratios with one another.

Your sex hormones—progesterone, testosterone, and the three estrogens (estradiol, estrone, and estriol)—are produced in both your genital organs and your adrenal glands, about half in each, until female menopause and male andropause, when they're all made mostly in the adrenal glands.

HOW DO HORMONE LEVELS CHANGE?

As you grow older, your hormone levels can drop by as much as 90 percent. This plummet plays a crucial role in the aging process—leading to impaired mood, muscle development, sleep patterns, memory, and sexual functions. For most men and women, sex hormones fall most rapidly in the 40s and 50s because of poor diet (that is, an excess of refined carbohydrates) and continual stress, both of which exhaust the adrenals. Low thyroid and hereditary factors can also play a part.

Sometimes excessively high levels of sex hormones can cause problems, too. Abnormally high levels of estrogen in both women and men can result from the use of hormone medications or supplements (including birth control pills), high-carbohydrate or high-soy diets, from the use of caffeine, tobacco, and alcohol, and even from contact with pesticides and common phytochemicals in substances like plastic.

In the brain, *estrogen* promotes the synthesis of mood-regulating neurotransmitters, particularly serotonin, making it a mighty antidepressant and sleep promoter, especially for women. Yet if estrogen levels are raised too high, because they increase cell proliferation, there is a much increased risk of developing certain cancers (such as uterine, breast, and prostate).

Progesterone promotes calmness, relaxation, healthy fetal development, and a normal ovulation pattern. Low progesterone can be a factor in infertility, anxiety, and PMS, while too much progesterone can lead to lethargy, weight gain, and depression, as women on synthetic progesterone (like the progestin Provera) often find.

Testosterone is a hormone critical for maintaining energy and a healthy sex drive; it also promotes muscle and bone development in both men and women. Low levels are linked to fatigue and depression and prostate cancer, but too much testosterone can prompt increased risk of heart disease, polycystic ovary syndrome, aggression and anger, hair loss, headaches, facial hair, oily skin, and acne.

Note: DHEA, an adrenal hormone, is the most plentiful hormone in your bloodstream and acts as the primary source material for the production of both estrogen and testosterone. DHEA can alleviate depression and senile dementia by protecting important brain neurons. But too much DHEA can trigger the symptoms of either too much testosterone or too much estrogen in both men and women.

Female Imbalances: Pre-, Peri-, and Postmenopause

Premenopausal Imbalances

Before you approach perimenopause (anytime after age 35), you may experience PMS or other signs of sex hormone imbalance.

PMS. Do you become "someone else" a week to ten days before your period? Someone those close to you would like to lock up? You could be mood-free by your next cycle with an improved diet and supplements. A diet of good-mood foods will eliminate PMS for most women under 35. If PMS persists, reduced serotonin activity is often the reason, and adding the aminos 5-HTP or tryptophan, at least during PMS days, to your good-mood diet can help. PMS moods can also erupt after a sudden drop in progesterone levels or with inadequate overall estrogen levels. The wonderful sex hormone home-testing kits discussed later can reveal exactly which hormonal peculiarities are causing your PMS, if it continues even after you start to eat well and try the aminos and your basic nutrient supplements.

Postpartum Depression

After childbirth, 80 percent of women suffer some depression that can go on for seven weeks. Of these, 20 percent have deeper and longer depressions. None of this is "normal." Levels of serotonin, omega-3 fats, and thyroid hormone can all drop too low by the end of a draining pregnancy, especially if you're nutritionally or hormonally deficient to begin with. If low serotonin is part of the problem, tryptophan supplements can help. (Avoid 5-HTP while nursing. If you aren't nursing, it's fine.) The omega-3 fats in your basic supplements may also be very helpful to you (and your nursing baby), as pregnancy depletes omega-3 levels known to protect us from this and other kinds of depression.[1] (And improves baby's intelligence, too!) Asking your physician to help you take a close look at your thyroid status (see the "Thyroid Tool Kit") is also in order, as low thyroid is another established cause of the postpartum blues.[2] It's a very good idea to test your sex hormones, too, to find out if an imbalance has developed there, particularly in progesterone levels, that should be corrected.[3] Be sure you're eating lots of good mood food, as well.

Perimenopausal Problems

After age 35, your sex hormone levels can often become progressively more imbalanced because your ovaries gradually make less of both estrogen and progesterone, until they run so low that your adrenals have to start extra production to compensate. Unfortunately, the adrenals may be too occupied with producing stress-coping hormones to do an adequate job with sex hormone production, too. The result: irregular periods, severe cramping, longer and more extreme PMS, hot flushes, and sleep problems. Here it is crucial to use saliva testing to assess these faltering sex hormone levels over your entire cycle, in addition to eating good-mood foods and taking your basic supplements.

Menopause

Menopause is traditionally defined as being without a period for one year. However, women sometimes continue to produce quite a bit of estrogen, progesterone, and testosterone and notice that cyclical symptoms (other than bleeding) such as tender breasts or moodiness continue for up to seven years after their last period. Some women feel as if they suddenly have PMS permanently, while other women have normal, uneventful transitions. If your sex hormone levels are significantly unbalanced, correction with herbs, a better diet, less stress, natural hormone replacement therapy (NHRT), and thyroid medication, if needed, can decrease or eliminate headaches, emotional fragility, hot flashes, vaginal dryness, and osteoporosis. It can also improve your mood, sleep, memory, and sex drive. NHRT, if done properly, may be very beneficial. If not done properly, though, it can cause serious problems. Proper testing is essential here. If you're still having monthly symptoms even after you've stopped bleeding, take a saliva test that monitors hormone levels for twenty-eight to thirty-five days (eighteen samples). If all your days are the same, get a blood test for one day and one to eleven saliva samples. And, of course, eat well!

Male Hormonal Cycles

As you age, the testes begin to produce less and less testosterone and estrogen, and progesterone levels can also fall. By the age of 60, a man's testosterone levels may reach only half of his youthful peaks and his estrogen levels rise to exceed a 60-year-old woman's, contributing to a drop in both sexual interest and erection frequency along with increases in weight gain, mood swings, irritability, depression, reduced vitality, and depleted muscle mass. Diabetes, poor cardiovascular health, circulatory disorders, adrenal and thyroid imbalances, and other health problems can also develop. How does this happen?

- Consuming too many high-carbohydrate foods (sweets and starches) and/or too much caffeine, alcohol, and tobacco for too long.
- Too much stress, which wears out the adrenals, the major testosterone-producing glands after age 40.

TESTING AND REBALANCING YOUR SEX HORMONES

Consulting Holistic Doctors and Finding Testing Labs and Compounding Pharmacies

Always consult with an experienced health care professional to order tests of your sex hormone levels and for help in interpreting your test results and formulating a hormone-rebalancing program. Make sure that your health professional is trained and experienced in the interpretation and application of these test results. Hormone-level test results can be complex and require a high standard of professional expertise to interpret effectively.

Some of the hormones needed for rebalancing are available only by prescription, so try to find an M.D., N.D., D.O., or nurse practitioner to work with. It may take hard work to find a holistic gynecologist or holistic general practitioner who has experience with natural hormone balancing. Use the suggestions in the "Resource Tool Kit." If the practitioners you find use only Premarin, Provera, or soy-based hormones, you may need to keep looking. The following information is based on approaches used by clinicians who are expert in hormone balancing.

Note: Acupuncturists also have ancient and accurate methods of diagnosing sex hormone imbalances and treating them with needles and herbs, often very effectively.

Reasons to Test Your Sex Hormone Levels

Don't try to *guess* about whether or not your hormones are adequate and balanced. Here's why:

1. Testing can explain why women have abnormal menstrual cycles and increases the chances for a healthy ovulation in women wishing to become pregnant by revealing the imbalances or deficiencies responsible for infertility.
2. Testing can explain the depression and insomnia in both men and women caused by imbalances between estrogens, progesterone, and testosterone, or deficient or excess cortisol and lead to effective hormone-rebalancing therapy.

3. Some studies have shown that high levels of estrone or estradiol are associated with breast and prostate cancer. Other studies show that low estriol and melatonin are associated with breast cancer. Testing can give early warnings.

4. If you've taken hormone replacement of any kind (including the birth control pill, DHEA, or pregnenolone), testing can monitor your hormone levels, helping you keep them in safe ranges. Most hormone-troubled women (and men) have never had their hormone levels tested, even the ones who are seeing specialists and are on potent hormone replacement therapy!

5. High cortisol and low estrogen, progesterone, testosterone, and DHEA can all contribute to bone loss and cardiovascular disease or insomnia. Identification of the specific hormone imbalance and correction with diet, exercise, and/or hormone supplementation could help prevent the development of cardiovascular disease and osteoporosis.

6. A woman can still be producing significant amounts of estrogen, progesterone, and testosterone even years after her last menses. Such a woman might assume she's now deeply postmenopausal and begin hormone replacement therapy. This can create an estrogen and/or progesterone dominance, putting a woman at risk for cancer and other serious health conditions. (This is probably as much a danger with natural HRT as with synthetic HRT.)

7. Body builders and weightlifters may be using steroid hormones or analogues. Testing can reveal if usage is safe or not.

8. If you've experienced little or no relief in your symptoms after two months on a natural hormone-balancing program, you need to know why. Specific *targeted* hormone retesting can usually reveal the reason.

Saliva and Blood Tests

Saliva testing is a simple, stress-free, and noninvasive way to determine your sex hormone levels. Substantial clinical and scientific research shows that the levels of hormones in saliva equate reliably to the bioavailable levels of hormones in the blood.[4] In fact, most research on hormones is now done using saliva testing. Saliva tests reveal the levels of free, "unbound" hormones in the system—those directly available to cells in your body. *Blood analysis* usually measures hormones that are both active *and* protein-bound (that is, not as biologically active). Skilled practitioners, like Elizabeth Vliet, M.D., author of *Women, Weight and Hormones,* can find real value in blood testing for sex hormones, but such practitioners are hard to find. Blood testing is done only for a single day, while saliva testing can map an entire twenty-eight-to-thirty-five-day period with all its fluctuations. The safest route is to test for both blood and salivary hormone levels.

Be sure to retest three to six months after you start taking any hormones and then every six months, until your levels are normal and you feel great. Retest any time you have new symptoms of hormonal imbalance. Continue to retest at least annually after age 40.

All labs listed in the "Resource Tool Kit" can provide saliva testing for reproductive hormone and adrenal hormone levels, as well as for levels of melatonin and other kinds of hormones. All conventional labs can test for blood levels.

Note: The hormones in saliva are stable, but I suggest that you send your samples by overnight mail, especially in hot weather.

When to Test Your Adrenal and Thyroid Functions

Thyroid malfunctions are associated with many symptoms of sex hormone imbalance, from premature (before age 12) or late (after age 13) menstruation, to heavy menstrual bleeding, to infertility, to postpartum depression, to menopausal weight gain. Look at the low-thyroid symptoms on page 67, and order the five blood tests described in the "Thyroid Tool Kit" if you have a number of the symptoms listed there. Correcting thyroid function can sometimes correct sex hormone imbalances, all by itself.

Too much stress can cause *adrenal malfunction*, exhausting your adrenals and leading to sex hormone (and mood) imbalances, particularly after age 35, in both men and women. If your levels of the stress-coping hormones cortisol and DHEA test low, this could be the real key to your sex hormone problems. It's a sign that your adrenals may be too exhausted by stress to make adequate amounts of estrogen, progesterone, or testosterone. Remember that in perimenopause and menopause, your adrenals are supposed to take over as your ovaries or testes stop producing as much of these hormones. Dealing with stress always takes priority, and sex hormone production can be put on indefinite hold by your adrenals.

Have salivary adrenal testing done at the same time as sex hormone testing, especially if you are over 35. Nutritionally supporting and rebuilding healthy adrenal function may be vital to restoring balance to your sex hormones and your overall health. See the "Adrenal Tool Kit" for information on adrenal salivary testing and restoring adrenal health.

Examples of How the Right Testing
Leads to the Right Hormone Balancing

The following examples of hormone testing and hormone rebalancing, based on test results, are meant to give you an idea of how a practitioner might address some common imbalance problems. But every case must be addressed individually, based on symptoms and test results. (In the following cases, only saliva testing was used.)

In Premenopause

If you are a menstruating woman with moderate to severe PMS or other uncomfortable hormonal problems, it is best to "map" your entire monthly cycle by providing a small saliva sample every other day for one cycle. Some labs call this the "premenopause hormone profile." Estradiol and progesterone levels are measured in each sample along with at least one sample of testosterone (and sometimes DHEA). The whole cycle is then charted and graphed to reveal the rhythm, timing, and balance of the sex hormones, particularly estradiol and progesterone. (Be sure to keep a daily diary while collecting.)

The premenopausal profiles are vitally important in the prevention, identification, and treatment of the most common and serious health conditions facing young women, including PMS, infertility, endometriosis, polycystic ovary syndrome, dysmenorrhea, fibrocystic and malignant breast and uterine disease, and breast cancer. Once abnormal patterns are detected, an effective, customized (and usually brief) treatment plan can be developed to restore a woman's natural hormonal balance. This profile can also serve as an invaluable tool for monitoring the effectiveness of hormone therapy and safeguarding against excessive or unbalanced hormone levels caused by birth control pills and the unmonitored use of hormones (for instance, progesterone cream tends to build excessive levels).

An Example of Rebalancing a Menstruating Woman: Diane, a 30-year-old schoolteacher with regular menstrual cycles, complained of ten days of PMS: breast tenderness, headaches, mood swings, chocolate cravings, and fluid retention. Saliva testing showed her luteal phase (second half of cycle) progesterone levels were low relative to her estrogen levels, which were high-normal. Following supplementation with progesterone skin cream during the last three to four days of her luteal phase (⅛ teaspoon for three to four days only, just before menses), her troublesome symptoms vanished. Retesting after three months showed that, as her disappearing symptoms indicated, her progesterone levels had normalized. Diane then discontinued use of the progesterone skin cream. *Fertility note:* Since she hoped to become pregnant, it was doubly important for Diane to raise her levels of progesterone, the hormone that allows women to hold on to a fertilized egg.

In Perimenopause (Anytime from Age 35 to Menopause)

If you are transitioning into menopause but are still menstruating, a premenopausal hormone profile would also be the best test choice for you and can probably explain any adverse symptoms you may be experiencing. (Be sure to test your cortisol and DHEA levels, too.)

Low Progesterone: Mary Beth was just turning 40. She had always had regular monthly cycles, but gradually she'd developed really severe PMS and menstrual discomfort. She complained of two weeks of fatigue, headaches, abdominal bloating, severe uterine cramping, irritability, mood swings, and craving for sweets, with breast tenderness and swelling. Saliva testing revealed low adrenal function as well as low progesterone levels throughout the luteal phase (the second half of her cycle). Mary Beth began to reduce stress and improve her diet with nutritional support (as per the "Adrenal Tool Kit") and use oral progesterone drops (1.2 milligrams each drop). Mary Beth's schedule looked like this:

Days fourteen and fifteen—4 drops progesterone just after breakfast.

Days sixteen and seventeen—6 drops progesterone just after breakfast.

Days eighteen through twenty-two—8 drops progesterone just after breakfast.

Days twenty-three and twenty-four—6 drops progesterone just after breakfast.

Days twenty-five and twenty-six—4 drops progesterone just after breakfast.

Note: Higher doses may be needed for infertility.

She responded almost immediately, with her PMS symptoms quickly abating. Retesting after three months revealed adrenal hormones were now normal, with progesterone being at just below normal levels. She stopped adrenal support supplementation and cut her progesterone drops in half. Testing two months later showed normal progesterone levels. She then completely stopped the progesterone drops.

Women vary widely in their ability to maintain adequate hormone levels after rebuilding when they go off natural HRT. That's why follow-up testing, especially where signs of imbalance are evident, is so important. If a woman stays on natural HRT, this monitoring is crucial to prevent excess.

Rebalancing in a Case of Progesterone and Estrogen Insufficiency: At 46, Ruth suddenly developed cravings for carbohydrates, and her cycle became erratic. She was skipping periods and then having several abbreviated periods in a month. Ruth also began experiencing fatigue, depression, insomnia, occasional night sweats, and compulsive overeating.

Her saliva testing showed overall low cortisol, estrogen, and progesterone. She was given adrenal support, natural progesterone pellets, and black cohosh. (Ruth took the progesterone pellets twice daily on days fourteen through twenty-six of her cycle.) This comprehensive approach eliminated her troublesome symptoms, and her periods gradually returned to a twenty-eight-day cycle. Later testing showed marked improvements in all three formerly deficient hormones, and she gradually stopped using her supplements. As Ruth was perimenopausal, follow-up testing of her hormones was recommended twice a year or with the return of any problem symptoms.

Postmenopause

Especially if you still have fluctuating hormonal symptoms (such as moodiness, food cravings, or tender breasts), collect saliva samples every other day for twenty-two days, eleven total samples. Include a measurement of cortisol and DHEA levels as well, to assess your adrenal function at the same time.

Test results usually reveal one of two patterns. First, if you still have some natural hormone production, adequate levels of estrogen and progesterone will be present and natural HRT may not be needed or needed very little. Second, if you are not producing many hormones, a flat pattern will be present with consistently low levels of estradiol and estriol (the two forms of estrogen usually tested) and/or progesterone. This suggests the need for supplementation with natural hormones (and of course for evaluation and support of the adrenal glands) to get levels somewhat closer to what the body would normally produce while still menstruating and asymptomatic.

Rebalancing in Postmenopause: Sarah, at age 52, had stopped menstruating two years before and was experiencing a host of symptoms unlike anything in her past: crying for no reason, tension, anxiety, reduced memory and concentration, weight gain, chills and hot flushes, racing heart, migraines, painful intercourse, insomnia, extreme fatigue, and intense food cravings. Testing revealed Sarah to be low in the sex hormones estradiol and progesterone (estriol and testosterone were not quite as low), as well as in her adrenal stress-coping hormones cortisol and DHEA. Adrenal support supplementation was initiated, including 10 milligrams pregnenolone and 15 milligrams DHEA twice daily. Sarah's doctor also prescribed a natural source combination estradiol, estriol, and progesterone product, which was cycled three weeks on and one week off. Sarah's symptoms began to disappear. Follow-up testing after two months showed that her cortisol and DHEA levels were normal, so adrenal support supplementation was stopped. But her sex hormone levels, although improved, were still low. Progesterone/estrogen augmentation therapy continued, as did regular retesting and less discomfort. *Note:* Sarah's doctor did not prescribe testosterone supplements, because he knew that her DHEA supplement would probably raise her testosterone levels, and it did!

Andropause: Male Menopause

Rebalancing in a Case of Testosterone/DHEA Deficiency: Sam, at 58, was a shipping executive who complained of significant fatigue, loss of libido, weight gain, and moodiness. His test showed estrogen to be in the high normal range, but his free testosterone and DHEA were both found to be low, an imbalance that seems to encourage both depression and prostate

---

Hormone Horrors

A 27-year-old woman, about to marry the love of her life, had low DHEA, no energy, and no sex drive. On DHEA she was in-line skating after work within a week and happily impressing her fiancé with a great libido. After a month, though, she reported acne and constant, severe headaches. Her testosterone levels had shot too high. At our suggestion, she stopped taking DHEA and kept her benefits but lost the side effects. Four weeks of DHEA was all she needed! This is an example of why I want you to work regularly with a health practitioner if you start taking any hormone supplements, natural or synthetic, including soy products, and test your sex hormones. Any of their levels could rise too high, creating new, uncomfortable, or even dangerous imbalances: hair loss in men, growth of facial hair in women, or mood deterioration in both are common examples. Sex-hormone-related cancers could also result.

cancer. (His cortisol was also low.) Reducing the caffeine, alcohol, and sweets and starches in his diet, increasing protein and vegetables, and taking 50–100 milligrams zinc, DHEA, and (prescription) testosterone resulted in a reduction in estrogen and an increase in testosterone. Follow-up testing after three months revealed levels that had improved but were still lower than ideal. A third test six months later showed adequate levels had been achieved. Both DHEA and testosterone supplements were reduced, and Sam's hormone levels were monitored.

Note: It's important for men over 40 to test for low progesterone levels too, especially if stress and insomnia are problems, as well as for DHT, LH, FSH, free PSA, and sex-hormone-binding globulin to assess their prostate health.

Synthetic Hormone Replacement

In addition to the millions of premenopausal women taking synthetic estrogen and progestin-containing birth control pills, at or near menopause about one-third of women in the United States begin to take synthetic hormones as replacement therapy. The most common prescription combines Premarin (made with estrogen derived from pregnant mare's urine) and Provera (not progesterone, but the synthetic replica progestin). Both can have many unpleasant side effects, due primarily to the fact that neither is enough like the human hormone. In the late 1970s, studies showed women taking Premarin alone were at a higher risk for endometrial cancer. Provera was then added to help protect the endometrial lining. But about two-thirds of women stop Provera, often in the first year, as it can mimic the worst of PMS symptoms, including irritability, bloating, and depression.

Some women seem to do well on these synthetic female hormones. These women are satisfied as their energy, sleep, and mental clarity improve. But many other women find that synthetic hormones cause a new set of problems and have hazardous side effects. The most common adverse symptoms reported are mood swings, food cravings, and weight gain. But much more serious, even life-threatening, changes can be set in motion by these drugs. We know from two studies involving fifty thousand postmenopausal women that the use of HRT and birth control pills containing unnatural estrogen, with or without progestin, is responsible for a 20 to 85 percent increased risk of breast cancer[5] and *no* improved risk of heart disease. In fact, in another large study, the rate of heart disease and stroke increased so dramatically in the HRT (Prempro) taking group that the study was halted in 2002 and all subjects were told to stop taking Premarin and Provera immediately.[6]

Using birth control pills also increases the risk of stroke and heart disease. The "pill" can raise levels of certain hormones too high as well as cause the body's production of its own hormone levels to drop. The pill can cause weight gain and a greater risk for uterine fibroids and breast cancer. The synthetic estrogen and progestins in the pill alter natural estrogen (especially estriol) and progesterone levels, which protect against fibroid and tumor growth. Taking the birth control pill can add to or create a hormonal imbalance—even years after going off the pill. Staying on the pill for more than ten years can raise the risk of breast cancer as well as yeast overgrowth.

The Natural Alternatives

Caution: All hormones are quite powerful and have tremendously broad effects on the whole body. This is as true for natural plant-based hormones as for synthetically derived ones. Natural hormones are favored simply because fewer side effects occur with their use. But natural plant-based hormones are very potent, too, and can also be overused. Creams are especially apt to build up excessively high levels of hormones. We've seen many cases where progesterone levels tested thousand of times above normal. Testing labs see this frequently, most noticeably with progesterone cream overuse. Be sure to retest your hormone levels every three to six months while experimenting with natural HRT. Check with your practitioner, who should have you stop using any hormone if any of your hormone levels rise too high or you begin to get adverse effects (in which case retest immediately).

Herbs for PMS. If you suffer from PMS, try an herbal formula that includes the herbs angelica and dong quai (used to regulate hormone levels in women in China for thousands of years), along with other herbs with long histories of hormonal helpfulness for women (like blue cohosh and sarsaparilla). Our clinic uses the Systemic Formulas Bio Function brand Female Plus, for example, which combines many of these herbs.

Herbs for Menopause. Our clients have successfully used many herbal formulations that feature dong quai, black cohosh, and maca. They are easy to find in health stores, and they often eliminate hot flashes, insomnia, and other adverse menopausal symptoms. But these herbs may *not* fully normalize hormone levels. Test yourself and find out.

Natural Hormones. You can buy natural progesterone, DHEA, and pregnenolone in creams, drops, pills, or pellets over the counter, from your health professional or local health food store, or from compounding pharmacies. Pregnenolone strengthens the adrenal glands and may be converted in the body to any of the other sex hormones, particularly progesterone and cortisol. Natural estrogen and testosterone are available only by prescription through compounding and some other pharmacists.

Compounding pharmacists can make a blend of naturally occurring estrogens, usually estradiol and estriol, to your doctor's specifications and add progesterone or testosterone if needed. There is some controversy over what the best proportions and safest delivery should be. The hormone 17 beta-estradiol alone as a low-potency patch has quite a good track record but combining it, as the body does, with some estriol as a liver-sparing patch may be ideal. (See "Resource Tool Kit" for information on finding a compounder.)

Most compounding pharmacists are holistically oriented. You'll need to find a physician (M.D., N.D., or D.O.) who will prescribe from a compounder. The pharmacies can make referrals and consult with you and your physician by phone about what and how much of any hormone to use, depending on your symptoms and test results. Be ready to call the compounding pharmacist yourself first, since so many physicians don't seem to be aware that these compounders and their valuable hormonal products and advice exist. I have seen women switch successfully from synthetic hormonal medications to natural hormones with the help of compounding pharmacists. But beware compounders who do not advise hormone testing *before* prescribing or who advocate only soy-based formulations or progesterone. (See chapter 9 for facts on soy and the "Resource Tool Kit" for more on locating compounders.)

Armed with your symptoms and actual test results, you can move very carefully into balancing your hormones. Natural hormones are identical to those produced within our bodies. They are fully absorbable in micronized (microscopic) form.

Note: Though gels and creams are, like patches, preferable to oral hormones because they bypass the liver, they can affect bedmates. Apply in the morning after rising.

Natural HRT for Men

If cortisol, DHEA, testosterone, and estrogen are all low, you can try DHEA (an over-the-counter supplement), which converts to testosterone and estrogen and also shores up your adrenal stress response. *Note on DHEA*: Watch your reaction carefully. DHEA can convert to excess estrogen or to excess testosterone. Retest to stay in safe ranges. *Natural testosterone* is available only by prescription. Avoid synthetic methyltestosterone, which is very hard on the liver. If your progesterone levels are too low, you can use natural progesterone.

If Your Levels of Any Hormones Are Too High. The following will help you reduce excess hormones in your body:

➤ Stop taking any foods, herbs, or supplemental hormones that might be encouraging the excess (hormone creams or soy foods are especially suspect).
➤ Increase the amount of vitamin C you are taking to 5 grams per day for a few months.
➤ Increase the amount of pure water (not tap water) to help wash out the excess hormones. Drink at least ten full glasses daily.
➤ Use a gentle fiber, like citrus pectin, daily. Mix it in plenty of water. Be sure to also eat plenty of fiber-containing foods—fruit, beans, crunchy vegetables, seeds, and whole grains.
➤ Saw palmetto is an herb that may reduce testosterone levels.
➤ Explore medications if natural methods fail.

RECOMMENDED READING

Ahlgrimm, Marla, R.P.H. *The HRT Solution* (New York: Avery, 1999).

Collins, Joseph, N.D. *What's Your Menopause Type?* (Roseville, Calif.: Prima Publishing, 2000).

Vliet, Elizabeth, M.D. *Women, Weight and Harmony* (New York: M. Evans, 2001).

Klaiber, Edward L. *Hormones and the Mind* (New York: HarperCollins, 2001).

Sellman, Sherill, M.A. *Hormone Heresy* (Honolulu: Get Well International, 1998).

Shippen, Eugene, M.D. *The Testosterone Syndrome* (New York: M. Evans, 1998).

Food Craving Tool Kit

≈⁓

Are You Addicted to Sweets, Starches, or Fats?

Sodas, chocolates, ice cream, biscuits, potato crisps, bread, fries, and pasta are "hard drugs" for many people. If they are for you, please stop berating yourself for having weak willpower and respect the fact that you're actually physically addicted. The next thing to do is breathe a sigh of relief, because help is right around the corner.

The following is an eight-part questionnaire developed for my first book, *The Diet Cure*. It gives a quick symptom picture of each of the eight imbalances that can cause cravings for sweet or starchy carbohydrates or for rich, fatty foods. By your score in each section, as compared to the ideal score, you'll see which imbalances you have. After each section, I've summarized the nutritional or other strategies that our clinic has found can stop the cravings caused by that particular imbalance. All strategies include the basic supplements and good-mood foods. I recommend that you buy and read *The Diet Cure* (Penguin, 2000) for additional guidance.

I. Is depleted brain chemistry the source of your cravings?

4 Sensitivity to emotional (or physical) pain; cry easily
4 Eat as a reward or for pleasure, comfort, or numbness
4 Worry, anxiety, phobia, or panic
4 Difficulty getting to sleep or staying asleep
3 Difficulty with focus, attention deficits
2 Low energy, drive, and arousal
4 Obsessive thinking or behavior
4 Inability to relax after tension, stress
3 Depression, negativity
4 Low self-esteem, lack of confidence
4 More mood and eating problems in winter or at the end of the day
3 Irritability, anger
4 Use alcohol or drugs to improve mood

Total Score _____ *Is your score over 10?*

If you crave sweets or starches to stop particular bad moods, the four amino acids that I discuss in chapters 2 through 5 will usually stop your cravings just as quickly as they take care of your moods.

➤ *5-HTP* (or *tryptophan*) if you eat to eliminate the low-serotonin dark cloud symptoms: try 50–100 mg 5-HTP,* afternoon and at bedtime.

➤ *Tyrosine* if you are a blah type who uses food for relief from low-energy depression and poor concentration: try 500–1,000 mg on arising and in midmorning.

➤ *GABA* if you eat to calm your stressed-out feelings: try 100–500 mg as needed. See the "Adrenal Tool Kit" if GABA is not enough.

➤ *DLPA* if you eat to soothe oversensitive feelings and eliminate comfort-food cravings: try 500–1,000 mg on arising and in mid-morning.

_____
*Or 500–1,000 mg tryptophan as per Action Steps, chapter 2.

continued

2. Are you craving because of low-calorie dieting?

4   Increased cravings for and focus on food after dieting
4   Regain weight after dieting, more than was lost
3   Increased moodiness, irritability, anxiety, or depression
3   Less energy and endurance
3   Usually eat less than 2,100 calories a day
3   Skip meals, especially breakfast
3   Eat mostly low-fat carbohydrates (bagels, pasta, frozen yogurt, and others)
2   Think constantly about weight
2   Use aspartame (NutraSweet) daily
2   Take Prozac or similar serotonin-boosting drugs
2   Have become vegetarian
3   Have decreased self-esteem
4   Have become bulimic, anorectic, or overexerciser

Total Score _____ *Is your score over 12?*

You probably have dieter's malnutrition, which, oddly enough, speeds up cravings, overeating, and unneeded weight gain. Be brave, quit starving yourself, and follow the good-mood eating recommendations in chapter 9. Also take the basic supplements. Get *The Diet Cure* and read its chapters 2 and 10. If you're a chronic dieter, this information will explain why dieting is so counterproductive.

3. Are your cravings due to stress or blood sugar instability?

4   Crave a lift from sweets or alcohol, but later experience a drop in energy and mood after ingesting them
3   Dizzy, weak, or headachy, especially if meals are delayed
4   Family history of diabetes, hypoglycemia, or alcoholism
3   Nervous, jittery, irritable on and off throughout the day; calmer after meals

continued

3 Crying spells, mood swings
3 Mental confusion, decreased memory
3 Heart palpitations, rapid pulse
4 Frequent thirst
3 Night sweats (not menopausal)
5 Sores on legs that take a long time to heal

Total Score _____ *Is your score over 12?*

If blood sugar swings cause your carb cravings, try the following nutrients:

➤ *L-glutamine* 500–1,500 mg on awakening, in midmorning, and in midafternoon.
➤ *Chromium* 200 mg with breakfast, lunch, dinner, and at bedtime.

Reduce carbs. Emphasize protein, fat, and vegetables.

4. Do you have unrecognized low thyroid function?

4 Low energy
4 Easily chilled (especially hands and feet)
4 Other family members have thyroid problems
4 Can gain weight without overeating; hard to lose excess weight
3 Have to force yourself to do even moderate exercise
4 Find it hard to get going in the morning
3 High cholesterol
3 Low blood pressure
4 Weight gain began near the start of menses, a pregnancy, or menopause
3 Chronic headaches
3 Use food, caffeine, tobacco, and/or other stimulants to get going

Total Score _____ *Is your score over 15?*

continued

See the "Thyroid Tool Kit" for directions on how to test for and treat a thyroid problem if you eat for an energy boost that tyrosine doesn't provide.

5. Are you addicted to foods you are actually allergic to?

3 Crave milk, ice cream, yogurt, cheese, or doughy foods (pasta, bread, cookies, among others) and eat them frequently
3 Experience bloating after meals
4 Gas, frequent belching
3 Digestive discomfort of any kind
3 Chronic constipation and/or diarrhea
4 Respiratory problems, such as asthma, postnasal drip, congestion
3 Low energy or drowsiness, especially after meals
4 Allergic to milk products or other common foods
3 Undereat or often prefer beverages to solid food
3 Avoid food or throw up food because bloating after eating makes you feel fat or tired
4 Can't gain weight
3 Hyperactivity or manic-depression
3 Severe headaches, migraines
4 Food allergies in family

Total Score _____ *Is your score over 12?*

If you're addicted to grains or dairy products, turn to page 140 of chapter 7 for a simple home test for suspect foods. Then eliminate any foods that fail the test, and leave your cravings (and other allergy symptoms) behind.

continued

6. Are your hormones unbalanced?

4   Premenstrual mood swings
4   Premenstrual or menopausal food cravings
4   Irregular periods
3   Experienced a miscarriage, an abortion, or infertility
4   Use(d) birth control pills or other hormone medication
3   Uncomfortable periods—cramps, lengthy or heavy
     bleeding, or sore breasts
4   Peri- or postmenopausal discomfort (hot flushes, sweats,
     insomnia, or mental dullness)
3   Skin eruptions with period

Total Score _____ *Is your score over 6?*

Sex hormone imbalances can set up intense food cravings. If you have cravings only briefly before your periods, the basic supplements and good-mood foods should take care of your problem. See the "Sex Hormone Tool Kit" for how to test for and treat any more serious imbalances that you may have.

7. Do you have yeast overgrowth triggered by antibiotics, cortisone, or birth control pills?

4   Often bloated, abdominal distention
3   Foggy-headed
2   Depressed
4   Yeast infections
4   Used antibiotics extensively (at any time in life)
4   Used cortisone or birth control pills for more than one
     year
4   Have chronic fungus on nails or skin or athlete's foot
3   Recurring sinus or ear infections as an adult or child

continued

3   Achy muscles and joints
3   Chronically fatigued
4   Rashes, itching
3   Stool unusual in color, shape, or consistency

Total Score _____ *Is your score is over 13?*

If you have a yeast, fungal, or parasitic overgrowth, you'll need to kill the little monsters. Natural killers like oil of oregano can help. So can certain medicines in brief courses. I suggest that you order both a stool test (see the "Resource Tool Kit") , to specifically identify the type of yeast, fungus, or parasite affecting you, and the specific herbal or pharmaceutical protocols our clinic clients have used to successfully eradicate whichever bugs you turn out to be infested by. Call 800-733-9293, or see our Web site, www.diet.cure.com.

8. Are you fatty-acid deficient?

4   Crave crisps, cheese, and other rich foods more than, or in addition to, sweets and starches
4   Have ancestry that includes Irish, Scottish, Welsh, Scandinavian, or coastal Native American
3   Alcoholism or depression in the family history
*4   Feel heavy, uncomfortable, and "clogged up" after eating fatty foods
*4   History of hepatitis or other liver or gallbladder problems
*4   Light-colored stool
*4   Hard or foul-smelling stool
*1   Pain on right side under your rib cage
*2   Have lost your gallbladder or had gallstones

Total Score _____ *Is your score over 12?*

continued

If your basic fish oil supplement dose and the good-mood fats you'll be eating don't stop your cravings for starchy foods or other symptoms, try taking extra fish oil capsules.

If you crave fats because your liver or gallbladder are not processing them correctly (if you checked off more than one starred item), try taking the fat-digesting enzyme lipase with meals, along with the herb *milk thistle* for your liver (300 mg at breakfast and 300 mg at dinner.)

If you have *no gallbladder*, the lecithin in egg yolks should become your best friend to help you break down fats (add them to salad dressings, smoothies, and so on). Try a digestive enzyme that contains ox bile with all meals. Use three soy lecithin capsules with fatty meals that don't contain egg yolk, if you can tolerate soy.

Notes

Chapter 1. Are Your Emotions True or False?

1. Hibbeln, Joseph, M.D., NIH, in "Fats for Mental Health," an interview with Cory Ser-Vaas and Patrick Perry. *Sat Eve Post*, 1999 Mar 3.
2. Skaer, Tracy L. "Anxiety Disorders in the USA, 1990–1997." *Clin Drug Investigation* 2000;20(4):237–44.
3. Mark Olfson, et al. "National trends in the outpatient treatment of depression." *JAMA* 2002;287:203–09.
4. Thurman, Chuck. "High Anxiety." *The Pacific Sun* 2001 Jan 24:29–31.
5. *Report of the Surgeon General's Conference on Children's Mental Health.* Department of Health and Human Services, 1999 Dec.
6. UNILO (United Nations International Labor Organization). "Job Stress: The 20th Century disease." UN Conference, Oct 2000, as reported by Reuters Medical News.
7. Brown, Raymond J, Ph.D., Blum, Kenneth, Ph.D., and Trachtenberg, Michael C., Ph.D. "Neurodynamics of relapse prevention: A neuronutrient approach to outpatient DUI offenders." *J of Psychoactive Drugs* 1990 Apr–Jun;22(2).
8. First Conference on "Reward Deficiency Syndrome": Genetic Antecedents and Clinical Pathways, November 12, 2000, San Francisco. Abstracts published in *Molecular Psychiatry* 2001 Feb;6(suppl 1):57–58.

Chapter 3. Lifting the Dark Cloud

1. Kellerman, Gottfried, Ph.D. Prepublication research data on 2200 subjects and controls given urinary neurotransmitter level testing at Pharmasan Labs, Minneapolis, 1996–2002.
2. Garrison R and Somer E. *Nutrition Desk Reference* (New Canaan, Conn.: Keats, 1995), p. 226.
3. Wells AS, Read NW, Laugharne JD, and Ahluwalia NS. "Alterations in mood after changing to a low-fat diet." *Br J Nutr* 1998 Jan;79(1):23–30.
4. Whitaker-Azmitia, Patricia, and Peroutka, Stephen, eds. *The Neuropharmacology of Serotonin* (New York: NY Academy of Sciences, 1990), p. 429.

5. Blum, Kenneth, Ph.D., Rassner, Michael, D.D.S., and Payne, James E. "Neuro-nutrient therapy for compulsive disease: Rationale and clinical evidence." *Addiction and Recovery* 1990 Aug.

6. Kasper S, Wehr TA, Bartko JJ, et al. "Epidemiological findings of seasonal changes in mood and behavior." *Arch Gen Psychiatry* 1989;46:823–33.

7. "Current perspectives on the management of seasonal affective disorder." *J Am Pharm Assoc* 39(6):822–29.

8. Gallin PF, Terman M, Reme CE, et al. "Ophthalmologic examination of patients with seasonal affective disorder before and after bright light therapy." *Am J Ophthalmol* 1995;119:202–10.

9. Kogan AO and Guilford PM. "Side effects of short-term 10,000 lux light therapy." *Am J Psychiatry* 1998;155:293–94.

10. Pinchasov BB, Shurgaja AM, Grishin OV, and Putilov AA. "Mood and energy regulation in seasonal and non-seasonal depression before and after midday treatment with physical exercise or bright light." *Psychiatry Res* 2000;94:29–42.

11. Germano, Carl, R.D. *Nature's Pain Killers* (New York: Kensington, 1999), p. 76.

12. Van Hiele JJ. "L-5-hydroxytryptophan in depression: The first substitution therapy in psychiatry?" *Neuropsychobiology* 1980;6:230–40. (Found in Michael Murray's marvelous book, *5-HTP*.)

13. Poldinger W, PhD. "A functional-dimensional approach to depression: Serotonin deficiency as a target syndrome in a comparison of 5-hydroxytryptophan (5-HTP) and fluvoxamine." *Psychopathology* 1991;24:53–81.

14. Ibid.

15. Ibid.

16. Benkert O. "Effect of parachlorophenylalanine and 5-hydroxytryptophan on human sexual behavior." *Monographs in Neural Sciences* 1976;3: 88–93.

17. ———. "Studies on pituitary hormones and releasing hormones in depression and sexual impotence." *Progress in Brain Research* 1975;42: 25–36.

18. Young S, PhD. "Behavioral effects of dietary neurotransmitter precursors: Basic and clinical aspects." 1976 summer;20(2):313–23.

19. Van der Does AJ. "The effects of tryptophan depletion on mood and psychiatric symptoms." *J Affect Disord* 2001 May;64(2–3):107–19.

20. Steinberg S, Annable L, Young SN, and Belanger MC. "Tryptophan in the treatment of late luteal phase dysphoric disorder: A pilot study." *J Psychiatry Neurosci* 1994 Mar;19(2):114–19.

21. Russell IJ, Michalek JE, Viparo GA, Fletcher EM, and Wall K. "Serum amino acids in fibrositis/fibromyalgia syndrome." *J Rheumatol Suppl* 1989 Nov:19:158–63.

22. Savory CJ, Mann JS, and MacLeod MG. "Incidence of pecking damage in growing bantams in relation to food form, group size, stocking density, dietary tryptophan concentration and dietary protein source." *British Poultry Science* 1999;40:597–84.

23. Durstin SM, Devarajan S, and Kutcher S. "The 'dalhousie serotonin cocktail' for treatment-resistant major depressive disorder." *J Psychopharmacol* 2001 Jun;15(2): 136–38.

24. Levitan RD, Shen JH, Jindal R, Driver HS, Kennedy SH, and Shapiro CM. "Preliminary randomized double-blind placebo-controlled trial of tryptophan combined with fluoxetine to treat major depressive disorder: Antidepressant and hypnotic effects." *Psychiatry Neurosci* 2000 Sep;25(4):337–46.

25. Brenner R, Azbel V, Madhusoodanan S, and Pawlowska M. "Comparison of an extract of hypericum (LI 160) and sertraline in the treatment of depression: A double-blind, randomized pilot study." *Clin Ther* 2000;22:411–19.
26. Volz HP and Laux P. "Potential treatment for subthreshold and mild depression: A comparison of Saint-John's wort extracts and fluoxetine." *Compr Psychiatry* 2000 Mar–Apr; 41(2 suppl 1):133–37.

Chapter 4. Blasting the Blahs

1. Cooper, Jack, Ph.D., Bloom, Floyd, Ph.D., and Roth, Robert, Ph.D. *The Biochemical Basis of Neuropharmacology* (New York: Oxford University Press, 1996), pp. 269, 309–10.
2. Koob GF. "The role of the striatopallidal and extended amygdala systems in drug addiction." *Ann NY Acad Sci* 1999;877:445–60.
3. Raucoules D, Azorin JM, Barre A, and Tissot R. "Plasma levels and membrane transports in red blood cells of tyrosine and tryptophane in depression: Evaluation at baseline and recovery." *Encephale* 1991;17:197–201.
4. Agharanya JC, Alonso R, and Wurtman RJ. "Tyrosine loading enhances catecholamine excretion by rats." *J Neural Transm* 1980;49:31–43.
5. Lehnert H, Reinstein DK, Strowbridge BW, and Wurtman RJ. "Neurochemical and behavioral consequences of acute, uncontrollable stress: Effects of dietary tyrosine." *Brain Res* 1984;303:215–23.
6. Gelenberg AJ, Wojcik JD, Gibson CJ, and Wurtman RJ. "Tyrosine for depression." *J Psychiatr Res* 1982;17:175–80.
7. Amen, Daniel, M.D. *Healing ADD* (New York: Putnam, 2001).
8. Owasoyo JO, Neri DF, and Lamberth JG. "Tyrosine and its potential use as a countermeasure to performance detriment in military sustained operations." *Aviat Space Environ Med* 1992;63:364–369.
9. Blum K, et al. "Reward deficiency syndrome." *American Scientist* 1996 Mar–Apr.
10. Kaats G, Blum K, et al. "Effects of chromium picolinate supplementation on body composition." *Current Therapeutic Research* 1996;57(10).
11. Divi RL, Chang HC, and Doerge DR. "Anti-thyroid isoflavones from soybean: isolation, characterization, and mechanisms of action." *Biochem Pharmacol* 1997 Nov 15;54(10):1087–96.
12. Gohler L, Hahnemann T, Michael N, Oehme P, Steglich HD, Conradi E, Grune T, and Siems WG. "Reduction of plasma catecholamines in humans during clinically controlled severe underfeeding." Clinics of Physical Medicine and Rehabilitation, University Hospital Charite, Humboldt University, Berlin, Germany. *Prev Med* 2000 Feb; 30(2):95–102.
13. Baldessarini RJ and Tarsy D. "Dopamine and the pathophysiology of dyskinesias induced by antipsychotic drugs." *Ann Rev Neurosci* 1980;3:23–41.
14. Braverman, Eric, M.D. *Healing Nutrients Within* (New Canaan: Conn.: Keats, 1997), p. 70.
15. Amen, Daniel, M.D. *Change Your Brain, Change Your Life* (New York: Three Rivers Press/Crown, 2000).
16. Cooney CA, Wise CK, Poirier LA, and Ali SF. "Methamphetamine treatment affects blood and liver S-adenosylmethionine (SAM) in mice: Correlation with dopamine depletion in the striatum." *Ann NY Acad Sci* 1998;844:191–200.

17. Shekim WO, Antun F, Hanna GL, McCracken JT, and Hess EB. "S-adenosyl-L-methionine (SAM) in adults with ADHD, RS: Preliminary results from an open trial." *Psychopharmacol Bull* 1990;26: 249–53.
18. Arem, Ridha, M.D. *The Thyroid Solution* (New York; Ballantine, 1999).
19. Ishizuki, Y, et al. "The effect on the thyroid gland of soy beans administered experimentally in healthy subjects." *Nippon Naibunpi gakkai Zasshi* 1991; 67:622–29.
20. Wang, S. "Traumatic stress and attachment." *Acta Physiologica Scandinavica* 1997;161 (suppl 640):164–69.
21. Revis NW, McCauley P, Bull R, and Holdsworth G. "Relationship of drinking water disinfectants to plasma cholesterol and thyroid hormone levels in experimental studies." *Proc Natl Acad Sci* USA 1986;83:1485–89.
22. Revis NW, McCauley P, and Holdsworth G. "Relationship of dietary iodide and drinking water disinfectants to thyroid function in experimental animals." *Environ Health Perspect* 1986;69:243–46.
23. Zeighami EA, Watson AP, and Craun GF. "Chlorination, water hardness and serum cholesterol in forty-six Wisconsin communities." *Int J Epidemiol* 1990;19:49–58.
24. Mullenix PJ. "Fluoride and the brain: Hidden 'halo' effects." XXII Conference of the International Society of Fluoride Research, 1998; www.nofluoride.com.
25. Langer, Stephen, M.D. *Solved: The Riddle of Illness* (New Canaan, Conn.: Keats, 1984), p. 156.

Chapter 5. All Stressed Out

1. Zorilla EP, DeRubeis RJ, and Redei E. "High self-esteem, hardiness and affective stability." *Psychoneuroendocrinology* 1995; 20:591–601.
2. Jefferies, William, M.D. *Safe Uses of Cortisol* (Springfield, Ill.: Thomas Books, 1996).
3. Rydvall A, Brandstrom AK, Banga R, Asplund K, Backlund U, and Stegmayr BG. "Plasma cortisol is often decreased in patients treated in an intensive care unit." *Intensive Care Med* 2000 May;26(5):545–51.
4. Rosmond R and Bjorntorp P. "The hypothalamic-pituitary-adrenal axis activity as a predictor of cardiovascular disease, type 2 diabetes and stroke." *J Intern Med* 2000 Feb;247(2):188–97.
5. Sephton SE, Sapolsky RM, Kraemer HC, and Spiegel D. "Diurnal cortisol rhythm as a predictor of breast cancer survival." *J Natl Cancer Inst* 2000 Jun 21;92(12):994–1000.
6. Kellerman, Gottfried, Ph.D. Prepublication research data on 2200 subjects and controls given urinary neurotransmitter level testing, Pharmasan Labs, Minneapolis, 1996–2002.
7. American Institute of Stress Statistics, posted in 2000.
8. Mitchell S, Ph.D. *I'd Kill for a Cookie* (New York: Dutton/Plume, 1998), p. 17.
9. U.S. Census Bureau statistic reported in *The New York Times*, May 15, 2001, pp. A1 and A10.
10. Belfiglio G. "Approaches to Depression Care." *Healthplan* 2001;42(2):12–17.
11. *Report of the Surgeon General's Conference on Children's Mental Health.* Department of Health and Human Services, 1999 Dec.
12. Frey WH. "Crying behavior in the human adult." *Interactive Psychiatry* 1983;1:94–100.
13. Wardle J, Steptoe A, Oliver G, and Lipsey Z. "Stress, dietary restraint and food intake." *J Psychosom Res* 2000 Feb;48(2):195–202.
14. Jefferies, William, M.D., F.A.C.P. *Safe Uses of Cortisol*, 2nd ed. (Springfield, Ill.: Thomas Books, 1996), p. 100.

15. Braverman, Eric, M.D. *Healing Nutrients Within* (New Canaan: Conn.: Keats, 1997), pp. 166–67.

16. Owasoyo JO, Neri DF, and Lamberth JG. "Tyrosine and its potential use as a countermeasure to performance decrement in military sustained operations." *Aviat Space Environ Med* 1992;63:364–69.

17. Banderet LE and Lieberman HR. "Treatment with tyrosine, a neurotransmitter precursor, reduces environmental stress in humans." *Brain Res Bull* 1989;22:759–62.

18. Zinder O and Dar DE. "Neuroactive steroids: Their mechanism of action and their function in the stress response." *Acta Physiol Scand* 1999;167:181–88.

19. Yehuda R, Bierer LM, Schmeidler J, Aferiat DH, Breslau I, and Dolan S. "Low cortisol and risk for PTSD in adult offspring of holocaust survivors." *Am J Psychiatry* 2000; 157:252–59.

Chapter 6. Too Sensitive to Life's Pain?

1. Rodriquez de Fonseca F, Rocio M, Carrera A, Navarro M, Koob GF, and Weiss F. "Activation of corticotropin-releasing factor in the limbic system during cannabinoid withdrawal." *Science* 1997 Jun 27;276:2050–54.

2. Krishnan-Sarin S, Rosen MI, and O'Malley SS. "Naloxone challenge in smokers: Preliminary evidence of an opioid component in nicotine dependence." *Arch Gen Psychiatry* 1999 Jul;56(7):663–68.

3. Drewnowski A, Krahn DD, Demitrack MA, Naim K, and Gosnell BA. "Progress in human nutrition." *Physiol Behav* 1992 Feb;51(2):371–79.

4. Van Furth WR, Wolterink G, and van Ree JM. "Regulation of masculine sexual behavior: Involvement of brain opioids and dopamine." *Brain Res Rev* 1995 Sep; 21(2):162–84.

5. Kim SW, Grant JE, Adson DE, and Shin YC. "Double-blind naltrexone and placebo comparison study in the treatment of pathological gambling." *Biol Psychiatry* 2001 Jun 1;49(11):914–21.

6. Gray L, Watt L, and Blass EM. "Skin-to-skin contact is analgesic in healthy newborns." *Pediatrics* 2000 Jan;105(1):e14.

7. Harte JL, Eifert GH, and Smith R. "The effects of running and meditation on beta-endorphin, corticotropin-releasing hormone and cortisol in plasma, and on mood." *Biol Psychol* 1995 Jun;40(3):251–65.

8. Hennig J, Laschefski U, and Opper C. "Biopsychological changes after bungee jumping: Beta-endorphin immunoreactivity as a mediator of euphoria?" *Neuropsychobiology* 1994;29(1):28–32.

9. Genazzani AR, Nappi G, Fachinetti F, Michieli G, Petraglia F, Bono G, Monittola C, and Savoldi F. "Progressive impairment of CSF beta-endorphin levels in migraine sufferers." *Pain* 1984;127–33.

10. Brandon DD, Markwick AJ, Chrousos GP, and Loriaux DL. "Glucocorticoid resistance in humans and nonhuman primates." *Cancer Res* 1989 Apr 15;49(8 suppl):2203s–13s.

11. Coiro V, Passeri M, Volpi R, Marchesi M, Bertoni P, Fagnoni F, Schianchi L, Bianconi L, Marcato A, and Chiodera P. "Different effects of aging on the opioid mechanisms controlling gonadotropin and cortisol secretion in man." *Horm Res* 1989;32(4):119–23.

12. Baker DG, West SA, Orth DN, Hill KK, Nicholson WE, Ekhator NN, Bruce AB, Wortman MD, Keck PE Jr, and Geracioti TD Jr. "Cerebrospinal fluid and plasma beta-endorphin in combat veterans with post-traumatic stress disorder." *Psychoneuroendocrinology* 1997 Oct;22(7):517–29.

13. Baker DG, West SA, Nicholson WE, Ekhator NN, Kasckow JW, Hill KK, Bruce AB, Orth DN, and Geracioti TD Jr. "Serial CSF corticotropin-releasing hormone levels and adrenocortical activity in combat veterans with posttraumatic stress disorder." *Am J Psychiatry* 1999;156: 585–588.
14. Volpicelli J, Balaraman G, Hahn J, Wallace H, and Bux D. "The role of uncontrollable trauma in the development of PTSD and alcohol addiction." *Alcohol Res Health* 1999;23(4):256–62.
15. Hatfield BD, Goldfarb AH, Sforzo GA, and Flynn MG. "Serum beta-endorphin and affective responses to graded exercise in young and elderly men." *J Gerontol* 1987 Jul;42(4):429–31.
16. Meyer WR, Muoio D, and Hackney TC. "Effect of sex steroids on beta-endorphin levels at rest and during submaximal treadmill exercise in anovulatory and ovulatory runners." *Fertil Steril* 1999 Jun;71(6):1085–91.
17. Leibenluft E, Fiero PL, and Rubinow DR. "Effects of the menstrual cycle on dependent variables in mood disorder research." *Arch Gen Psychiatry* 1994 Oct;51(10):761–81 [erratum in *Arch Gen Psychiatry* 1995 Feb;52(2):144;comment in *Arch Gen Psychiatry* 1995 Jul;52(7):605–06.
18. Miller MM, Bennett HP, Billiar RB, Franklin KB, and Joshi D. "Estrogen, the ovary, and neutotransmitters: Factors associated with aging." *Exp Gerontol* 1998 Nov–Dec; 33(7–8):729–57.
19. Giannini AJ, Melemis SM, Martin DM, and Folts DJ. "Symptoms of premenstrual syndrome as a function of beta-endorphin: Two subtypes." *Prog Neuropsychopharmacol Biol Psychiatry* 1994 Mar;18(2):321–27.
20. Stomati M, Monteleone P, Casarosa E, Quirici B, Puccetti S, Bernardi F, Genazzani AD, Rovati L, Luisi M, and Genazzani AR. "Six-month oral dehydroepiandrosterone supplementation in early and late postmenopause." *Gynecol Endocrinol* 2000 Oct;14(5):342–63.
21. Priest CA and Roberts JL. "Estrogen and tamoxifen differentially regulate beta-endorphin and cFos expression and neuronal colocalization in the arcuate nucleus of the rat." *Neuroendocrinology* 2000 Nov;72(5):293–305.
22. Leuschen MP, Willett LD, Bolam DL, and Nelson RM Jr. "Plasma beta-endorphin in neonates: effect of prematurity, gender, and respiratory status." *J Clin Endocrinol Metab* 1991 Nov;73(5):1062–6.
23. Ritter MM, Sonnichsen AC, Mohrle W, Richter WO, and Schwandt P. "Beta-endorphin plasma levels and their dependence on gender during an enteral glucose load in lean subjects as well as in obese patients before and after weight reduction." *Int J Obes* 1991 Jun;15(6):421–7.
24. Sabelli HC, Fawcett J, Gusovsky F, Javaid JI, Wynn P, Edwards J, Jeffriess H, and Kravitz H. "Clinical studies on the phenylethylamine hypothesis of affective disorder: Urine and blood phenylacetic acid and phenylalanine dietary supplements." *J Clin Psychiatry* 1986;47:66–70.
25. Ehrenpreis, Seymour, Ph.D. *Degradation of Endogenous Opioids: Its Relevance in Human Pathology and Therapy* (New York: Raven, 1983).
26. Fox, Arnold, M.D. *DLPA to End Chronic Pain and Depression* (New York: Pocket Books, 1985), p. 168.
27. Masala A, Satta G, Alagna S, Zolo TA, Rovasio PP, and Rassu S. "Suppression of electro-acupuncture (EA)-induced beta-endorphin and ACTH release by hydrocortisone

in man: Absence of effects on EA-induced anaesthesia." *Acta Endocrinol* (Copenh) 1983 Aug;103(4):469–72.

28. Bonica JJ, Liebskind JC, Albe-Fessard DG, eds. *Advances in Pain Research and Therapy*, vol. 3 (New York: Raven Press, 1978), pp. 479–88.

29. Donzelle G, Bernard L, Deumier R, Lacome M, Barre M, Lanier M, and Mourtada MB. "Curing trial of complicated oncologic pain by D-phenylalanine" (author's transl). *Anesth Analg* (Paris) 1981;38:655–58.

30. Ehrenpries S. "Pharmacology of enkephalinase inhibitors: Animal and human studies." *Acupunct Electrother Res* 1985;10(3):203–08.

31. Beckmann H, Athen D, Olteanu M, and Zimmer R. "DL-phenylalanine versus imipramine: A double-blind controlled study." *Arch Psychiatr Nervenkr* 1979;227:49–58.

32. Heller B. "Pharmacological and clinical effects of D-phenylalanine in depression and Parkinson's disease." In *Modern Pharmacology-Toxicology, Concatecholic Phenylethylamines, Part 1*, Mosnalm AD and Wolf ME eds. (New York: Marcel Dekker, 1978), pp. 397–417.

33. Ibid.

34. Beckmann H, Strauss MA, and Ludolph E. "DL-Phenylalanine in depressed patients: An open study." *J Neural Transm* 1977;41:123–34.

35. Russell AL and McCarty MF. "DL-phenylalanine markedly potentiates opiate analgesia: An example of nutrient/pharmaceutical up-regulation of the endogenous analgesia system." *Med.Hypotheses* 2000;55:283–88.

36. Genazzani AR, et al. "Effects of 5-HTP with and without carbidopa on plasma beta-endorphin and pain perception." *Cephalalgia* 1986;6:642–45.

37. Benton D, Haller J and Fordy J. "Vitamin supplementation for 1 year improves mood." *Neuropsychobiology* 1995;32(2):98–105.

38. Liu HT, Hollmann MW, Liu WH, Hoenemann CW, and Durieux ME. "Modulation of NMDA receptor function by ketamine and magnesium: Part 1." *Anesth Analg* 2001 May;92(5):1173–81.

39. Koinig H, Wallner T, Marhofer P, Andel H, Horauf K, and Mayer N. "Magnesium sulfate reduces intra- and postoperative analgesic requirements." *Anesth Analg* 1998 Jul;87(1):206–10.

40. Ovechkin AM, Gnezdilov AV, Kukushkin ML, Morozov DV, Syrovegin AV, Khmel'kova EI, and Gubkin IM. "Prevention of postoperative pain: Pathogenetic bases and clinical aspects." [Article in Russian] *Anesteziol Reanimatol* 2000 Sep–Oct;(5):71–6.

41. Peikert A, Wilimzig C, and Kohne-Volland R. "Prophylaxis of migraine with oral magnesium. Results from a prospective, multi center, placebo-controlled and double-blind randomized study." *Cephalalgia* 1996 Jun;16(4):257–63.

42. De Souza MC, Walker AF, Robinson PA, and Bolland K. "A synergistic effect of a daily supplement for 1 month of 200 mg magnesium plus 50 mg vitamin B_6 for the relief of anxiety-related premenstrual symptoms: A randomized, double-blind, crossover study." *J Women's Health Gend Based Med* 2000 Mar;9(2):131–39.

43. Demirkaya S, Vural O, Dora B, and Topcuoglu MA. "Efficacy of intravenous magnesium sulfate in the treatment of acute migraine attacks." *Headache* 2001 Feb;41(2):171–77.

44. Mocci F, Canalis P, Tomasi PA, Casu F, and Pettinato S. "The effect of noise on serum and urinary magnesium and catecholamines in humans." *Occup Med* (Lond) 2001; 51:56–61.

45. Thys-Jacobs S. "Micronutrients and the premenstrual syndrome: The case for calcium." *J Am Coll Nutr* 2000 Apr;19(2):220–27.
46. Evangelou A, Kalfakakou V, Georgakas P, Koutras V, Vezyraki P, Iliopoulou L, and Vadalouka A. "Ascorbic acid (vitamin C) effects on withdrawal syndrome of heroin abusers." *In Vivo* 2000 Mar–Apr;14(2):363–66.
47. Pert, Candace, Ph.D. *Molecules of Emotion* (New York: Scribners, 1997), p. 104.
48. Drewnowski A, Hann C, Henderson SA, and Gorenflo D. "Both food preferences and food frequency scores predict fat intakes of women with breast cancer." *J Am Diet Assoc* 2000 Nov;100(11):1325–33.
49. Zioudrou C, et al. "Opiod peptides derived from food proteins: the exorphins." *J Biol Chem* 1979; 254:2379–80.
50. Cooper JR, Bloom FE, and Roth R. *The Biochemical Basis of Neuropharmacology* (Oxford: Oxford University Press, 1996), p. 431–32.

Chapter 7. Out with the Bad-Mood Foods

1. Pawlak DB, Bryson JM, Denyer GS, and Brand-Miller JC. "High glycemic index starch promotes hypersecretion of insulin and higher bodyfat in rats without affecting insulin sensitivity." *J Nutr* 2001 Jan;131(1):99–104.
2. Anderson RJ, Freedland KE, Clouse RE, and Lustman PJ. "The prevalence of comorbid depression in adults with diabetes: A meta-analysis." *Diabetes Care* 2001 Jun;24(6): 1069–78.
3. Forshee RA and Storey ML. "The role of added sugars in the diet quality of children and adolescents." *J Am Coll Nutr* 2001 Feb;20(1):32–43.
4. Addolorato G, Stefanini GF.; Capristo E, Caputo F, Gasbarrini A, and Gasbarrini G. "Anxiety and depression in adult untreated celiac subjects and in patients affected by inflammatory bowel disease: A personality 'trait' or a reactive illness?" *Hepatogastroenterology* 1996;43:1513–17.
5. Hallert C, Allenmark S, Larsson-Cohn U, and Sedvall, G. "High level of pyridoxal 5'-phosphate in the cerebrospinal fluid of adult celiac patients." *Am J Clin Nutr* 1982; 36:851–54.
6. Farrell R and Kelly CP. "Celiac sprue, a review article." *New England J Med* 2002 Jan17;346(3):180–88.
7. Rapp, Doris J. *Is This Your Child? Discovering and Treating Unrecognized Allergies* (New York: William Morrow & Co., 1992).
8. Kalita, Dwight, M.D. *Brain Allergies* (New Canaan, Conn.: Keats 1987).
9. Ciacci C, Iavarone A, Mazzacca G, and De Rosa A. "Depressive symptoms in adult celiac disease." *Scand J Gastroenterol* 1998;33:247–50.
10. Sategna-Guidetti C, Volta U, Ciacci C, Usai P, Carlino A, De Franceschi L, Camera A, Pelli A, and Brossa C. "Prevalence of thyroid disorders in untreated adult celiac disease patients and effect of gluten withdrawal: An Italian multicenter study." *Am J Gastroenterol* 2001 Mar;96(3):751–57.
11. Tarcisio Not, of Clinica Pediatrica, I.R.C.C.S., Trieste, and colleagues: "Celiac Disease Linked to Autoimmune Thyroid Disease." *Digestive Diseases and Sciences* 2/2000; 45:403–06.
12. Economic Research Service/USDA Per Capita Consumption Data System *Table 14 Added Food Fats and Oils 1909–1998.*
13. Chang MC, Contreras MA, Rosenberger TA, Rintala JJ, Bell JM, and Rapoport SI. "Chronic valproate treatment decreases the in vivo turnover of arachidonic acid in

brain phospholipids: A possible common effect of mood stabilizers." *J Neurochem* 2001 May; 77(3):796–803.

14. Oken RJ. "Obsessive-compulsive disorder: A neuronal membrane phospholipid hypothesis and concomitant therapeutic strategy." *Med Hypotheses* 2001 Apr;56(4):413–15.

15. Harymi, Okuyama, Ph.D. "Choice of n-3 monounsaturated and trans-fatty acid-enriched oils for the prevention of excessive linoleic acid syndrome" *Workshop on the Essentiality of and Dietary Reference Intakes (DRIs) for Omega-6 and Omega-3 Fatty Acids*. The Cloisters National Institutes of Health.

16. USDA. Per Capita Fat Supply for the U.S., 1909–1998.

17. Pietinen P, Ascherio A, Korhonen P, Hartman AM, Willett WC, Albanes D, and Virtamo J. "Intake of fatty acids and risk of coronary heart disease in a cohort of Finnish men." The Alpha-Tocopherol, Beta-Carotene Cancer Prevention Study. *Am J Epidemiol* 1997 May 15;145(10):876–87.

18. Chang MC, Contreras MA, Rosenberger TA, Rintala JJ, Bell JM, and Rapoport SI, *op. cit.*

19. "Limit use of soy infant formula." New Zealand Ministry of Health Pamphlet Information taken from *Food Chemical News*, 1998 Nov 9: 4–5.

20. Freni-Titulaer IW, Cordero JF, Haddock I, Lebron G, Martinez R, and Mills JL. "Premature thelarche in Puerto Rico." *Am J Dis Child* 1986 Dec;140(12):1263–67.

21. Fort P, Lanes R, Dahlem S, Recker B, Weyman-Daum M, Pugliese M, and Lifshitz F. "Breast feeding and insulin-dependent diabetes mellitus in children." *J Am Coll Nutr* 1986;5(5):439–41.

22. Jabbar MA, Larrea J, and Shaw RA. "Abnormal thyroid function tests in infants with congenital hypothyroidism: The influence of soy-based formula." *J Am Coll Nutr* 1997 Jun;16(3):280–82.

23. Sarwar G. "Influence of tryptophan supplementation of soy-based infant formulas on protein quality and on blood and brain tryptophan and brain serotonin in the rat model." *Plant Foods Hum Nutr* 2001;56(3):275–84.

24. "Soy Concentrate for Weaning Pigs." On www.centralsoya.com, click on "animal nutrition," then "animal uses," then "swine." Scroll down to article.

25. Divi RL, Chang IIC, and Doerge DR. "Anti-thyroid isoflavones from soybean: Isolation, characterization, and mechanisms of action." *Biochem Pharmacol* 1997 Nov 15;54(10):1087–96.

26. Fort P, Moses N, Fasano M. Goldberg T, and Lifshitz F. "Breast and soy-formula feedings in early infancy and the prevalence of autoimmune thyroid disease in children." *J Am Coll Nutr* 1990;9:164–97.

27. Allred CD, Allred KF, Ju YH, Virant SM, and Helferich WG. "Soy diets containing varying amounts of genistein stimulate growth of estrogen-dependent (MCF-7) tumors in a dose-dependent manner." *Cancer Res* 2001 Jul 1;61(13):5045–50.

28. McMichael-Phillips DF, Harding C, Morton M, Roberts SA, Howell A, Potten CS, and Bundred NJ. "Effects of soy-protein supplementation on epithelial proliferation in the histologically normal human breast." *Am J Clin Nutr* 1998 Dec;68(6 suppl):1431s–35s.

29. Benson JE, Engelhart-Fenton KA, and Eisenman PA. "Nutritional aspects of amenorrhea in the female athlete." *Triad International J of Sports Nutr* 1996:134–45.

30. Nagata C, Inaba S, Kawakami N, Kakizoe T, and Shimizu H. "Inverse association of soy product intake with serum androgen and estrogen concentrations in Japanese men." *Nutr Cancer* 2000;36(1):14–18.

31. White LR, Petrovich H, Ross GW, and Masaki KH. "Association of mid-life consumption of tofu with late life cognitive impairment and dementia: The Honolulu-Asia Aging Study." *Fifth International Conference on Alzheimer's Disease*, #487, 1996 July 27, Osaka, Japan.

32. Margolis S and Rabins PV. "Depression and Anxiety." *The Johns Hopkins White Papers* 1995;16.

33. Melchior JC, Rigaud D, Colas-Linhart N, Petiet A, Girard A, and Apfelbaum M. "Immunoreactive beta-endorphin increases after an aspartame chocolate drink in healthy human subjects." *Physiol Behav* 1991 Nov;50(5):941–44.

34. Roberts, H.L., M.D. *Aspartame: Is It Safe?* (Philadelphia: Charles Press, 1990).

35. Walton RG, Hudak R, and Green-Waite RJ. "Adverse reactions to aspartame: Double blind challenge." *Biol Psychiatry* Jul 1–15;34(1–2):13–7.

36. Christensen L. "The roles of caffeine and sugar in depression." *The Nutrition Report* 1991:9(13):17, 24.

37. Rowe KS and Rowe KJ. "Synthetic food coloring and behavior: A dose-response effect in a double-blind, placebo-controlled, repeated-measures study." *J Pediatr* 1994;125(5 Pt 1):691–98.

38. Bhatia MS. "Allergy to tartrazine in psychotropic drugs." *J Clin Psychiatry* 2000 Jul;61(7):473–76.

39. Taylor, John, Ph.D. *Helping Your ADD Child* (Roseville, Calif.: Prima Publishing, 2001).

40. Schwartz G, M.D. *In Bad Taste: The M.S.G. Syndrome* (New York: Signet, 1988).

41. Bazylewicz-Walczak B. "Behavioral effects of occupational exposure to organophorous pesticides in female greenhouse planting workers." *Neurotoxicology* 1999 Oct;20(5): 819–26.

42. Hodge L, Yan KY, and Loblay RL. "Assessment of food chemical intolerance in adult asthmatic subjects." *Thorax* 1996 Aug;51(8):805–09.

43. Rapp, Doris J. *Is This Your Child? Discovering and Treating Unrecognized Allergies* (New York: William Morrow & Co, 1992).

44. Postley, John E. *The Allergy Discovery Diet* (New York: Doubleday, 1990).

Chapter 8. Your Good-Mood Food Master Plan

1. Stoll, Andrew L, M.D., *The Omega-3 Connection* (New York: Simon & Schuster, 2001), p. 108–15.

2. AHA Dietary Guidelines Revised for the New Millennium, *Clinician Reviews* 2001;11(8):58, 61–63.

3. Ibid.

4. Chalon S, Delion-Vancassel S, Belzung C, Guilloteau D, Leguisquet AM, Besnard JC, and Durand G. "Dietary fish oil affects monoaminergic neurotransmission and behavior in rats." *J Nutr* 1998 Dec;128(12):2512–19.

5. Brunner J, Parhofer KG, Schwandt P, and Bronisch T. "Cholesterol, omega-3 fatty acids, and suicide risk: Empirical evidence and pathophysiological hypotheses" *Fortschr Neurol Psychiatr* 2001 Oct;69(10):460–67. Review. German.

6. Stoll, Andrew. *The Omega Connection* (New York: Simon & Schuster, 2001).

7. Kidd PM. "Attention deficit/hyperactivity disorder (ADHD) in children: Rationale for its integrative management." *Altern Med Rev* 2000 Oct;5(5):402–28. Review.

8. Pawlosky RJ and Salem N, Jr. "Ethanol exposure causes a decrease in docosahexaenoic acid and an increase in docosapentaenoic acid in feline brains and retinas." *Am J Clin Nutr* 1995 Jun;61(6):1284–89.

9. Corrigan FM, Horrobin DF, Skinner ER, Besson JA, and Cooper MB. "Abnormal content of n-6 and n-3 long-chain unsaturated fatty acids in the phosphoglycerides and cholesterol esters of parahippocampal cortex from Alzheimer's disease patients and its relationship to acetyl CoA content." *Int J Biochem Cell Biol* 1998 Feb;30(2): 197–207.

10. Assies J, Lieverse R, Vreken P, Wanders RJ, Dingemans PM, and Linszen DH. "Significantly reduced docosahexaenoic and docosapentaenoic acid concentrations in erythrocyte membranes from schizophrenic patients compared with a carefully matched control group." *Biol Psychiatry* 2001 Mar 15;49(6):510–22.

11. Wainwright P. "Nutrition and behaviour: The role of n-3 fatty acids in cognitive function." *Br J Nutr* 2000 Apr;83(4):337–39.

12. *Harv Heart Lett* 2001 Nov;12(3):1–2. "Go fish: A good choice for preventing strokes."

13. Segal-Isaacson CJ and Wylie-Rosett J. "The cardiovascular effects of fish oils and omega-3 fatty acids." *Heart Dis* 1999 Jul–Aug;1(3):149–54.

14. Yuan JM, Ross RK, Gao YT, and Yu MC. "Fish and shellfish consumption in relation to death from myocardial infarction among men in Shanghai, China." *Am J Epidemiol* 2001 Nov 1;154(9):809–16.

15. Simopoulos AP. "Human requirement for N-3 polyunsaturated fatty acids." *Poult Sci* 2000 Jul;79(7):961–70.

16. Pietinen P, Ascherio A, Korhonen P, Hartman AM, Willett WC, Albanes D, and Virtamo J. "Intake of fatty acids and risk of coronary heart disease in a cohort of Finnish men. The alpha-tocopherol, beta-carotene cancer prevention study." *Am J Epidemiol* 1997 May 15;145(10):876–87.

17. Gillman MW, Cupples LA, Millen BE, Ellison RC, and Wolf PA. "Inverse association of dietary fat with development of ischemic stroke in men." *JAMA* 1997 Dec 24–31; 278(24):2145–50. Comment in *JAMA* 1997 Dec 24–31;278(24):2185–86. *JAMA* 1998 Apr 15;279(15):1171–72; discussion 1172–73.

18. Bibby DC and Grimble RF. "Tumour necrosis factor-alpha and endotoxin induce less prostaglandin E2 production from hypothalami of rats fed coconut oil than from hypothalami of rats fed maize oil." *Clin Sci* (Lond) 1990 Dec;79(6):657–62.

19. Tappia PS and Grimble RF. "Complex modulation of cytokine induction by endotoxin and tumour necrosis factor from peritoneal macrophages of rats by diets containing fats of different saturated, monounsaturated and polyunsaturated fatty acid composition." *Clin Sci* (Lond) 1994 Aug;87(2):173–78.

20. Wilson MD, Hays RD, and Clarke SD. "Inhibition of liver lipogenesis by dietary polyunsaturated fat in severely diabetic rats." *J Nutr* 1986 Aug; 116(8):1511–18.

21. Westman Eric C., M.D. "Low-carb diet offers second tier therapy for type II diabetics." *Journal of the American College of Nutrition* 1998;17:595–600.

22. USDA. Per Capita Fat Supply for the U.S., 1909 and 1998.

23. Singh RB and Niaz MA. "Genetic variation and nutrition in relation to coronary artery disease." *J Assoc Physicians India* 1999 Dec;47(12):1185–90.

24. Sani BP, Allen RD, Moorer CM, and McGee BW. "Interference of retinoic acid binding to its binding protein by omega-6 fatty acids." *Biochem Biophys Res Commun* 1987 Aug 31;147(1):25–30.

25. Taubes, Gary. "Nutrition: The soft science of dietary fat." *Science* 2001 Mar.

26. McGee D, Reed D, Stemmerman G, Rhoads G, Yano K, and Feinleib M. "The relationship of dietary fat and cholesterol to mortality in 10 years: The Honolulu heart program." *Int J Epidemiol* 1985 Mar;14(1):97–105.

27. Scanlon SM, Williams DC, and Schloss P. "Membrane cholesterol modulates serotonin transporter activity." *Biochemistry* 2001 Sep 4;40(35):10507–13.

28. Thomas EA, Carson MJ, and Sutcliffe JG. "Oleamide-induced modulation of 5-hydroxytryptamine receptor-mediated signaling." *Ann NY Acad Sci* 1998;861:183–89.

29. Boger DL, Patterson JE, and Jin Q. "Structural requirements for 5-HT2A and 5-HT1A serotonin receptor potentiation by the biologically active lipid oleamide." *Proc Natl Acad Sci USA* 1998;95:4102–07.

30. Renaud SC. "Diet and stroke." *J Nutr Health Aging* 2001;5(3):167–72.

31. Nidecker, Anna, senior writer. "Dietary fat may play role in psychiatric illness." *Clinical Psychiatry News* 1998;26(11):10. International Medical News Group.

32. Godfrey PS, Toone BK, Carney MW, et al. "Enhancement of recovery from psychiatric illness by methylfolate." *Lancet* 1990;336:392–95.

33. Reiter, Russel, Ph.D. *Melatonin* (New York: Bantam, 1996), pp. 193–94.

34. Vega WA, Kolody B, Aguilar-Gaxiola S, Alderete E, Catalano R, and Caraveo-Anduaga J. "Lifetime prevalence of DSM-III-R psychiatric disorders among urban and rural Mexican Americans in California." *Arch Gen Psychiatry* 1998 Sep;55(9):771–78. Comment in *Arch Gen Psychiatry* 1998 Sep;55(9):781–82.

Chapter 10. Your Master Supplement Plan

1. Young VR and Scrimshaw NS. "Genetic and biological variability in human nutrient requirements." *Am J of Clinical Nutr* 1979:32;486–500.

2. Lazarou J, M.Sc., Pomeranz BH, M.D., Ph.D., and Corey PN, Ph.D. "Incidence of adverse drug reactions in hospitalized patients: A meta-analysis of prospective studies." *JAMA* 1998 April;279(15):1200–05.

3. Benton D and Donohoe RT. "The effects of nutrients on mood." *Public Health Nutr* 1999;2:403–09.

4. Fugh-Berman A and Cott JM. "Dietary supplements and natural products as psychotherapeutic agents." *Psychosom Med* 1999;61:712–28.

5. Heseker H, Kubler W, Pudel V, and Westenhoffer J. "Psychological disorders as early symptoms of a mild-to-moderate vitamin deficiency." *Ann NY Acad Sci* 1992 Sep 30; 669:352–57.

6. Macready, Norra. "Vitamins associated with lower colon-cancer risk." *Lancet* 1997 Nov;15:1452.

7. Vieth R. "Vitamin D supplementation, 25-hydroxyvitamin D concentrations, and safety." *Am J Clin Nutr* 1999 May;69(5):842–56. Comment in *Am J Clin Nutr* 1999 May;69(5):825–26.

8. Balon R and Ramesh C. "Calcium channel blockers for anxiety disorders?" *Ann Clin Psychiatry* 1996;8:215–20.

9. De Souza MC, Walker AF, Robinson PA, and Bolland K. "A synergistic effect of a daily supplement for 1 month of 200 mg magnesium plus 50 mg vitamin B_6 for the relief of anxiety-related premenstrual symptoms: A randomized, double-blind, crossover study." *J Women's Health Gend Based Med* 2000;9:131–39.

10. Helmeste DM and Tang SW. "The role of calcium in the etiology of the affective disorders." *Jpn J Pharmacol* 1998;77:107–16.

11. Yamawaki S, Kagaya A, Okamoto Y, Shimizu M, Nishida A, and Uchitomi Y. "Enhanced calcium response to serotonin in platelets from patients with affective disorders." *J Psychiatry Neurosci* 1996;21:321–24.

12. Johnson S. "The multifaceted and widespread pathology of magnesium deficiency." *Med Hypotheses* 2001;56:163–70.
13. Young LT, Robb JC, Levitt AJ, Cooke RG, and Joffe RT. "Serum Mg2+ and Ca2+/Mg2+ ratio in major depressive disorder." *Neuropsychobiology* 1996;34:26–28.
14. Vieth R, Chan PC, and MacFarlane GD. "Efficacy and safety of vitamin D_3 intake exceeding the lowest observed adverse effect level." *Am J Clin Nutr* 2001 Feb;73(2):288–94.
15. Benjamin J, Agam G, Levine J, Bersudsky Y, Kofman O, and Belmaker RH. "Inositol treatment in psychiatry." *Psychopharmacol Bull* 1995;31:167–75.
16. Levitt AJ and Joffe RT. "Folate, B_{12}, and life course of depressive illness." *Biol Psychiatry* 1989;25:867–72.
17. Reynolds EH, Carney MW, and Toone BK. "Methylation and mood." *Lancet* 1984;2: 196–98.
18. Deijen JB, van der Beek EJ, Orlebeke JF, and van den BH. "Vitamin B_6 supplementation in elderly men: Effects on mood, memory, performance and mental effort." *Psychopharmacology* (Berl) 1992;109:489–96.
19. Benton D, Griffiths R, and Haller J. "Thiamine supplementation mood and cognitive functioning." *Psychopharmacology* (Berl) 1997;129:66–71.
20. Dillon PF, Root-Bernstein RS, Sears PR, and Olson LK. "Natural electrophoresis of norepinephrine and ascorbic acid." *Biophys J* 2000;79:370–76.
21. Rice ME. "Ascorbate regulation and its neuroprotective role in the brain." *Trends Neurosci* 2000;23:209–16.
22. Feingold IB, Longhurst PA, and Colby HD. "Effects of adrenocorticotropic hormone and dexamethasone on adrenal and hepatic alpha-tocopherol concentrations." *Free Radic Biol Med* 1999;26:633–38.
23. Pawlosky RJ, Hibbeln JR, Novotny JA, and Salem N, Jr. "Physiological compartmental analysis of alpha-linolenic acid metabolism in adult humans." *J Lipid Res* 2001 Aug;42(8):1257–65.
24. Newcomer LM, King IB, Wicklund KG, and Stanford JL. "The association of fatty acids with prostate cancer risk." *Prostate* 2001 Jun 1;47(4):262–68.

Chapter 11. Moods and Meds

1. Cotterchio M, Kreiger N, Darlington G, and Steingart A. "Antidepressant medication use and breast cancer risk." *Am J Epidemiol* 2000 May 15;151(10):951–57.
2. Kelly JP, Rosenberg L, Palmer JR, Rao RS, Strom BL, Stolley PO, Zauber AG, and Shapiro S. "Risk of breast cancer according to use of antidepressants, phenothiazines, and antihistamines." *J Epidemiol* 1999 Oct 15;150(8):861–68.
3. Wallace WA, Baisitis M, and Harrison BJ. "Male breast neoplasia in association with selective serotonin re-uptake inhibitor therapy: A report of three cases." *Eur J Surg Oncol* 2001 Jun;27(4):429–31.
4. Wood A, et al. "Making medicines safer: The need for an independent drug safety board." *New Eng J Med* 1998 Dec 17;25:1851–54.
5. Moore TJ, et al. "Time to act on drug safety." *JAMA* 1998 May 20;279(19): 1571–73.
6. Donovan S, et al. "Deliberate self-harm and antidepressant drugs." *Brit J Psychiatry* 2000;177:551–56.
7. Tracy AB. *Prozac: Panacea or Pandora?* (Salt Lake City: Cassia Publications, 1994, updated 2001), p. 9 ("Our Serotonin Aftermath").
8. Kessler D (FDA chief). "Introducing MedWatch." *JAMA* 1993;2765–68.

9. The FDA's own list of Adverse Drug Reactions to Prozac 1987–96, released by its Freedom of Information staff in 1996 to the Prozac Survivors Support Group, Inc.
10. Sternbach H. "The Serotonin Syndrome." *Am J Psychiatry* 1991 June;148(6):705–13.
11. Steiner W and Fontaine R. "Toxic reaction following the combined administration of fluoxetine and L-tryptophan: five case reports." *Bio Psychiatry* 1986;21:1067–71.
12. Levitan RD, Shen JH, Jindal R, Driver HS, Kennedy SH, and Shapiro CM. "Preliminary randomized double-blind placebo-controlled trial of tryptophan combined with fluoxetine to treat major depressive disorder: Antidepressant and hypnotic effects." *J Psychiatry Neurosci* 2000 Sep;25(4):337–46.
13. Radomski JW, Dursun SM, Reveley MA, and Kutcher SP. "An exploratory approach to the serotonin syndrome: An update of clinical phenomenology and revised diagnostic criteria." *Med Hypotheses* 2000 Sep;55(3):218–24.
14. Gorman, Jack M., M.D. *The Essential Guide to Psychiatric Drugs* (New York: St. Martin's Press, 1995).
15. Radomski JW, op. cit.
16. Boseley, Sarah. "Drug firm issues addiction warning." *The Guardian* 2002 Jan 23.
17. Glenmullen, Joseph, M.D. *Prozac Backlash* (New York: Simon & Schuster, 2000), pp. 72–76.
18. Dreshfield-Ahmad LJ, Thompson DC, Schaus JM, and Wong DT. "Enhancement in extracellular serotonin levels by 5-hydroxytryptophan loading after administration of WAY 100635 and fluoxetine." *Life Sci* 2000 Apr 14;66(21):2035–41.
19. Poldinger W, Calanchini B, and Schwarz W. "A functional-dimensional approach to depression: Serotonin deficiency as a target syndrome in a comparison of 5-hydroxytryptophan and fluvoxamine." *Psychopathology* 1991;24:53–81.
20. Van der Does AJ. "The effects of tryptophan depletion on mood and psychiatric symptoms." *J Affect Disord* 2001 May;64(2–3):107–19.
21. Bond AJ, Wingrove J, and Critchlow DG. "Tryptophan depletion increases aggression in women during the premenstrual phase." *Psychopharmacology* (Berl) 2001 Aug;156 (4):477–80.
22. Schrader E. "Equivalence of Saint-John's wort extract (Ze 117) and fluoxetine: A randomized, controlled study in mild-moderate depression." *Int Clin Psychopharmacol* 2000 Mar;15(2):61–8.
23. Brenner R, Azbel V, Madhusoodanan S, and Pawlowska M. "Comparison of an extract of hypericum (LI 160) and sertraline in the treatment of depression: A double-blind, randomized pilot study." *Clin Ther* 2000 Apr;22(4):411–19.
24. Babyak M, Blumenthal JA, Herman S, Khatri P, Doralswamy M, Moore K, Craighead WE, Baldewicz TT, and Krishnan KR. "Exercise treatment for major depression: Maintenance of therapeutic benefit at 10 months." *Psychosom Med* 2000 Sep–Oct;62 (5):633–38.
25. Ruhrmann S, Kasper S, Hawellek B, et al. "Effects of fluoxetine versus bright light in the treatment of seasonal affective disorder." *Psychol Med* 1998;28:923–33.
26. Benkert O. "Effect of parachlorophenylalanine and 5-hydroxytryptophan on human sexual behavior," *Monographs in Neural Sciences* 1976;3:88–93.
27. ———. "Studies on pituitary hormones and releasing hormones in depression and sexual impotence." *Progress in Brain Research* 1975;42:25–36.
28. Fuller, RW. "Role of serotonin in therapy of depression and related disorders." *J Clin Psychiatry* 1991 May; 52(suppl):52–57.

29. Smith TD, Kuczenski R, George-Friedman K, Malley JD, and Foote SL. "In vivo microdialysis assessment of extracellular serotonin and dopamine levels in awake monkeys during sustained fluoxetine administration." *Synapse* 2000 Dec 15;38(4):460–70.

30. Virkkunen M, DeJong J, Bartko J, Goodwin FK, and Linnoila M. "Relationship of psychobiological variables to recidivism in violent offenders and impulsive fire setters." *Archv Gen Psychiatry* 1989;44:241–47.

31. Mann, Jin, et al. "Serotonin and suicidal behavior." *Ann of NY Acad of Sci* 1990; +600: 446–85.

32. Yokogoshi H, Iwata T, Ishida K, and Yoshida A. "Effect of amino acid supplementation to low protein diet on brain and plasma levels of tryptophan and brain 5-hydroxyindoles in rats." *J Nutr* 1987 Jan;117(1):42–47.

33. Van Praag HM, et al. "In search of the mode of action of antidepressants: 5-HTP/tyrosine mixtures in depression." *Advances in Biological Psych* 1983;10:148–59.

34. Grimes MA, Cameron JL, and Fernstrom JD. "Cerebrospinal fluid concentrations of tryptophan and 5-hydroxyindoleacetic acid in Macaca mulatta: Diurnal variations and response to chronic changes in dietary protein intake." *Neurochem Res* 2000 Mar;25(3):413–22.

35. Botez MI, Young SN, Bachevalier J, and Gauthier S. "Thiamine deficiency and cerebrospinal fluid 5-hydroxyindoleacetic acid: A preliminary study." *J Neurol Neurosurg Psychiatry* 1982 Aug;45(8):731–33.

36. Dursun SM, Devarajan S, and Kutcher S. "The 'dalhousie serotonin cocktail' for treatment-resistant major depressive disorder." *J Psychopharmacol* 2001 Jun; 15(2):136–38.

37. Levitan RD, et al., op. cit.

38. E-mail correspondence from Dr. R. D. Levitan, Feb 22, 2002.

39. Shergill SS and Katona CL. "Pharmacological choices after one antidepressant fails: A survey of UK psychiatrists." *J Affect Disord* 1997 Mar;43(1):19–25.

40. Ichikawa J and Meltzer HY. "Effects of antidepressants on striatal and accumbens extracellular dopamine levels." *European J of Pharmacology* 1995 Aug 15;281(3):255–61.

41. Korf J, van den Burg W, and van den Hoofdakker RH. "Acid metabolites and precursor amino acids of 5-hydroxytryptamine and dopamine in affective and other psychiatric disorders." *Psychiatr Clin* (Basel) 1983;16(1):1–16.

42. Arem, Ridha, M.D. *The Thyroid Solution* (New York: Ballantine, 1999), pp. 87–96.

43. Howland RH. "Thyroid dysfunction in refractory depression: Implications for pathophysiology and treatment." *J of Clin Psychiatry* 1993;54(2):47–54.

44. Arem, Ridha, M.D., op. cit., p. 119.

45. Prange AJ, Jr. "Novel uses of thyroid hormones in patients with affective disorders." *Thyroid* 1996;6:537–43.

46. Yu PH. "Effect of the Hypericum perforatum extract on serotonin turnover in the mouse brain." *Pharmacopsychiatry* 2000 Mar;33(2):60–65.

47. Di Matteo V, Di Giovanni G, Di Mascio M, and Esposito E. "Effect of acute administration of hypericum perforatum-CO2 extract on dopamine and serotonin release in the rat central nervous system." *Pharmacopsychiatry* 2000 Jan; 33(1):14.

Chapter 12. Sleep and Your Moods

1. Munson, Becky Lien. ". . . About Sleep Deprivation." *Nursing* 2000 July.
2. Crespi F, Ratti E, and Trist DG. "Melatonin, a hormone monitorable in vivo by voltammetry?" *Analyst* 1994;119(10):2193–97.
3. Schneider-Helmert D and Spinweber CL. "Evaluation of L-tryptophan for treatment of insomnia: A review." *Psychopharmacology* (Berl) 1986;89(1):1–7.
4. Demisch K, Bauer J, and Georgi K. "Treatment of severe chronic insomnia with L-tryptophan and varying sleeping times." *Pharmacopsychiatry* 1987 Nov;20(6):245–48.
5. Autret A, Minz M, Beillevaire T et al. "Clinical and polygraphic effects of dl 5HTP on narcolepsy-cataplexy." *Biomedicine* 1997;27:200–03.
6. Reiter, Russel, Ph.D. *Melatonin: Your Body's Natural Wonder Drug* (New York: Bantam, 1995).
7. Byerley WF, et al. "Biological effect of bright light." *Progress in Neuro-Psychopharmacology and Biological Psychiatry* 1989;13(5):683–86.
8. Vgontzas AN, Bixler EO, Lin HM, et al. "Chronic insomnia is associated with nyctohemerul activation of the hypothalamic-pituitary-adrenal axis: clinical implications." *J Clin Endocrinol Metab* 2001; 86(8):3787–94.
9. Reiter, Russel, op. cit., pp. 125–26.
10. O'Keeffe ST, Gavin K, and Lavan JN. "Iron status and restless legs syndrome in the elderly." *Age Ageing* 1994 May;23(3):200–03.
11. Lee KA, Zaffke ME, and Baratte-Beebe K. "Restless legs syndrome and sleep disturbance during pregnancy: The role of folate and iron." *J Women's Health Gend Based Med* 2001 May;10(4):335–41.
12. Giller, Robert, M.D. *Natural Prescriptions* (New York: Ballantine, 1995).
13. Hudgel DW, Gordon EA, and Meltzer HY. "Abnormal serotonergic stimulation of cortisol production in obstructive sleep apnea." *Am J Respir Crit Care Med* 1995 Jul; 152(1):186–92.
14. Schmidt HS. "L-tryptophan in the treatment of impaired respiration in sleep." *Bull Eur Physiopathol Respir* 1983 Nov–Dec;19(6):625–29.
15. Lissoni P, Resentini M, and Fraschini F "Effects of Tetrohydrocannabinol on Melotonin secretion in man." Hormone and Metabolic Research 1986;18:77–78.

Chapter 13. Nutritional Rehab

1. Valliant, George, M.D. *The Natural History of Alcoholism* (Cambridge, Mass.: Harvard University Press: 1983).
2. Brown, Raymond J, Ph.D., Blum, Kenneth, Ph.D., and Trachtenberg, Michael C., Ph.D. "Neurodynamics of relapse prevention: A neuronutrient approach to outpatient DUI offenders." *J of Psychoactive Drugs* 1990 Apr–Jun;22(2).
3. O'Malley SS, Krishnan-Sarin S, Farren C, and O'Connor PG. "Naltrexone-induced nausea in patients treated for alcohol dependence: Clinical predictors and evidence for opioid-mediated effects." *J Clin Psychopharmacol* 2000 Feb;20(1):69–76.
4. Navarro M, Carrera MR, Fratta W, Valverde O, Cossu G, Fattore L, Chowen JA, Gomex R, del Arco I, Villanua MA, Maldonado R, Koob GF, and de Fonesca FR. "Functional interaction between opioid and cannabinoid receptors in drug self-administration." *J Neurosci* 2001 Jul 15;21(14):5344–50.
5. Krishnan-Sarin S, Rosen MI, and O'Malley SS. "Naloxone challenge in smokers: Preliminary evidence of an opioid component in nicotine dependence." *Arch Gen Psychiatry* 1999 Jul;56(7):663–68.

6. Evangelou A, Kalfakakou V, Georgakas P, Koutras V, Vezyraki P, Iliopoulou L, and Vadalouka A. "Ascorbic acid (vitamin C) effects on withdrawal syndrome of heroin abusers." *In Vivo* 2000 Mar–Apr; 14(2):363–66.
7. Timofeer M.F. "Effects of ampinotate and an agonist of opiate receptors on heroin dependent patients." *Amer J Chinese Med* 1999; 27(2):143–48.
8. Milam, James. *Under the Influence* (Seattle: Madrone Press, 1981).

Thyroid Tool Kit

1. Barnes, Broda O., M.D. "Basal Temperature versus Basal Metabolism." *Jour Amer Med Assoc* 1942;119:1072.
2. Sacher, Ronald. *Widmann's Clinical Interpretation of Laboratory Tests*, 10th ed. (Philadelphia: F. A. Davis Company, 1991), p. 583.
3. Press release by the AACE in New York, Jan 18, 2001.
4. Shomon, Mary. *Living Well with Hypothyroidism* (New York: Avon Books, 2000), p. 94. See her book for more on TRH testing and many other helpful tips. Also see her Web sites: www.thyroid-info.com and http://thyroid.about.com.
5. Weetman AP. "Clinical Review: Fortnightly review; hypothyroidism; screening and subclinical disease." *BMJ* 1997(19 Apr);314:1175.
6. Sategna-Guidetti G, Volta U, Ciacci C, Usal P, Carlino A, De Franceschi L, Camera A, Pelli A, and Brossa C. "Prevalence of thyroid disorders in untreated adult celiac disease patients and effect of gluten withdrawal." *Am J Gastroenterol* 2001; 96:751–57.

Adrenal Tool Kit

1. Hedaya, Robert, M.D. *The Antidepressant Survival Guide* (New York: Three Rivers Press, 2000), pp. 187–88.
2. Jeffries, William. *Safe Uses of Cortisol* (Springfield, Ill.: Charles C. Thomas, 1996), p. 100.

Sex Hormone Tool Kit

1. Stoll A. M.D. *The Omega 3 Connection* (New York: Simon & Schuster, 2001), pp. 100–04.
2. Lazarus JH. "Clinical manifestations of postpartum thyroid disease." *Thyroid* 1999; 9:685–89.
3. Harris B, Lovett L, Newcombe RG, Read GF, Walker R, and Riad-Fahmy D. "Maternity blues and major endocrine changes: Cardiff puerperal mood and hormone study II." *BMJ* 1994 Apr 9;308(6934):949–53.
4. Walker RF, Read GF, Wilson DW, Riad-Fahmy D, and Griffiths K. "Chronobiology in laboratory medicine: Principles and clinical applications illustrated from measurements of neutral steroids in saliva." *Prog Clin Biol Res* 1990;341A:105–07.
5. Chen CL, Weiss NS, Newcomb P, Barlow W, and White E. "Hormone replacement therapy in relation to breast cancer." *JAMA* 2002 Feb 13;287(6):734–41.
6. Grady D, Herrington D, Bittner V, et al. "Heart disease outcomes during 6.8 years of hormone therapy." *JAMA* 2002;200(1):49–57.

Index